Series Editors:
David R. Beukelman
Joe Reichle

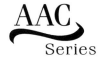

Autism Spectrum Disorders and AAC

Also in the Augmentative and
Alternative Communication Series:

- -

*Exemplary Practices for Beginning
Communicators: Implications for AAC*
edited by Joe Reichle, Ph.D.,
David R. Beukelman, Ph.D.,
and Janice C. Light, Ph.D.

- -

*Augmentative and Alternative Communication
for Adults with Acquired Neurologic Disorders*
edited by David R. Beukelman, Ph.D.,
Kathryn M. Yorkston, Ph.D.,
and Joe Reichle, Ph.D.

- -

*Communicative Competence for Individuals Who
Use AAC: From Research to Effective Practice*
edited by Janice C. Light, Ph.D.,
David R. Beukelman, Ph.D.,
and Joe Reichle, Ph.D.

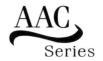

AAC
Series

Autism Spectrum Disorders and AAC

edited by

Pat Mirenda, Ph.D.
University of British Columbia
Canada

and

Teresa Iacono, Ph.D.
Monash University
Australia

with invited contributors

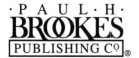

·P A U L·H·
BROOKES
PUBLISHING C⁰ ®

Baltimore • London • Sydney

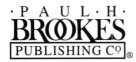

Paul H. Brookes Publishing Co.
Post Office Box 10624
Baltimore, Maryland 21285-0624
USA

www.brookespublishing.com

Typeset by Spearhead Global, Inc., Bear, Delaware.
Manufactured in the United States of America by
Sheridan Books, Inc., Chelsea, Michigan.

The names and identifying details of the family members described in
the vignettes and interviews recorded in this book have been changed to
protect their identities.

Library of Congress Cataloging-in-Publication Data

Autism spectrum disorders and AAC/edited by Pat Mirenda and
Teresa Iacono with invited contributors.
     p.   cm.–(Augmentative and alternative communication series)
  Includes bibliographical references and index.
  ISBN-13: 978-1-55766-953-7 (hardcover)
  ISBN-10: 1-55766-953-8
  1. Autistic children–Means of communication.   2. Autistic youth–
  Means of communication.
  I. Mirenda, Pat. II. Iacono, Teresa. III. Title. IV. Series: AAC
  series.
  [DNLM: 1. Autistic Disorder–rehabilitation. 2. Child Development
  Disorders, Pervasive–rehabilitation. 3. Adolescent. 4. Child.
  5. Communication Disorders–rehabilitation. 6. Communication.
  7. Disabled Children–education. WM 203.5 A93845   2009]
RJ506.A9A92385   2009
618.92′85882–dc22   2008042670

British Library Cataloguing in Publication data are available from the
British Library.

2012   2011   2010   2009   2008

10   9   8   7   6   5   4   3   2   1

Contents

Series Preface

The purpose of the *Augmentative and Alternative Communication Series* is to address advances in the field as they relate to issues experienced across the life span. Each volume is research-based and practical, providing up-to-date and ground-breaking information on recent social, medical, and technical developments. Each chapter is designed to be a detailed account of a specific issue. To help ensure a diverse examination of augmentative and alternative communication (AAC) issues, an editorial advisory board assists in selecting topics, volume editors, and authors. Prominent scholars, representing a range of perspectives, serve on the editorial board so that the most poignant advances in the study of AAC are sure to be explored.

In the broadest sense, the concept of AAC is quite old. Gestural communication and other types of body language have been widely addressed in the literature about communication for hundreds of years. Only recently, though, has the field of AAC emerged as an academic discipline that incorporates graphic, auditory, and gestural modes of communicating. The series concentrates on achieving specific goals. Each volume details the empirical methods used to design AAC systems for both descriptive groups and for individuals. By tracking the advances in methods, current research, practice, and theory, we will also develop a broad and evolutionary definition of this new discipline.

Many reasons for establishing this series exist, but foremost has been the number and diversity of the people who are affected by AAC issues. AAC consumers and their families, speech-language pathologists, occupational therapists, physical therapists, early childhood educators, general and special educators, school psychologists, neurologists, and professionals in rehabilitative medicine and engineering all benefit from research and advancements in the field. Likewise AAC needs are not delineated by specific age parameters; people of all ages who have developmental and acquired disabilities rely on AAC. Appropriate interventions for individuals across a wide range of disabilities and levels of severity must be considered.

Fundamentally, the field of AAC is problem driven. We, the members of the editorial advisory board, and all professionals in the field are dedicated to solving problems in order to improve the lives of people with disabilities. The inability to communicate effectively is devastating. As we chronicle the advances in the field of AAC, we hope to systematically dismantle the barriers that prevent effective communication for all individuals.

Volume Preface

Autism Spectrum Disorders and AAC was written for practicing professionals, graduate students, and others who are interested in learning more about current research and practice on this topic. It is not intended as an introduction to either autism spectrum disorders (ASDs) or AAC; rather, it is intended to be a text that supplements and expands on existing knowledge in these related areas. Chapters in the book represent a multidisciplinary perspective and were authored by leading researchers and clinicians from fields that include speech-language pathology, psychology, occupational therapy, and education.

The chapters are organized into four sections. In Part I, two introductory chapters provide overviews of AAC for individuals with an ASD and assessment issues related to this area. Specifically, in Chapter 1, Pat Mirenda reviews the history of AAC and ASDs, the importance of evidence-based practice, and current conundrums and controversies that challenge both researchers and practitioners. In Chapter 2, Teresa Iacono and Teena Caithness discuss approaches for assessing the distinct skill profiles and communication needs of individuals with an ASD and various models that can be used for such assessment, with emphasis on a Lifespan Model that is illustrated using a clinical example of an adult with ASD.

Part II contains four chapters focusing on communication modalities that are commonly used by people with ASDs. In Chapter 3, Charity M. Rowland reviews the research on presymbolic communication for this population, with an extensive section on intervention approaches that have an emerging evidence base. In Chapter 4, Oliver Wendt provides the results of a meta-analysis related to the use of both graphic symbols and manual signs with individuals with ASDs, with recommendations based on the existing research. In Chapter 5, Ralf W. Schlosser, Jeff Sigafoos, and Rajinder K. Koul review the evidence base on the use of speech-output and speech-generating devices with individuals with ASDs, with implications for research and clinical practice. Finally, in Chapter 6, Diane C. Millar discusses the research on the effects of AAC on the natural speech development of individuals with ASDs, using data from a larger study related to developmental disabilities in general as well as on additional research specific to ASDs. In total, this section of the book provides readers with a comprehensive overview of the current state of the art related to various types of symbols and AAC techniques with this population.

Part III contains seven chapters that provide information on AAC intervention or instructional approaches that are research-based. Chapter 7 provides a summary of the use of AAC for supporting communication and social development in individuals with ASDs within the SCERTS® Model, and was written by Emily Rubin, Amy C. Laurent, Barry M. Prizant, and Amy M. Wetherby. This multidisciplinary team provides numerous examples of AAC use, with illustrations of specific applications. In Chapter 8, MaryAnn Romski, Rose A. Sevcik, Ashlyn Smith, R. Micheal Barker, Stephanie Folan, and Andrea Barton-Hulsey discuss the System for Augmenting Language (SAL) and provide previously unpublished data on its effectiveness with a small group of toddlers who have ASDs. Chapter 9, authored by Kathryn D.R. Drager, Janice C. Light, and Erinn H. Finke, emphasizes the importance of AAC to promote social interaction, a core deficit in individuals with ASDs. With this goal in mind, the authors draw on research involving children with typical development to discuss a number of strategies for customizing and selecting appropriate AAC technologies. They also provide an overview of the principles that underlie a social-pragmatic approach to intervention, with a case study that illustrates use of these principles. This is followed, in Chapter 10, by an overview of the Picture Exchange Communication System (PECS) by Andy Bondy and Lori Frost, in which they discuss the use of PECS, as well as interventions that go beyond traditional PECS, and review the growing body of research related to its use. In Chapter 11, Pat Mirenda and Kenneth E. Brown discuss the role of AAC for augmented input and provide a review of visual supports that use AAC symbols, including visual schedules, contingency maps, visual-augmented social stories, video-enhanced activity schedules, and other applications. Finally, authors Jeff Sigafoos, Mark F. O'Reilly, and Giulio E. Lancioni (Chapter 12) and Krista M. Wilkinson and Joe Reichle (Chapter 13) turn their attention to AAC interventions that can be used to address problem behavior. In Chapter 12, Sigafoos and colleagues review the research on functional communication training and choice-making interventions in this regard; and in Chapter 13, Wilkinson and Reichle provide a detailed account of specific techniques for using aided AAC to replace unconventional communicative acts with more conventional behaviors. Overall, Part III of the book provides both researchers and clinicians with a rich and diverse set of chapters on current research and practical applications related to AAC intervention.

The focus of Part IV is on three issues that are directly related to AAC implementation: literacy, inclusive education, and supporting the participation of adolescents and adults with complex communication needs. David A. Koppenhaver and Karen A. Erickson discuss the research on ASDs, AAC, and literacy in Chapter 14, within a comprehensive model of reading, writing, and emergent literacy development and instruction. They provide both educational implications and directions for future research in this thoughtful summary. In Chapter 15, Michael McSheehan, Rae M. Sonnenmeier, and Cheryl M. Jorgenson discuss the use of AAC as one component of inclusive education for students with ASDs, with emphasis on the Beyond Access Model of collaboration and support that they have developed over the past several years. Finally, in Chapter 16, Teresa Iacono, Hilary Johnson, and Sheridan Forster remind us that children with ASDs grow up to become adolescents and adults with ASDs who are no less in need of AAC supports than their younger counterparts. In reviewing the limited research in this neglected area, these authors emphasize the needs of adults with complex communication needs and encourage both researchers and clinicians to address them.

As we developed the outline for this book and as we worked with the authors whose work is contained here, we were struck repeatedly by how much the research base related to ASDs and AAC has grown over the past decade. In fact, a decade ago, this book could not have been written because there simply was not sufficient research to support it. Combined, these chapters provide a much-needed map to guide the next generation of research that will close the gaps and further advance the knowledge base on ASDs and AAC in general. We are so very grateful to the authors—all of whom have multiple responsibilities and projects of their own to support!—for their (usually cheerful) contributions. Were it not for these individuals, we would know much, much less than we do in this important area.

About the Editors

Pat Mirenda, Ph.D., Professor, Department of Educational and Counseling Psychology, and Special Education, University of British Columbia, 2125 Main Mall, Vancouver, British Columbia V6T 1Z4, Canada

Dr. Mirenda earned her doctorate in behavioral disabilities from the University of Wisconsin–Madison. For 8 years, she was a faculty member in the Department of Special Education and Communication Disorders, University of Nebraska–Lincoln. From 1992 to 1996, she provided a variety of training, research, and support services to individuals with severe disabilities through CBI Consultants, Ltd., in Vancouver, British Columbia. She is now Professor in the Department of Educational and Counseling Psychology and Special Education at the University of British Columbia. From 1998 to 2001, she was editor of the journal *Augmentative and Alternative Communication.* In 2004, she was named a Fellow of the American Speech-Language-Hearing Association and was awarded the Killam Teaching Prize at the University of British Columbia. In 2008, she was named a Fellow of the International Society for Augmentative and Alternative Communication. Dr. Mirenda is the author of numerous book chapters and research publications; she lectures widely and teaches courses on augmentative and alternative communication, inclusive education, developmental disabilities, autism, and positive behavior support. Her current research focuses on describing the developmental trajectories of young children with autism and factors that predict the outcomes of early intervention.

Teresa Iacono, Ph.D., Associate Professor and Senior Research Fellow, Director of Research, Centre for Developmental Disability Health Victoria, Monash University, 270 Ferntree Gully Road Building 1, Notting Hill, Victoria, 3166, Australia

Dr. Iacono earned her doctorate in Special Education and Communication Disorders at the University of Nebraska–Lincoln. She is a speech-language pathologist, having received her B.App.Sc. and M.App.Sc.

degrees in speech pathology in Australia. For 9 years she was an academic member of Macquarie University, where she co-convened a Masters in Communication Disorders within the Department of Linguistics and taught within the Institute of Early Childhood; she also held an honorary position within Macquarie University Special Education Centre. Her clinical, teaching, and research work has focused on developmental disabilities and complex communication needs. In her position at the Centre for Developmental Disability Health Victoria, this focus has extended to physical and mental health issues of adults with developmental disabilities.

Dr. Iacono is the author of chapters and research publications concerning communication and health and well-being in developmental disabilities. She was editor of the journal *Augmentative and Alternative Communication* from 2002 to 2004. In 2007, she was a recipient of the inaugural National Health and Medical Research Council (Australia) Ethics Award for her work addressing ethical concerns of including people with developmental disabilities in research.

Contributors

R. Micheal Barker, M.A.
Doctoral Candidate
Georgia State University
One Park Place South, Suite 928
Atlanta, GA 30303

Andrea Barton-Hulsey, M.A.,
  CCC-SLP
Speech-Language Pathologist
Georgia State University
Post Office Box 4000
Atlanta, GA 30302

Andy Bondy, Ph.D.
Co-Founder
Pyramid Educational
  Consultants, Inc.
13 Garfield Way
Newark, DE 19713

Kenneth E. Brown, M.A.
Positive Behaviour Support
  Options
3878 Hamber Place
North Vancouver V7G 2K1,
  British Columbia
Canada

Teena Caithness, B.App.Sc.
Speech Pathologist/Senior
  Clinical Consultant
Statewide Behaviour Intervention
  Service
Department of Ageing, Disability
  and Home Care
Level 1, 242 Beecroft Road
Epping, New South Wales 2121
Australia

Kathryn D.R. Drager, Ph.D.
Associate Professor
The Pennsylvania State
  University
308 Ford Building
University Park, PA 16802

Karen A. Erickson, Ph.D.
Director, Center for Literacy
  & Disability Studies
321 South Columbia Street,
  Suite 1100
CB #7335
University of North Carolina
  at Chapel Hill
Chapel Hill, NC 27599

Erinn H. Finke, M.S.
Assistant Professor
Communication Sciences
  and Disorders
The University of Utah
390 South 1530 East
1213 Social and Behavioral
  Sciences Building
Salt Lake City, UT 84108

Stephanie Folan, B.A.
Graduate Student
Georgia State University
3911 Bretton Woods Road
Decatur, GA 30032

**Sheridan Forster, B.App.Sc.
  (Speech Pathology),
  GradDip (Special Ed.)**
Centre for Developmental
  Disability Health Victoria
Monash University
Building 1
270 Ferntree Gully Road
Notting Hill 3166
Australia

Lori Frost, M.S., CCC-SLP
Co-Founder
Pyramid Educational
  Consultants, Inc.
13 Garfield Way
Newark, DE 19713

Hilary Johnson, M.A., FSPAA
Manager
Scope
830 Whitehorse Road
Box Hill, Victoria 3128
Australia

Cheryl M. Jorgensen, Ph.D.
Project Director and Assistant
  Research Professor
Institute on Disability
University of New Hampshire
10 West Edge Drive, Suite 101
Durham, NH 03824

David A. Koppenhaver, Ph.D.
Professor
Language, Reading and
  Exceptionalities Department
Appalachian State University
RCOE, 124 Edwin Duncan
  Hall
Boone, NC 28608

Rajinder K. Koul, Ph.D.
Professor and Chairperson
Associate Dean (Research),
  School of Allied Health
  Sciences
Texas Tech University Health
  Sciences Center
3601 4th Street
Lubbock, TX 79430

Giulio E. Lancioni, Ph.D.
Professor
Department of Psychology
University of Bari
Via Quintino Sella 268
Bari 70100
Italy

**Amy C. Laurent, Ed.M.,
  OTR/L**
Private Practice Affiliate
Communication Crossroads
100 Juniper Drive
North Kingstown, RI 02852

Janice C. Light, Ph.D.
Distinguished Professor
Department of Communication
    Sciences and Disorders
The Pennsylvania State
    University
308 Ford Building
University Park, PA 16802

Michael McSheehan
Clinical Assistant Professor
Department of Communication
    Sciences and Disorders
Institute on Disability
University of New Hampshire
10 West Edge Drive, Suite 101
Durham, NH 03824

Diane C. Millar, Ph.D.
Associate Professor
Radford University
113 Waldron Hall
Radford, VA 24142

Mark F. O'Reilly, Ph.D.
Mollie Villeret Davis Professor in
    Learning Disabilities
Meadows Center for the
    Prevention of Educational Risk
College of Education
The University of Texas at Austin
1 University Station, D5300
Austin, TX 78712

**Barry M. Prizant, Ph.D.,
    CCC-SLP**
Director
Childhood Communication
    Services
Adjunct Professor
Brown University
2024 Broad Street
Cranston, RI 02905

Joe Reichle, Ph.D.
Professor
Departments of Speech-
    Language-Hearing Sciences
    and Educational Psychology
University of Minnesota
115 Shevlin Hall
164 Pillsbury Drive S.E.
Minneapolis, MN 55455

MaryAnn Romski, Ph.D.
Regents' Professor of
    Communication, Psychology,
    Educational Psychology, and
    Special Education
Associate Dean of Social and
    Behavioral Sciences
Georgia State University
38 Peachtree Center Avenue
Atlanta, GA 30303

Charity M. Rowland, Ph.D.
Associate Professor of Pediatrics
Oregon Health & Science
    University
Post Office Box 574
Portland, OR 97207

Emily Rubin, M.S., CCC-SLP
Director, Communication
    Crossroads
Lecturer, Yale University School
    of Medicine
Post Office Box 222171
Carmel, CA 93922

Ralf W. Schlosser, Ph.D.
Professor and Chair
Department of Speech-Language
    Pathology and Audiology
Northeastern University
106 Forsyth
Boston, MA 02115

Rose A. Sevcik, Ph.D.
Professor
Department of Psychology
Georgia State University
Urban Life, 11th Floor
140 Decatur Street
Atlanta, GA 30303

Jeff Sigafoos, Ph.D.
Professor
Victoria University of
    Wellington
Donald Street
Karori, Wellington 6005
New Zealand

Ashlyn Smith, M.A.
Doctoral Student
Georgia State University
One Park Place South, Suite 928
Atlanta, GA 30303

Rae M. Sonnenmeier, Ph.D.
Clinical Assistant Professor
Institute on Disability
University of New Hampshire
10 West Edge Drive
Durham, NH 03824

Oliver Wendt, Ph.D.
Assistant Professor of Speech,
    Language, and Hearing
    Sciences
Assistant Professor of Special
    Education
Purdue University
100 North University Street
West Lafayette, IN 47907

Amy M. Wetherby, Ph.D.
Director
FSU Autism Institute
Professor of Clinical Sciences
Laurel Schendel Professor of
    Communication Disorders
Florida State University
625B North Adams Street
Tallahassee, FL 32301

Krista M. Wilkinson, Ph.D.
Professor
Communication Sciences
    and Disorders
404 Ford Building
The Pennsylvania State
    University
University Park, PA 16802
(previously at Emerson College)

Acknowledgments

Special appreciation is due a number of individuals with whom we have been fortunate to work before and during the production of this book. These include the staff at Special Education Technology-BC (SET-BC), Vancouver, British Columbia, Canada; Sunny Hill Health Centre for Children in Vancouver, British Columbia, Canada; the Centre for Developmental Disability Health Victoria, Melbourne, Australia; and the Communication Resource Centre, Scope, Melbourne, Australia. These individuals have collaborated with us extensively over the years and have thus greatly contributed to our AAC experiences and knowledge. In addition, Pat Mirenda thanks Jackie Brown for her patience and support in all of its many forms over the years; and Teresa Iacono thanks Greg Graham for his unfaltering support, encouragement, and humor. We also appreciate the encouragement and cheerleading efforts of Janice C. Light and David R. Beukelman, who talked us into producing this book in the first place; and, of course, the support provided by the team at Brookes Publishing: Astrid Zuckerman, Johanna Cantler, Melanie Allred, and Janet Krejci. Finally, we thank the many people with ASDs who rely on AAC and have allowed us to work with them—they have taught us virtually everything we know about AAC and have provided us with both inspiration and motivation.

We dedicate this book to the many, many individuals with autism spectrum disorders who do not yet have access to professionals with the attitudes, knowledge, and skills that are needed for comprehensive and appropriate AAC interventions. May your silence remind us of the work we still have left to do.

I

Overview
and Assessment

1

Introduction to AAC for Individuals with Autism Spectrum Disorders

PAT MIRENDA

- - - - - Because some alternative nonspeech communication systems have become increasingly employed in cases of language deficiencies, it needs to be determined whether such systems hold promise for the autistic individual and which systems are most suitable.   (Schuler & Baldwin, 1981, p. 246)

Since Schuler and Baldwin made this proposal in 1981, both research and practice in the use of augmentative and alternative communication (AAC) for individuals with autism spectrum disorders (ASDs) have evolved rapidly—so much so that this edited volume is now possible, which was not the case even a decade ago! AAC does indeed "hold promise" for individuals with ASDs; in many places, it has become the cornerstone of interventions aimed at increasing communication and literacy skills and/or decreasing problem behavior. This chapter will provide 1) a brief history of AAC modality and assessment issues related to individuals with ASDs, 2) an overview of evidence-based practice and its relevance to ASDs, and 3) an overview of some of the key conundrums and controversies that affect AAC practice today.

ASDs AND AAC

Autism spectrum disorder is an increasingly popular term that refers to the pervasive developmental disorders described in the *Diagnostic and Statistical Manual of Mental Disorders, Fourth Edition, Text Revision* (American Psychiatric Association, 2000). The ASDs include the following:

- Autistic disorder (more commonly called *autism*)
- Pervasive developmental disorder-not otherwise specified, "a collection of features that resemble autism but may not be as severe or extensive" (Dunlap & Bunton-Pierce, 1999)
- Asperger syndrome, a diagnosis assigned to individuals who display the social criteria for autism but have intact language and cognitive abilities
- Rett syndrome, a degenerative genetic condition with neurological signs that affects only girls
- Childhood disintegrative disorder, a rare regressive disorder characterized by a loss of communication and other previously acquired skills

The symptoms of autism are evident within the first 3 years of life and include significant difficulties with social interaction, delayed or abnormal functioning in verbal and nonverbal communication, and unusual patterns of behavior (e.g., restricted interests, repetitive activities, stereotyped movements, unusual responses to sensory stimuli). The ASDs occur in all racial, ethnic, and socioeconomic groups and are 4 times more likely to occur in boys than in girls. A recent report by the Autism and Developmental Disabilities Monitoring Network indicated that about 1 in 150 eight-year-old children in multiple areas of the United States have been diagnosed with one of the ASDs (Centers for Disease Control and Prevention, 2007).

All disorders on the autism spectrum are characterized by communication impairments of some type, although the specific symptoms vary widely. The increased availability of early diagnosis and intervention over the past decade or more has been accompanied by changes in the prognosis for speech development (Tager-Flusberg, Paul, & Lord, 2005). Nonetheless, a significant proportion of individuals with ASDs of all ages are likely to require AAC for expressive communication, either temporarily (i.e., until speech develops) or permanently. In addition, many individuals with ASDs—even those with relatively intact speech and language—may benefit from AAC support to enhance comprehension (American Speech-Language-Hearing Association [ASHA], 2005).

AAC MODALITIES AND TECHNIQUES

A variety of both unaided and aided communication techniques have been implemented for individuals with ASDs over the years. Unaided communication does not require any equipment that is external to the body and involves the use of symbols such as manual signs, pantomimes, and gestures. Aided communication incorporates devices that are external to the individuals who use them (e.g., communication books, speech-generating devices) and involves the use of real objects or graphic symbols such as photographs, line drawings, letters, and written words. Most people, including those with ASDs, use a combination of unaided and aided communication techniques, depending on the context and the communication partner (Beukelman & Mirenda, 2005).

Chimps, Chips, Signs, and Lexigrams

For the most part, the individuals with ASDs for whom AAC techniques were first introduced lived in institutions or attended state schools for people with intellectual disabilities. They were presumed to be essentially subhuman and, if they were unable to speak, largely incapable of acquiring communication or language skills. Therefore, it is perhaps not surprising that many of the early AAC experiments with these individuals were based on research aimed at examining the extent to which various language elements could be taught to nonhuman primates (e.g., chimpanzees). The sad and distasteful logic inherent in these early AAC experiments was that if chimps could learn to communicate, perhaps people with autism also could.

Plastic Chips   One of the earliest descriptions of "nonspeech communication" with a child with autism is from Premack and Premack (1974). Prior to this, the Premacks taught Sarah, a female chimpanzee, to associate plastic pieces of various colors and shapes with more than 130 words in semantic categories that included nouns, verbs, adjectives, and prepositions, among others. Sarah not only understood the meanings of these plastic chips, but she also used them to both produce and respond to a variety of simple sentences and questions (Premack, 1971). The Premacks later extended this research to teach an 8-year-old boy with autism and severe visual impairment to use plastic chips to communicate, noting that "the plastic visual system is clearly preferable to no language at all, and it may also prove helpful in speeding the acquisition of natural language" (Premack & Premack, 1974, p. 375). The success of this intervention was followed by a number of additional research projects documenting the efficacy of the plastic chip system, which was later published and marketed as the Non-Speech Language Initiation Program (Non-SLIP; Carrier & Peak, 1975). Early research reports suggested that this could be a useful system of communication for at least some children with ASDs (deVilliers & Naughton, 1974; McLean & McLean, 1974).

Manual Signs   Simultaneous with the efforts of the Premacks, another pair of language researchers was teaching a chimp named Washoe to communicate using American Sign Language (Gardner & Gardner, 1969). Shortly thereafter, a few references to attempts at teaching gestural language to children with autism appeared in the published literature (e.g., Churchill, 1972); however, Margaret Creedon's (1973) presentation to the Society for Research in Child Development is generally acknowledged as the first public report of the successful use of a formal "simultaneous communication system" (i.e., speech plus manual signs) with these individuals. In her paper, Creedon described the outcomes of simultaneous communication instruction with 21 children with autism over a 3-year period. Later that same year, two published case studies described the results of quite different instructional approaches that were used to teach children with ASDs to both understand and communicate using a small number of manual signs paired with speech (Miller & Miller, 1973; Webster, McPherson, Sloman, Evans, & Kuchar, 1973).

Over the next decade, numerous research reports on the use of simultaneous communication (also referred to as *total communication*) were published (for a review, see Goldstein, 2002). By the mid-1980s, total communication in one form or another was the most commonly used AAC technique for individuals who were labeled as *autistic* or *severely/profoundly intellectually disabled* in the United States (Bryen & Joyce, 1985; Matas, Mathy-Laikko, Beukelman, & Legresley, 1985), the United Kingdom (Kiernan, 1983; Kiernan, Reid, & Jones, 1982), and Australia (Iacono & Parsons, 1986). In addition, this decade saw dissemination of the Makaton Vocabulary, a method for teaching British Sign Language that was originally developed for institutionalized deaf adults with intellectual disabilities in the United Kingdom (Cornforth, Johnson, & Walker, 1974). The Makaton method was expanded in the mid-1980s to incorporate pictorial Makaton symbols and speech in addition to manual signs; the method was used internationally with individuals with a wide range of developmental disabilities, including autism (Walker, 1987).

Lexigrams   A third pair of researchers initiated a longitudinal project (the Lana Project, named after its first subject) that was designed to teach chimpanzees to communicate using abstract lexigrams composed of nine geometric forms (Rumbaugh, 1977; Savage-Rumbaugh, Rumbaugh, & Boysen, 1978). The lexigrams were accessed through computer-linked, touch-sensitive display panels that produced illuminated symbols (in the early phases of the project) or synthetic speech (in later phases). The results of the Lana project were later applied successfully to 13 boys with severe cognitive impairments—two of whom had autism—in a project called the System for Augmenting Language, discussed further in Chapter 8 (Romski & Sevcik, 1996).

Written Words

Orthographic symbols (i.e., alphabet letters) were used with people with autism in the early days of AAC. Structured operant conditioning interventions were initiated by several researchers to demonstrate that at least some of these individuals could learn to associate printed words with their referents (e.g., Hewett, 1964; Marshall & Hegrenes, 1972; LaVigna, 1977; Ratusnik & Ratusnik, 1974). Interestingly, although these interventions proved at least as efficacious as the early demonstrations using other types of symbols, orthography was not widely used with this population for communication, even after a flurry of interest in the mid-1980s related to hyperlexia (i.e., the precocious, self-taught ability to read printed words that is seen in many individuals with autism; e.g., Frith & Snowling, 1983; Whitehouse & Harris, 1984). In recent years, the advent of balanced literacy practices and the availability of a wide range of technologies to support reading and writing have enabled many individuals with ASDs to participate meaningfully in literacy experiences alongside their typically developing peers, as discussed further in Chapter 14 (Kliewer & Biklen, 2001; Koppenhaver, 2000; Mirenda, 2003a).

Visual-Graphic Symbols

Reports of the successful use of visual-graphic pictorial systems with individuals with autism began to appear in the 1980s (Lancioni, 1983; Mirenda & Iacono, 1988; Mirenda & Santogrossi, 1985; Reichle & Brown, 1986). Over the next decade, their use became widespread and, at least in the published literature, has largely replaced manual signing as the predominant AAC approach used with individuals with ASDs today. Among the most popular approaches to teach these individuals to communicate with visual-graphic symbols is the Picture Exchange Communication System, which was first introduced in the mid-1990s (Bondy & Frost, 1994) and is discussed further in Chapter 10.

Speech Output

Speech output was first introduced to students with autism in the 1970s by Colby and his colleagues at Stanford University (Colby, 1973; Colby & Kraemer, 1975; Colby & Smith, 1974). Their goal was to "stimulate or catalyze a damaged or slow-developing natural process of language acquisition" (Colby, 1973, p. 259) by engaging children in exploratory games that enabled them to activate symbols on a computer screen (e.g., the letter *H*) paired with auditory stimuli (e.g., a voice saying "H"). They reported that 13 of 17 children began "voluntarily to use speech for social communication" (Colby, 1973, p. 259) after exposure to this treatment.

With the exception of a few additional early case reports (e.g., Hedbring, 1985), it was not until the 1990s that research in this area began in earnest (for a review, see Schlosser & Blischak, 2001). Some of this work was aimed at examining the use of speech output for individuals with autism in the context of computer-assisted learning (e.g., Bernard-Opitz, Ross, & Tuttas, 1990; Chen & Bernard-Opitz, 1993; Heimann, Nelson, Tjus, & Gillberg, 1995; Parsons & LaSorte, 1993; Tjus, Heimann, & Nelson, 1998). Other research involved the use of portable speech-generating devices (SGDs) in interventions designed to facilitate communicative interactions (Schepis, Reid, Behrmann, & Sutton, 1998), decrease problem behavior (Durand, 1999), or teach specific skills such as spelling (Schlosser, Blischak, Belfiore, Bartley, & Barnett, 1998). Over the past decade, research on the use of various technologies for individuals with developmental disabilities such as ASDs has expanded rapidly (e.g., Lancioni et al., 2007).

Facilitated Communication

Facilitated communication involves the use of a letterboard or keyboard on which messages are typed on a letter-by-letter basis. The typist's forearm, wrist, and (if necessary) index finger are physically supported by a facilitator, who also provides emotional and instructional support. Gradually, the supports provided by the facilitator are faded, with the goal of independent typing. Facilitated communication was first mentioned in a 1974 manual describing "effective teaching methods for autistic children" (Oppenheim, 1974). In Australia, facilitated communication was first used for individuals with ASDs by Rosemary Crossley in 1986 (see Crossley, 1993) and was later introduced to North America by Douglas Biklen (1990).

Facilitated communication is controversial, primarily because of the authorship question: Who is actually typing the message, the typist or the facilitator? The controversy stems from the fact that many facilitated typists are able to compose sophisticated messages that far exceed their perceived cognitive and language abilities, often in the absence of formal literacy instruction. In addition, whenever a facilitator supports the hand or arm of a typist, the potential exists for the facilitator to guide the typing process, albeit unintentionally.

Numerous publications have attempted to answer the authorship question through various research approaches. The vast majority of this research indicates that typists with ASDs are easily influenced by their facilitators when composing messages and that facilitators often influence typists' messages without realizing they are doing so (for reviews, see Jacobson, Mulick, & Schwartz, 1995; Mostert, 2001; and Simpson & Smith Myles, 1995). Given this, many professional organizations, including ASHA (1995), have issued position statements or resolutions recommending that facilitated communication not be used at all or that it be used very cautiously. Some typists, however, seem to compose messages without facilitator influence (Biklen & Cardinal, 1997). Other individuals began communicating through facilitated communication but are now able to communicate independently, without physical contact from a facilitator (Biklen, 2005; Biklen & Kliewer, 2006). Therefore, although facilitated communication remains controversial and is not accepted by most AAC clinicians or researchers, the issue is not as straightforward as it may seem (Mirenda, 2008).

AAC ASSESSMENT

One of the goals of an AAC assessment is to determine whether an individual requires AAC supports. This might appear to be an easy task, as it seems obvious that individuals who are unable to meet their daily communication needs through natural speech require AAC interventions. Nevertheless, in the 1970s and 1980s in particular, considerable controversy was generated about candidacy or eligibility criteria for AAC services. In many cases, individuals with ASDs were considered to be too "something" (e.g., too young; too old; too cognitively, behaviorally, or linguistically impaired) to qualify for AAC services. Other individuals were excluded from AAC services because they were perceived as having too many skills, especially with regard to natural speech. For example, AAC supports were often withheld from individuals with ASDs who could say a few words, in the hopes that their speech abilities would improve.

One of the most notable advancements in this field is the number of official documents that address the inappropriateness of such eligibility practices. For example, in 2005, ASHA noted that although there are no evidence-based procedures for determining whether a given individual is likely to benefit from AAC, "[n]o individuals should be denied this right, irrespective of the type and/or severity of communication, linguistic, social, cognitive, motor, sensory, perceptual, and/or other disability[ies] they may present" (p. 1). ASHA's statement is aligned with that of the National Joint Committee (NJC) for the

Communication Needs of Persons with Severe Disabilities (2003a, 2003b), which asserted that eligibility for communication services and supports should be based on communication needs alone, rather than on criteria such as discrepancies between cognitive and communication functioning, chronological age, diagnosis, absence of cognitive or other skills purported to be prerequisites, or other factors. Together, the ASHA and NJC statements are important advances in the AAC field because they emphasize that assessment can no longer be used as a gate-keeping mechanism for determining who may or may not receive AAC services. The question to be addressed by AAC assessment is *how* AAC interventions and supports can best be applied to a given individual rather than *if* an individual should have access to AAC interventions and supports. This advancement is especially important for many older individuals with ASDs, who may have access to AAC assessment and intervention for the first time as a result of these statements.

Another goal of AAC assessment is to identify discrepancies between an individual's communication needs and current capabilities to determine which AAC techniques may result in improved receptive and expressive communication. AAC assessment for individuals with ASDs is often quite challenging because of the effects of the social, language, sensory, and/or cognitive impairments they may experience. When conducting an AAC assessment, ASHA (2004) recommends the use of the Participation Model (Beukelman & Mirenda, 2005), which focuses on procedures aimed at identifying current and potential strengths and needs to guide the development of AAC interventions for both the present and the future. The use of this model was illustrated in a case study describing the process used by a school team to design AAC supports for a 6-year-old boy with autism (Light, Roberts, Dimarco, & Greiner, 1998). The authors used the general structure of the Participation Model to gather information about 1) the child's current and anticipated future communication needs; 2) his current abilities with regard to the sensory, receptive language, expressive communication, symbol representation, lexical organization, and motor skills needed for communication; 3) the communication opportunities that were available to him; and 4) the interaction strategies used by his frequent communication partners. The authors used a combination of parent and teacher interviews, a communication needs survey, ecological inventories, systematic observations, and both formal and informal (i.e., criterion-referenced) assessment tools to gather this information. They then designed a multimodal communication system that incorporated the child's existing natural speech, conventional gestures, a communication book and dictionary, and an SGD with software to support his writing and literacy development. This case study exemplifies the holistic, systematic assessment process that is required to make individualized AAC decisions for people with ASDs. See Chapter 2 for more information on assessment issues.

EVIDENCE-BASED PRACTICE

A relatively recent development in the field of AAC is an increased emphasis on evidence-based practice (EBP) for assessment, intervention planning, and implementation. EBP is "the integration of best and current research evidence with clinical/educational expertise and relevant stakeholder perspectives to facilitate decisions for assessment and intervention that are deemed effective and efficient for a given stakeholder" (Schlosser & Raghavendra, 2003, p. 263). EBP does *not* mean that either clinical reasoning or the perspectives of individuals who use AAC and their families are discounted during the AAC assessment or decision-making processes. Rather, in addition to these important elements, a third component—current research evidence—is added to the mix.

The EBP process, described by Schlosser and Raghavendra (2003), can be used to make decisions about the intervention components that are most likely to lead to positive outcomes for a given individual. The six steps of this process are

1. Ask a well-built question, such as "Should we use manual signing or should we use graphic symbols to teach requesting to this adolescent with autism?" or "Should we use an SGD to teach social interaction skills to this child with Rett syndrome?"

2. Select evidence sources (e.g., textbooks, research databases, journals).

3. Search the literature.

4. Examine the evidence systematically.

5. Apply the evidence to make decisions on behalf of the specific individual who requires AAC.

6. Evaluate the outcome of the decision over time.

One of the practical outcomes of the emphasis on EBP has been the generation of a number of integrative reviews of AAC research. In such reviews, authors examine research related to a specific type of AAC intervention (e.g., SGDs) with a specific population (e.g., children with ASDs), using either statistical or narrative techniques. They also provide summary statements regarding, for example, the benefits that have been shown to result from the use of a specific intervention or the optimum conditions for generating positive outcomes. Many authors in this book have used this process or a variation thereof to integrate existing research on specific aspects of AAC. In addition, integrative reviews on AAC for individuals with ASDs have addressed topics such as manual signing (Goldstein, 2002; Mirenda, 2001, 2003b; Wendt, Schlosser, & Lloyd, 2005), graphic symbols (Mirenda, 2001, 2003b; Wendt et al., 2005), SGDs and computers with speech output (Schlosser & Blischak, 2001; Wendt et al., 2005), functional communication training (Bopp, Brown, & Mirenda, 2004; Wendt et al., 2005), and visual schedules that use graphic symbols (Bopp et al., 2004).

Decision making that incorporates research evidence is important when designing AAC interventions for individuals with ASDs for a number of reasons. First, these individuals constitute an extremely heterogeneous group with regard to the social, cognitive, motivational, and motor abilities that underlie successful communication. Thus, AAC decisions must be made on the basis of individual skill and preference profiles, rather than on the basis of an ASD diagnosis alone. Researchers have therefore examined strategies for incorporating the modality preferences of individuals with ASDs into the decision-making process (Sigafoos, O'Reilly, Ganz, Lancioni, & Schlosser, 2005; Son, Sigafoos, O'Reilly, & Lancioni, 2006).

Second, the field of ASDs in general is "littered with the debris of dead ends, crushed hopes, ineffective treatments, and false starts" (Schreibman, 2005, p. 7). With regard to AAC, this was highlighted in 1970s by the wholesale adoption of total communication as "the answer" for all individuals with ASDs who were unable to speak; in the 1990s, a similar furor focused on facilitated communication. The tendency of many professionals and families to adopt the latest fad intervention, regardless of the quantity or quality of research evidence to support it, can be counteracted by the adoption of an EBP approach to decision making.

Third, for professionals in the field, EBPs are guaranteed to keep us humble by making us aware of just how much we still have to learn. The fact is that we do not know even more than we *do* know about AAC for individuals with ASD. We do not know how to select the combination of AAC modalities that will result in optimal communication for each individual; how to design comprehensive AAC instructional interventions that truly build on each person's abilities and strengths; or how to maximally support social, language, and literacy development through AAC. If it is indeed true that with humility comes wisdom, the systematic examination of research evidence for decision making is essential for the field to move forward.

CONUNDRUMS AND CONTROVERSIES

The Merriam-Webster Online Dictionary (2007) defines a *conundrum* as "an intricate and difficult problem." In the field of AAC, as in all other fields of scientific endeavor, a number of conundrums have come and gone over the years, while several have lingered and are still active today. Many of the currently controversial issues as they pertain to individuals with ASDs are examined in individual chapters of this book, including the use of SGDs for individuals with ASDs (Chapter 5) and how various AAC modalities affect the likelihood of speech production (Chapter 6). Additional chapters examine the use and effectiveness of both behavioral and social/developmental instructional approaches, including the Picture Exchange Communication System (Chapter 10; see also Frost & Bondy, 2002); the Social Communication, Emotional Regulation, and Transactional Support (SCERTS®) Model (Chapter 8; see also Prizant, Wetherby, Rubin, Laurent, & Rydell, 2005a, 2005b); and various aided language models (Chapters 7 and 9). Chapters on the use of AAC techniques for problem behavior (Chapters 12 and 13), literacy development (Chapter 14), and inclusive education (Chapter 15) also address conundrums that confront and challenge many families and AAC professionals who support individuals with ASDs. This chapter explores three additional controversial issues: 1) integrating AAC with other early intervention approaches for young children with ASDs, 2) deciding whether or not AAC is appropriate and choosing individualized AAC techniques, and 3) critically reexamining conventional assumptions about ASDs as they apply to AAC.

Early Intervention and AAC

The importance of early intervention for young children with ASDs is not a matter for debate. In a comprehensive, evidence-based report, the U.S. National Research Council (NRC) Committee on Educational Interventions for Children with Autism (2001) strongly recommended that entry into intervention programs should begin as soon as an ASD diagnosis is seriously considered, rather than waiting until it is confirmed. The NRC Committee also concurred that "active engagement in intensive instructional programming" (p. 219) should be provided to children at least up to age 8 years for a minimum of 25 hours per week on a year-round basis, and should consist of "repeated, planned teaching opportunities" (p. 219) conducted in both one-to-one and very small group sessions. They also recommended that emphasis be placed on the use of evidence-based instructional techniques in six main instructional areas: 1) functional, spontaneous communication using speech and/or AAC; 2) developmentally appropriate social skills with parents and peers; 3) play skills with peers; 4) various goals for cognitive development, with emphasis on generalization; 5) positive behavior supports for problem behaviors; and 6) functional academic skills, as appropriate.

The NRC Committee (2001) acknowledged that a wide range of instructional approaches may be used to accomplish these goals. These approaches include structured teaching based on the principles of applied behavior analysis such as discrete trial teaching (Smith, 2001), incidental teaching (McGee, Morrier, & Daly, 1999), applied verbal behavior (Sundberg & Partington, 1998), and pivotal response training (Koegel & Koegel, 2006). They also include social/developmental approaches such as the Developmental, Individual-Difference, Relationship-Based (DIR) model (Greenspan & Weider, 1999) and the SCERTS Model (Prizant et al., 2005a, 2005b). Although the NRC Committee did not recommend a specific curriculum or approach, they stressed the importance of goal-directed, evidence-based, individualized programs that meet the needs of both children with ASDs and their families.

Because of these recommendations, immediately after receiving a diagnosis for their child, families are faced with the daunting task of deciding what to do for their child with ASD and how best to do it. Some of their decisions may affect the extent to which AAC techniques of various types will be accepted and used (e.g., in an applied verbal behavior approach, manual signing may be accepted but graphic symbols may not be; see Mirenda, 2003b; Sundberg, 1993). Even when there is agreement about the techniques to implement, AAC practitioners will almost always need to work with other professionals whose views may be quite divergent from (and perhaps even incompatible with) their own. The potential for controversy is considerable and the potential for conflict is high; therefore, the ability to negotiate and collaborate is required of all involved.

To AAC or Not to AAC?

If the goal of an AAC system is to "enable individuals to efficiently and effectively engage in a variety of interactions and participate in activities of their choice" (Beukelman & Mirenda, 2005, p. 8), it is critical that AAC interventions be maximally individualized. This principle raises a number of contentious issues, the first and foremost of which is that many parents of young children (and some practitioners as well) are reluctant to implement AAC interventions out of concern that they will prevent speech production (Cress & Marvin, 2003). Despite credible research evidence to the contrary (Chapter 6; see also Millar, Light, & Schlosser, 2006), this reluctance continues to limit the extent to which individuals who can benefit from AAC have access to it. In addition, AAC is no less immune to "one-size-fits-all" thinking than is any other type of educational intervention. Some practitioners who ascribe to this way of thinking institute one or more AAC techniques with everyone whose social-communication interactions are lacking, regardless of whether AAC is actually required. Other practitioners espouse the superiority of a particular instructional technique over all others, regardless of the abilities and preferences of individuals with ASDs or their families. Still others may always prescribe the specific AAC modality with which they have experience, rather than considering the entire range of available options. For example, some practitioners claim that manual signing is the best AAC technique for all individuals with ASDs, based largely on theoretical arguments rather than on empirical evidence (Mirenda, 2003b). Regardless, this one-size-fits-all thinking invariably limits the communication options that are available to individuals with ASDs and can be avoided by adopting the general EBP approach that was described in a previous section of this chapter.

(Mis)conceptions About ASDs and AAC

Research has called into question at least two of the assumptions that most people accept about ASDs in general: 1) motor impairments are not part of the disorder and 2) in most cases, intellectual disability is. Mirenda (2008) noted that these two assumptions directly affect both the design and the goals of AAC interventions for many individuals with ASDs. Alternative access or instructional supports are rarely provided to compensate for the types of motor planning or coordination problems that appear to be more common than previously thought (e.g., Dziuk et al., 2007; Hardan, Kilpatrick, Keshavan, & Minshew, 2003; Ming, Brimacombe, & Wagner, 2007; Minshew, Sung, Jones, & Furman, 2004). AAC goals are often focused solely on basic requesting skills, under the assumption that most individuals with ASDs will be unable to acquire a broad range of communicative functions because of limited cognitive capacity. Edelson (2006) and others (e.g., Dawson, Soulières, Gernsbacher, & Mottron, 2007), however, have provided empirical evidence to challenge the conventional presumption that intellectual disability usually co-occurs with ASDs. In addition, some researchers have started to demonstrate that individuals with ASDs can become much more communicatively competent through the use of AAC than might be expected in the presence of intellectual disability (e.g., Light et al., 2005). Given all of this, Mirenda (2008) urged AAC clinicians and researchers to "question what we think we know about people with ASD in general and how we support those individuals whose speech does not develop to communicate through AAC in particular." It remains to be seen whether the AAC community will take up this challenge both to reconceptualize ASDs in general and to design innovative AAC interventions that push traditional boundaries and presume the potential for competence.

CONCLUSION

Decision making related to AAC interventions for individuals with ASDs is a complex and challenging endeavor. Because of the wide heterogeneity of this population, decisions about appropriate AAC techniques cannot and should not be made in the abstract; rather, they must be made for specific learners, in specific contexts, to meet specific needs (Beukelman & Mirenda, 2005). It is clear that that the success or failure of any AAC intervention is not simply a matter of choosing symbols or devices; instructional variables are also critically important. Indeed, when AAC fails to result in spontaneous, functional communication, this failure usually reflects limitations in the procedures and methods used for instruction rather than an inherent problem with AAC itself. In the end, the combination of research-based modality selection, excellent instruction, and goodness-of-fit (Bailey et al., 1990) with regard to environments, communication partners, and communication needs are all needed to maximize the possibility of successful communication for individuals with ASDs.

REFERENCES

American Psychiatric Association. (2000). *Diagnostic and statistical manual of mental disorders* (4th ed., text rev.). Washington, DC: Author.

American Speech-Language-Hearing Association. (1995, March). Position statement on facilitated communication. *ASHA Supplement, 37*(14), 22.

American Speech-Language-Hearing Association. (2004). Roles and responsibilities of speech-language pathologists with respect to augmentative and alternative communication: Technical report. *ASHA Supplement, 24*, 1–17.

American Speech-Language-Hearing Association. (2005). Roles and responsibilities of speech-language pathologists with respect to augmentative and alternative communication: Position statement. *ASHA Supplement, 25*, 1–2.

Bailey, B.D., Simeonsson, R.J., Winton, P.J., Huntington, G.S., Comfort, M., Isbell, P., et al. (1990). Family-focused intervention: A functional model for planning, implementing and evaluating individualized family services in early intervention. *Journal of the Division for Early Childhood, 10*, 156–171.

Bernard-Opitz, V., Ross, K., & Tuttas, M.L. (1990). Computer assisted instruction for autistic children. *Annals of the Academy of Medicine, 19*, 611–616.

Beukelman, D.R., & Mirenda, P. (2005). *Augmentative and alternative communication: Supporting children and adults with complex communication needs* (3rd ed.). Baltimore: Paul H. Brookes Publishing Co.

Biklen, D. (1990). Communication unbound: Autism and praxis. *Harvard Educational Review, 60*, 291–314.

Biklen, D. (2005). *Autism and the myth of the person alone*. New York: New York University Press.

Biklen, D., & Cardinal, D. (1997). *Contested words, contested science: Unraveling the facilitated communication controversy*. New York: Teachers College Press.

Biklen, D., & Kliewer, C. (2006). Constructing competence: Autism, voice and the "disordered" body. *International Journal of Inclusive Education, 10*, 169–188.

Bondy, A., & Frost, L. (1994). The Picture Exchange Communication System. *Focus on Autistic Behavior, 9*, 1–19.

Bopp, K., Brown, K., & Mirenda, P. (2004). Speech-language pathologists' roles in the delivery of positive behavior support for individuals with developmental disabilities. *American Journal of Speech-Language Pathology, 13*, 5–19.

Bryen, D., & Joyce, D. (1985). Language intervention with the severely handicapped: A decade of research. *Journal of Special Education, 19*, 7–39.

Carrier, J., Jr., & Peak, T. (1975). *Non-SLIP (Non-speech language initiation program)*. Lawrence, KS: H & H Enterprises.

Centers for Disease Control and Prevention. (2007, February). Prevalence of autism spectrum disorders—Autism and Developmental Disabilities Monitoring Network, six sites, United States, 2000. *Morbidity and Mortality Weekly Report, 56*(SS-1), 1–40.

Chen, S.H.A., & Bernard-Opitz, V. (1993). Comparison of personal and computer-assisted instruction for children with autism. *Mental Retardation, 31i(6)*, 368–376.

Churchill, D.W. (1972). The relation of infantile autism and early childhood schizophrenia to developmental language disorders of childhood. *Journal of Autism and Childhood Schizophrenia, 2*, 182–197.

Colby, K.M. (1973). The rationale for computer-based treatment of language difficulties in non-speaking autistic children. *Journal of Autism and Childhood Schizophrenia, 3*, 254–260.

Colby, K.M., & Kraemer, H. (1975). An objective measurement of nonspeaking children's performance with a computer-controlled program for the stimulation of language behavior. *Journal of Autism and Childhood Schizophrenia, 5*, 139–146.

Colby, K.M., & Smith, D.C. (1974). Computers in the treatment of nonspeaking autistic children. In J.H. Masserman (Ed.), *Current psychiatric therapies*. New York: Grune & Stratton.

Cornforth, A.R.T., Johnson, K., & Walker, M. (1974). Teaching sign language to the deaf mentally handicapped. *Apex, 2*(1), 23–25.

Creedon, M.P. (1973, March). *Language development in nonverbal autistic children using a simultaneous communication system*. Paper presented at the Society for Research in Child Development meeting, Philadelphia.

Cress, C., & Marvin, C. (2003). Common questions about AAC services in early intervention. *Augmentative and Alternative Communication, 19*, 254–272.

Crossley, R. (1993). *Flying high on paper wings*. Retrieved March 18, 2007, from http://home.vicnet.net.au/~dealcc/Flying.htm

Dawson, M., Soulières, I., Gernsbacher, M.A., & Mottron, L. (2007). The level and nature of autistic intelligence. *Psychological Science, 18*, 657–662.

deVilliers, J., & Naughton, J. (1974). Teaching a symbol language to autistic children. *Journal of Consultation in Clinical Psychology, 42,* 111–117.

Dunlap, G., & Bunton-Pierce, M. (1999). Autism and autism spectrum disorder. In *ERIC Digest #E583.* Washington, DC: Education Resources Information Center. (ERIC Document Reproduction Service No. ED436068)

Durand, V.M. (1999). Functional communication training using assistive devices: Recruiting natural communities of reinforcement. *Journal of Applied Behavior Analysis, 32,* 247–267.

Dziuk, M., Gidley, J., Larson, J., Apostu, A., Mahone, E., Denckla, M., et al. (2007). Dyspraxia in autism: Association with motor, social, and communicative deficits. *Developmental Medicine & Child Neurology, 49,* 734–739.

Edelson, M.G. (2006). Are the majority of children with autism mentally retarded? A systematic evaluation of the data. *Focus on Autism and Other Developmental Disabilities, 21,* 66–83.

Frith, U., & Snowling, M. (1983). Reading for meaning and reading for sound in autistic and dyslexic children. *British Journal of Developmental Psychology, 1,* 329–342.

Frost, L., & Bondy, A. (2002). *Picture Exchange Communication System training manual* (2nd ed.). Newark, DE: Pyramid Education Products.

Gardner, R., & Gardner, B. (1969). Teaching sign language to a chimpanzee. *Science, 165,* 664–672.

Goldstein, H. (2002). Communication intervention for children with autism: A review of treatment efficacy. *Journal of Autism and Developmental Disorders, 32,* 373–396.

Greenspan, S., & Weider, S. (1999). A functional developmental approach to autism spectrum disorders. *Journal of The Association for Persons with Severe Handicaps, 24,* 147–161.

Hardan, A., Kilpatrick, M., Keshavan, M., & Minshew, N. (2003). Motor performance and anatomic magnetic resonance imaging (MRI) of the basal ganglia in autism. *Journal of Child Neurology, 18,* 317–324.

Hedbring, C. (1985). Computers and autistic learners: An evolving technology. *Australian Journal of Human Communication Disorders, 13,* 169–188.

Heimann, M., Nelson, K.E., Tjus, T., & Gillberg, C. (1995). Increasing reading and communication skills in children with autism through an interactive multimedia computer program. *Journal of Autism and Developmental Disorders, 25(5),* 459–480.

Hewett, F. (1964). Teaching reading to an autistic boy through operant conditioning. *Reading Teacher, 17,* 613–618.

Iacono, T., & Parsons, C. (1986). A survey of the use of signing with the intellectually disabled. *Australian Communication Quarterly, 2,* 21–25.

Jacobson, J.W., Mulick, J.A., & Schwartz, A.A. (1995). A history of facilitated communication: Science, pseudoscience, and antiscience. *American Psychologist, 50,* 750–765.

Kiernan, C. (1983). The use of nonvocal communication techniques with autistic individuals. *Journal of Child Psychology and Psychiatry, 24,* 339–375.

Kiernan, C., Reid, B., & Jones, M. (1982). *Signs and symbols: Use of non-vocal communication systems.* London: Heinemann.

Kliewer, C., & Biklen, D. (2001). "School's not really a place for reading": A research synthesis of the literacy lives of students with severe disabilities. *Journal of The Association for Persons with Severe Handicaps, 26*, 1–12.

Koegel, R., & Koegel, L.K. (2006). *Pivotal response treatments for autism: Communication, social, and academic development.* Baltimore: Paul H. Brookes Publishing Co.

Koppenhaver, D.A. (2000). Literacy in AAC: What should be written on the envelope we push? *Augmentative and Alternative Communication, 16*, 270–279.

Lancioni, G.E. (1983). Using pictorial representations as communication means with low-functioning children. *Journal of Autism and Developmental Disorders, 13*, 87–105.

Lancioni, G.E., O'Reilly, M., Cuvo, A., Singh, N., Sigafoos, J., & Didden, R. (2007). PECS and VOCAs to enable students with developmental disabilities to make requests: An overview of the literature. *Research in Developmental Disabilities, 28*, 468–488.

LaVigna, G. (1977). Communication training in mute autistic adolescents using the written word. *Journal of Autism & Childhood Schizophrenia, 17*, 115–132.

Light, J., Drager, K., Curran, J., Hayes, E., Kristiansen, L., Lewis, W., et al. (2005). *AAC interventions to maximize language development in young children.* Retrieved on November 3, 2007, from http://www.aac-rerc.com/index.php?option=com_content&task=view&id=135&Itemid=152

Light, J., Roberts, B., Dimarco, R., & Greiner, N. (1998). Augmentative and alternative communication to support receptive and expressive communication for people with autism. *Journal of Communication Disorders, 31*, 153–180.

Marshall, N., & Hegrenes, J. (1972). The use of written language as a communication system for an autistic child. *Journal of Speech and Hearing Disorders, 2*, 258–261.

Matas, J., Mathy-Laikko, P., Beukelman, D., & Legresley, K. (1985). Identifying the nonspeaking population: A demographic study. *Augmentative and Alternative Communication, 1*, 17–31.

McGee, G., Morrier, M., & Daly, T. (1999). An incidental teaching approach to early intervention for toddlers with autism. *Journal of The Association for Persons with Severe Handicaps, 24*, 133–146.

McLean, L., & McLean, J. (1974). A language training program for nonverbal autistic children. *Journal of Speech and Hearing Disorders, 39*, 186–193.

Merriam-Webster Online Dictionary. (2007). Definition of "conundrum" retrieved March 11, 2007, from http://www.m-w.com/dictionary

Millar, D., Light, J.C., & Schlosser, R.W. (2006). The impact of augmentative and alternative communication on the speech production of individuals with developmental disabilities: A research review. *Journal of Speech, Language, and Hearing Research, 49*, 248–264.

Miller, A., & Miller, E.E. (1973). Cognitive-developmental training with elevated boards and sign language. *Journal of Autism and Childhood Schizophrenia, 3*, 65–85.

Ming, X., Brimacombe, M., & Wagner, G. (2007). Prevalence of motor impairment in autism spectrum disorders. *Brain & Development, 29*, 565–570.

Minshew, N., Sung, K., Jones, B., & Furman, J. (2004). Underdevelopment of the postural control system in autism. *Neurology, 63,* 2056–2061.

Mirenda, P. (2001). Autism, augmentative communication, and assistive technology: What do we really know? *Focus on Autism and Other Developmental Disabilities, 16,* 141–151.

Mirenda, P. (2003a). "He's not really a reader....": Perspectives on supporting literacy development in individuals with autism. *Topics in Language Disorders, 23,* 270–281.

Mirenda, P. (2003b). Toward functional augmentative and alternative communication for students with autism: Manual signs, graphic symbols, and voice output communication aids. *Language, Speech, and Hearing Services in Schools, 34,* 202–215.

Mirenda, P. (2008). A back door approach to autism and AAC. *Augmentative and Alternative Communication, 24,* 219–233.

Mirenda, P., & Iacono, T. (1988). Strategies for promoting augmentative and alternative communication in natural contexts with students with autism. *Focus on Autistic Behavior, 3*(4), 1–16.

Mirenda, P., & Santogrossi, J. (1985). A prompt-free strategy to teach pictorial communication system use. *Augmentative and Alternative Communication, 1,* 143–150.

Mostert, M. (2001). Facilitated communication since 1995: A review of published studies. *Journal of Autism and Developmental Disorders, 31,* 287–313.

National Joint Committee for the Communication Needs of Persons with Severe Disabilities. (2003a). Position statement on access to communication services and supports: Concerns regarding the application of restrictive "eligibility" policies. *ASHA Supplement, 23,* 19–20.

National Joint Committee for the Communication Needs of Persons with Severe Disabilities (2003b). Supporting documentation for the position statement on access to communication services and supports: Concerns regarding the application of restrictive "eligibility" policies. *ASHA Supplement, 23,* 73–81.

National Research Council, Committee on Educational Interventions for Children with Autism, Division of Behavioral and Social Sciences and Education. (2001). *Educating children with autism.* Washington, DC: National Academies Press.

Oppenheim, R. (1974). *Effective teaching methods for autistic children.* Springfield, IL: Charles C Thomas.

Parsons, C., & La Sorte, D. (1993). The effect of computers with synthesized speech and no speech on the spontaneous communication of children with autism. *Australian Journal of Human Communication Disorders, 21,* 12–31.

Premack, D. (1971). Language in a chimpanzee? *Science, 172,* 808–822.

Premack D., & Premack, A. (1974). Teaching visual language to apes and language-deficient persons. In R. Schiefelbusch & L.L. Lloyd (Eds.), *Language perspectives—Acquisition, retardation, and intervention* (pp. 347–376). Baltimore: University Park Press.

Prizant, B.M., Wetherby, A.M., Rubin, E., Laurent, A.C., & Rydell, P.J. (2005a). *The SCERTS® Model: A comprehensive educational approach for children with autism spectrum disorders. Vol. 1: Assessment.* Baltimore: Paul H. Brookes Publishing Co.

Prizant, B.M., Wetherby, A.M., Rubin, E., Laurent, A.C., & Rydell, P.J. (2005b). *The SCERTS® Model: A comprehensive educational approach for children with autism spectrum disorders. Vol. 2: Intervention.* Baltimore: Paul H. Brookes Publishing Co.

Ratusnik, C., & Ratusnik, D. (1974). A comprehensive communication approach for a ten-year-old nonverbal autistic child. *American Journal of Orthopsychiatry, 43,* 396–403.

Reichle, J., & Brown, L. (1986). Teaching the use of a multipage direct selection communication board to an adult with autism. *Journal of The Association for Persons with Severe Handicaps, 11,* 68–73.

Romski, M.A., & Sevcik, R. (1996). *Breaking the speech barrier: Language development through augmented means.* Baltimore: Paul H. Brookes Publishing Co.

Rumbaugh, D. (1977). *Language learning in the chimpanzee: The LANA Project.* New York: Academic Press.

Savage-Rumbaugh, S., Rumbaugh, D., & Boysen, S. (1978). Symbolic communication between two chimpanzees *(Pan troglodytes). Science, 201,* 641–644.

Schepis, M., Reid, D., Behrmann, M., & Sutton, K. (1998). Increasing communicative interactions of young children with autism using a voice output communication aid and naturalistic teaching. *Journal of Applied Behavior Analysis, 31,* 561–578.

Schlosser, R., & Blischak, D. (2001). Is there a role for speech output in interventions for persons with autism? A review. *Focus on Autism and Other Developmental Disabilities, 16,* 170–178.

Schlosser, R., Blischak, D., Belfiore, P., Bartley, C., & Barnett, N. (1998). Effects of synthetic speech output and orthographic feedback in a student with autism: A preliminary study. *Journal of Autism and Developmental Disorders, 28,* 309–319.

Schlosser, R., & Raghavendra, P. (2003). Toward evidence-based practice in AAC. In R. Schlosser (Ed.), *The efficacy of augmentative and alternative communication* (pp. 260–297). New York: Elsevier.

Schreibman, L. (2005). *The science and fiction of autism.* Cambridge, MA: Harvard University Press.

Schuler, A., & Baldwin, M. (1981). Nonspeech communication and childhood autism. *Language, Speech, and Hearing Services in Schools, 12,* 246–257.

Sigafoos, J., O'Reilly, M., Ganz, J., Lancioni, G., & Schlosser, R. (2005). Supporting self-determination in AAC interventions by assessing preference for communication devices, *Technology and Disability, 17,* 143–153.

Simpson, R., & Smith Myles, B. (1995). Effectiveness of facilitated communication with children and youth with autism. *Journal of Special Education, 28,* 424–439.

Smith, T. (2001). Discrete trial training in the treatment of autism. *Focus on Autism and Other Developmental Disabilities, 16,* 86–92.

Son, S.-H., Sigafoos, J., O'Reilly, M., & Lancioni, G. (2006). Comparing two types of augmentative and alternative communication systems for children with autism. *Pediatric Rehabilitation, 9,* 389–395.

Sundberg, M. (1993). Selecting a response form for nonverbal persons: Facilitated communication, pointing systems, or sign language? *The Analysis of
Verbal Behavior, 11,* 99–116.

Sundberg, M., & Partington, J. (1998). *Teaching language to children with autism
and other developmental disabilities* (version 7.1). Pleasant Hill, CA: Behavior
Analysts.

Tager-Flusberg, H., Paul, R., & Lord, C. (2005). Language and communication
in autism. In F.G. Volkmar, R. Paul, A. Klin, & D. Cohen (Eds.), *Handbook of
autism and pervasive developmental disorders* (Vol. 1, pp. 335–364). Hoboken,
NJ: John Wiley & Sons.

Tjus, T., Heimann, M., & Nelson, K. (1998). Gains in literacy through the use of
a specially developed multimedia computer strategy: Positive findings from
13 children with autism. *Autism, 2,* 139–156.

Walker, M. (1987, March). *The Makaton Vocabulary: Uses and effectiveness.* Paper
presented at the First International AFASIC Symposium, University of Reading, England.

Webster, C.D., McPherson, H., Sloman, L., Evans, M.A., & Kuchar, E. (1973).
Communicating with an autistic boy by gestures. *Journal of Autism and Childhood Schizophrenia, 3,* 337–346.

Wendt, O., Schlosser, R., & Lloyd, L.L. (2005, November). *How effective are AAC
interventions for children with autism? A meta-analysis of research outcomes.*
Paper presented at the annual convention of the American Speech-
Language-Hearing Association, San Diego.

Whitehouse, D., & Harris, J. (1984). Hyperlexia in infantile autism. *Journal of
Autism & Developmental Disorders, 14,* 281–289.

2

Assessment Issues

TERESA IACONO AND TEENA CAITHNESS

The function and principles of assessment relevant to people with autism spectrum disorders (ASDs) are the same as for any other group with developmental disabilities. This similarity is true also when considering assessment that will inform augmentative and alternative communication (AAC) interventions. There are differences, however, in the particular challenges that face people with ASD. Such differences relate to their individual strengths and weaknesses, as well as the effectiveness of their support systems, which enhance communication in reciprocal interactions.

Assessment is a comprehensive, dynamic, and ongoing process based on a transactional model of communication interaction. For children, the assessment process involves the family, other people who provide primary support to the child, and the recognition of their concerns and preferences within approaches that are family-centered. Assessment extends beyond the testing of skills to gathering information about the child's functioning in terms of communication and related areas across environments or social contexts. It includes discovering the preferences of a child with ASD on what and how to learn and, over time, gaining an understanding of his or her perspective. In this chapter, these principles are extended to adults with ASDs, particularly those for whom a clear diagnosis has never been obtained or for whom the information has not been seen as particularly relevant because of an overriding intellectual disability. For these adults, family-centered practice may merge with person-centered practice, as well as consideration of AAC within supported community-based settings (e.g., group homes) and family homes.

Much has been written about diagnostic assessments of children with suspected ASDs (American Speech-Language-Hearing Association, 2006; Lord & Risi, 2000; Paul, 2005). This literature provides characteristics that differentiate ASD from other developmental disabilities. Once diagnosis is confirmed, however, the need for assessment continues as a means of informing interventions. This chapter focuses on the function of assessment to inform interventions that involve AAC to address discrepancies between current communication functioning and the communication needs of people with ASDs. In particular, this chapter presents assessment principles and strategies from both AAC and ASD literature, a review of learner characteristics in ASD, and a proposed lifespan model of assessment.

MODELS FOR ASSESSMENT

In this section, the participation model and family- and person-centered planning approaches are introduced, both of which are often used as foundations for AAC assessment.

Participation Model

AAC assessment informs planning for intervention to address communication needs over a person's lifetime. The participation model provides a guide to AAC assessment (Beukelman & Mirenda, 2005) by focusing on an area addressed by the International Classification of Functioning, Disability and Health (World Health Organization, 2001). It provides a process to identify participation restrictions while also addressing the levels of impairment and activity restrictions through such criteria as assessment of capabilities and current activities. Using the participation model, information is gathered from a wide range of sources to gain an understanding of an individual's current communication patterns, participation patterns, and opportunities for participation. Distilling this information allows intervention to meet the individual's current needs through AAC systems, which will prepare the person to meet future communication needs (Beukelman & Mirenda, 2005; Mirenda, 2001).

Family- and Person-Centered Approaches

Family involvement in the assessment and intervention process receives the most attention in early childhood intervention literature. Within the context of family-centered approaches, the fact that the child is part of a family unit, which is in turn a part of a larger community, has been acknowledged (Crais & Calculator, 1998; Dunst, Johanson, Trivette, & Hamby, 1991). Building on an argument by Beukelman and Mirenda (2005) about consensus building in AAC assessment, Crais and Calculator (1998) argued that caregivers must be made integral to the assessment and intervention of young children through collaboration with professionals in problem identification, determining the purpose of assessment, assessment planning and conduct, and development of intervention goals and strategies. Facilitating such an integral role of caregivers is thought to strengthen family functioning (Dunst et al., 1991).

Limited research is available on the impact of cultural differences on the role of families in their child's development, as well as perspectives about disability, professionals, and the use of services. Lynch and Hanson (2004) argued that learning about the cultural group represented within a community and working with a cultural mediator or guide can provide an understanding of factors that influence a caregiver's level of involvement in their child's assessment and intervention, as well as culturally acceptable approaches and strategies. Such an understanding will strengthen the professional's collaboration with the family.

Within the participation model, involving both the individual who is the focus of the assessment and the individual's family is a means of obtaining comprehensive information, promoting ownership of interventions by the person and the family, developing trust between participants, and allowing the individual and family members to become part of the team (Beukelman & Mirenda, 2005). For adults with ASD who may not live in a family unit, support workers are often their main communication partners. Unfortunately, support workers may not want to be involved in the process (Iacono, Forster, Bryce, & Bloomberg, 2004) or may lack the necessary skills to facilitate the person's communicative interactions (Bloomberg, West, & Iacono, 2003). However, recent research by Iacono and colleagues (Iacono et al., 2004; Forster & Iacono, 2007) suggests that with prolonged engagement, support workers can come to see themselves as being communication partners and supports to adults with disabilities in their care.

Involvement of the individual with ASD in the assessment and intervention process also extends the notion of family-centered practice to person-centered approaches, whereby the individual is seen as a valued and included member of society. Of particular relevance for adults with developmental disabilities and complex communication needs, including those with ASDs, is the need for careful consideration of how best to determine that person's needs and preferences, rather than only those of caregivers and other support people. Strategies that address this need fall under the umbrella of person-centered planning approaches, which have developed during the last 30 years (O'Brien & O'Brien, 2002). According to O'Brien and O'Brien (2002), these approaches share the characteristics of 1) seeing people, rather than diagnostic labels, first; 2) avoiding professional jargon in favor of everyday language; 3) actively identifying a person's gifts and capacities within community life; and 4) ensuring that the voice of the person is heard, both directly and through others who know the person well, to evaluate present conditions and identify desirable changes.

Person-centered planning has particular relevance to assessment of adults for the development of AAC interventions. In focusing on the perspectives of the individual, there is a need to determine how communication can be enhanced with preferred interaction partners, in preferred contexts, and using preferred modalities, including extant modes of communication. In addition, these approaches reflect family-centered approaches by considering the perspectives and resources provided by the family and others who take on facilitator roles (Sanderson, 2000).

IDENTIFICATION OF SKILL PROFILES AND LEARNER CHARACTERISTICS

For people with ASDs, the assessment of capabilities presents particular challenges that arise from their impairment in social functioning. The profiling of skills is essential because the characteristics of people with ASD differ from those of people with other developmental disabilities; these characteristics also contribute to learning styles and methods of processing information. According to Abbeduto and Boudreau (2004), a learner's previous experiences and developmental achievements will influence the capability to acquire new information and approaches to effective intervention. Knowledge of a learner's profile gives insight into previous potential learning experiences. In addition, because the patterns of strengths and weaknesses differ between individuals (Mundy & Sigman, 1989; Wetherby, Prizant, & Hutchinson, 1998) and may change from childhood to adulthood (Howlin, Goode, Hutton, & Rutter, 2004), a comprehensive assessment of social and communication skills is warranted. When planning AAC interventions, such profiles of learner characteristics and capabilities inform the development of AAC systems and strategies, which support continued skill development and enhance social interactions.

Distinct Communication Profiles

ASD is characterized by core deficits in joint attention, symbolic capacity, and social-affective behavior (e.g., Wetherby, Prizant, & Schuler, 2000). These core deficits influence the communication profiles of individuals with ASDs as they progress from early childhood to adulthood.

Early Childhood In their preschool years, the early communicative behaviors of children with ASDs tend to be limited to regulating behavior rather than engaging social interaction or referencing joint attention. Mundy, Sigman, and Kasari (1990) found that children with autism showed a specific deficit in 1) the use of early gestures to coordinate attention between objects or events and another person, 2) sharing experiences with others by drawing their attention to objects or events, 3) following another person's gaze or pointing, and 4) using gaze to shift another person's attention. These deficits lead to asynchronies in the development of early pragmatic functions, particularly the increased use of intentional communication behaviors to signal requests rather than comments (Wetherby, Yonclas, & Bryan, 1989). This pattern is thought to arise from fundamental impairments in social cognition (Mundy et al., 1990), including an awareness that other people have a state of mind that is separate from the child's own.

Young children with ASDs also show delays in symbolic capacity, as reflected in the limited use of symbolic gestures and symbolic play (Wetherby et al., 2000), which contrast with apparent strengths in constructive play (Rogers, Cook, & Meryl, 2005). Along with skills in joint attention, symbolic play has been found to be associated with language performance (e.g., Mundy, Sigman, Ungerer, & Sherman, 1987). Wetherby et al. (2000) argued that as a result of their impairment in symbolic communication, children with ASDs learn to rely on idiosyncratic, unconventional, or undesirable behavior to achieve communicative functions such as gaining attention, escaping situations, or protesting against unexpected changes to routines.

Related to weaknesses in joint attention and symbolic communication are difficulties with social-affective signaling (Greenspan & Wieder, 1997; Wetherby et al., 2000), defined as "the use of gaze shifts between person and object, expression of positive affect with directed eye gaze, and episodes of negative affect" (Wetherby et al., 1998, p. 84). Social-affective signaling is integral to the development of communication in that it impacts the extent to which a child engages with the social environment through meaningful interactions, including shared routines that allow a child to make sense of the world (Carpenter & Tomasello, 2000). As a result of impaired social interaction, children with ASDs have difficulties with receptive language (Greenspan & Wieder, 1997) and integrating linguistic input with real world knowledge, which lead to deficits in pragmatic skills. These deficits, in turn, result in difficulty understanding rules and the nuances that govern social interactions (Lord & Paul, 1997).

Problems with sensory modulation have also been identified in young and school-age children with ASDs. Baranek, Parham, and

Bodfish (2005) noted that sensory problems have been described in various ways, including hypo- or hypersensitivity and preoccupation with different types of sensory input. In addition, some children have shown motor deficits, including difficulties with motor imitation (Baranek et al., 2005; Rogers et al., 2005). According to a review by Rogers et al. (2005), research has failed to identify the primary mechanism underlying imitation problems, although dyspraxia has been nominated as a cause. Despite differences in terms of research findings, Baranek et al. (2005) stated that variations in sensory and motor difficulties across children contribute to the heterogeneity of this group. Furthermore, they argued the need to consider potential differences in learning experiences across children that may arise from sensory or motor difficulties. Such information may assist in the determination of appropriate intervention strategies and preferences for augmented input and production.

Later Childhood   Lord and Paul (1997) noted frequent reports that 50% of children with autism fail to develop spoken communication after the age of 5 years. For those children with ASD who do develop functional speech, it is often characterized by immediate and delayed echolalia, which may have interactive or noninteractive pragmatic functions (Prizant & Duchan, 1981), arise from high constraint communicative contexts (Rydell & Mirenda, 1994), or be indicative of limited linguistic skills (Roberts, 1989, 1999). In addition, McEvoy, Loveland, and Landry (1988) found that reductions in the frequency of echolalia were associated with increased levels of expressive language in children with ASD. Roberts (1999) found that an increase in immediate echolalia with a concomitant increase in the percentage of echolalia that was changed in some way (i.e., mitigated), was associated with an increase in receptive language skills.

For children with functional spoken communication, few problems are experienced in terms of linguistic form. A longitudinal study by Tager-Flusberg et al. (1990) indicated that six young children with ASDs (ages 3 years 4 months to 7 years 7 months) showed the same general patterns in their grammatical and lexical skill development during a 12- to 26-month period as a group of language-matched children with Down syndrome. Other studies have provided support for normal developmental patterns in semantic, grammatical, and syntactic language skills, although they may be delayed (see Tager-Flusberg, 1997).

An important skill to consider for AAC is reading, given the potential to develop a system using written words and text (Paul, 2005). Research into the reading skills of children with ASDs has focused on apparent hyperlexia, in which skill in word decoding occurs without comprehension (Nation, Clarke, Wright, & Williams, 2006), which is surprising because of the cognitive and language impairment seen in individuals with autism or intellectual disability (Snowling & Frith, 1986). Nation et al. (2006) noted that although hyperlexia occurs in children other than those with ASDs, it has been associated mostly with this group. Much of the research is based on single case studies (e.g., Atkin & Perlman Lorch, 2006) or small groups (e.g., Snowling & Frith, 1986).

Research has indicated that the poor reading comprehension seen in children and adults with ASD has been associated with poor verbal language skills, particularly receptive language (Nation et al., 2006; Snowling & Frith, 1986). The implication is that apparent word reading skills may not sustain engagement and progress in academic activities, which are reliant on the ability to comprehend connected text as a mechanism for reading to learn (Westby, 1999).

Nation et al. (2006) warned that the focus on hyperlexia in ASD reflects an assumption that reading is an area of strength for this group, in some cases being considered a savant skill (see Atkin & Perlman Lorch, 2006). Their own research with 41 children with ASDs, ages 6–15 years, demonstrated a wide variety of skills. Nine children were nonreaders. Of the remaining 32 children, some showed the hyperlexic pattern of strong word reading but poor reading comprehension of text; others were poor at reading words and nonwords, or nonwords only, despite strong word reading skills. In addition, although they demonstrated strong relationships amongst component skills of reading (e.g., word or nonword reading and text reading), the correlations were smaller than have been demonstrated for a normative sample. Such heterogeneity points to the need for comprehensive reading assessments that include phonemic awareness, word and nonword reading, comprehension of text, and receptive language profiles, including semantic and syntactic skills.

Adolescents and Adults   In contrast to the large body of literature addressing communication and learning characteristics of young children, research addressing adolescents and adults is limited (Howlin et al., 2004). The few follow-up studies of children with ASDs have indicated variable outcomes; many adults, even those with high IQs, remain dependent on family and fail to gain open (i.e., in a general, not a special, setting) employment (see Chapter 16; Howlin, 2004; Howlin et al., 2004).

Literature addressing adults with ASDs has focused on continued behavioral difficulties. Ballaban-Gil, Rapin, Tuchman, and Shinnar (1996) noted high rates of behavior problems in adolescents and young adults with ASDs that appear to be associated, at least to some extent, with continued limitations in language skills. Therefore, although research has indicated that early difficulties with responding to others' communication may ameliorate with time (Lord & Risi, 2000), ongoing limitations in language skills and ritualistic behaviors continue to present significant obstacles to adolescents and adults, particularly in their attempts to achieve independence and form friendships (Howlin, 2004; Howlin et al., 2004). For people with intellectual disabilities, such ritualistic behaviors are overlaid with severe communication impairments, which, in turn, exacerbate problem behaviors (Sigafoos, Arthur, & O'Reilly, 2003).

Learning Styles

The relationship between core deficits and communication profiles appears to be complex and mediated to a large extent by social-cognitive learning styles that are specific to ASD. Wetherby et al. (2000), for example, noted that young children with ASDs use trial-and-error methods rather than observational learning or other strategies that involve social interaction. This preference would explain their strengths in constructive rather than symbolic play, predominance of early requests rather than comments, and difficulty with motor imitation (Rogers et al., 2005). Developing an understanding of these styles can be achieved through appropriate assessment strategies and may facilitate the development of effective communication interventions (Wetherby, Schuler, & Prizant, 1997), including AAC systems (Mirenda & Schuler, 1988).

AAC interventions may be particularly suitable for individuals with ASDs because they require processing of visual information that can be made nontransient (e.g., use of static graphic displays or holding a sign constant), which these individuals find easier to process than the auditory transient information of speech (Mirenda & Schuler, 1988). In addition, Prizant (1983) argued that individuals with ASDs process information in a gestalt fashion—that is, they process both visual and auditory information as unanalyzed wholes rather than as sequential units of information. This theory provided both researchers and clinicians with a way of understanding the basis for echolalia. With such an understanding, the need to explore patterns of echolalia becomes apparent.

APPROACHES TO COMMUNICATION PROFILING

Dynamic Assessment

Dominating the literature on assessment of children with ASDs is a model of dynamic assessment, described by Kublin, Wetherby, Crais, and Prizant (1998) as comparing "a child's assisted and unassisted performances, thereby locating learning within the social context of the help provided and offering hypotheses about the child's learning in situations beyond the assessment" (p. 287). In this way, a child's *zone of proximal development* (Vygotsky, 1934/1986, cited in Kublin et al., 1998) can be identified as a means of fine tuning the assistance that practitioners provide, allowing children to realize their learning potential.

Dynamic assessment has particular relevance to AAC interventions that address the cognitive and language delays of children with ASDs. Unfortunately, few examples of the use of dynamic assessment for developing AAC interventions are evident in the literature. An exception is a strategy suggested by Nigam (2001), whereby symbols are included in a milieu approach to teaching symbol combinations to children with autism. Unfortunately, no data were provided to support the use of the strategy.

Despite the lack of data specific to AAC, strategies to assess a person's potential to increase skills and abilities, as well as the use of systems and devices to assess a person's current communication needs within the participation model (Beukelman & Mirenda, 2005), are consistent with dynamic assessment. This consistency was exampled in a case study by Light, Roberts, Dimarco, and Greiner (1998) of a 6-year-old boy with autism. With the goal of enhancing the child's functional communication across his daily contexts, the assessment included 1) identification of his communication needs, 2) assessment of his skills, 3) identification of useful strategies used by his facilitators, and 4) planning intervention. Dynamic assessment was used to determine the extent to which augmented input, in the form of written information, assisted him in understanding spoken instructions. This strategy was used in conjunction with formal testing and observation of the child in his classroom.

Transactional Model

The case study provided in the previous section by Light et al. (1998) highlights the need to conduct assessments in a person's daily environments (home and school) and to consider meaningful interactions. This approach is consistent with a transactional model, whereby communication is thought to develop within interactions between the child and communication partners (McLean & Snyder-McLean, 1978). Support for this model comes from studies demonstrating the bidirectional nature of communication, with mutual influence on behaviors, in mother–child dyads involving both children without (e.g., Akhtar, Dunham, & Dunham, 1991) and with disabilities (McCathren, Warren, & Yoder, 1996).

Kublin et al. (1998) applied the transactional model as a means of extending the dynamic assessment approach. They argued that the trial of strategies to scaffold communication should occur within interactive child–adult contexts, both unstructured and structured, to examine a child's initiations, readability of signals, and responsiveness to others. In addition, the style of the communication partner can be observed, as well as the child's response to the dynamic assessment component provided in the form of various scaffolds, such as modeling, providing directions, and expanding on the child's behaviors.

A Lifespan Model

Recent literature on the assessment of individuals with ASDs for the purpose of intervention planning converge on the need to profile current social communication skills, identify learning objectives and priorities, and examine the influence of communication partners and learning environments (American Speech-Language-Hearing Association, 2006; Kublin et al., 1998; Paul, 2005; Prizant, Wetherby, & Rydell, 2000). Such a holistic approach is also consistent with the participation model.

Strategies for how to conduct such a comprehensive assessment of social communication skills have appeared in the literature according to the development stage of a child with ASD, but the focus has been on children, with a noticeable neglect of adults with ASDs (e.g., Paul, 2005). The principles of assessment identified previously are relevant across the lifespan, as they are to various types of disabilities. In this section, a lifespan model of assessment is presented incorporating these principles, with a discussion of available assessment tools and strategies that are appropriate according to the life stages of early childhood, later childhood, and adolescence and adulthood. The principles of the lifespan assessment model and their implications from early childhood to adulthood in people with ASD are presented in Table 2.1. The use of tools and strategies that can be used in an AAC assessment according to life stages are discussed in the following sections.

Young Children The principles of assessment outlined by Kublin et al. (1998) are fundamental to SCERTS®, a comprehensive educational approach for prelinguistic children with ASDs and associated social-communicative disorders (see Chapter 7; Prizant et al., 2000, 2005). The aim of this approach is to enhance the social communication, emotional regulation, and transactional supports of children and their families. According to Prizant et al. (2000, 2005), key elements of SCERTS are that intervention addresses core deficits of ASD through

Table 2.1. A lifespan model of assessment

Principle	Application across the lifespan
Communication occurs within interactive contexts that are meaningful for the individual.	Assessment is conducted across various situations and environments and includes key people who interact on a regular or semiregular basis with the individual. For children, contexts will include home and early childhood or school settings with caregivers (usually parents), teachers, siblings, and peers. For adults, these contexts will include home (with family or in supported community accommodation), respite care, employment or day activity centers, and community settings (e.g., sports centers, local shops or shopping centers).
Primary caregivers and support people play an integral and collaborative role in the assessment process.	For children, members of the team include parents or other primary caregivers and teachers. For adults, members of the team include parents or other family members, advocates and key support people from supported community accommodation, employment settings and day activity centers. These people provide information about the individual with ASD relating to their relationships, role in each context, expectations and challenges being faced, and about their own concerns, goals, and preferences for the individual. Their knowledge and understanding of and attitudes towards the person with ASD's use of informal and formal communication, including various AAC modalities are also explored.
The assessment provides the opportunity for the individual with ASD to indicate preferences.	For children, information is gathered about learning style and interests that assist in identifying goals and teaching strategies. For adults, strategies are used to gather information about preferences and learning style, as well as preferred activities, dreams, and motivations. This information is gathered in both typical and new contexts that provide the opportunity to respond both to what is known and that which may be unfamiliar. This process includes the provision and support to use various AAC modalities across environments and social interaction contexts to allow the person to indicate preferences (using conventional or unconventional modes of communication) and the extent to which they meet his or her learning styles.
The focus is on identifying strengths in communication and related areas.	For children, the assessment yields information to provide a profile of strengths and areas that show delay across communicative functions, means (gestural and vocal), reciprocity, social-affective signaling, verbal and nonverbal symbolic behavior, receptive and expressive linguistic skills, and conversational pragmatics. Similarly, for adults, assessment provides information relating to areas of strengths in terms of gestural and vocal communication, reciprocity, social-affective signaling, and level of intentional communication. For both children and adults, a variety of tools are used to gather data, including those relying on informant reports, communication sampling procedures that range in degree of structure, and involve various communication partners, formalized tests, and ecological or environmental inventories. Within these interactions, the extent to which various communication modalities are used, including AAC, is determined.

(Continued)

Table 2.1. *(continued)*

Principle	Application across the lifespan
The assessment is a dynamic process.	For both children and adults, assessment includes the trial of strategies that scaffold learning, which informs intervention. Trials of such scaffolds continue as the individual moves through an ongoing cycle of assessment and intervention, and of hypothesis formulation and testing. Scaffolds include the use of various AAC systems, both aided and unaided
Information is gathered about factors that both facilitate and impede performance and responses to learning opportunities.	For both children and adults, interview and observational data are gathered about factors that may reduce the individual's capacity to learn, including health issues, hearing and vision status, medications, dietary restrictions or preferences, tendency to fatigue, and sensitivities to various stimuli in the environment. In addition, data are gathered so as to sample environments and times of day.
Information from the assessment is shared with team members in ways that are meaningful and allow each member to participate in the collaborative process of setting goals, and planning intervention.	The results are presented in reports that are accessible to and culturally appropriate for each member of the team, using language without jargon. They contain information about an individual's profile of skills and areas of deficit, learning styles and preferences, and strategies that scaffold communication and social interaction. These reports are used by the team to identify members who will take responsibility for key roles in the intervention process and the supports or assistance they will need to do so. They also provide the basis for discussing concerns about the implementation of strategies, including the use of AAC, and the supports and resources each team member requires. Reports are likely to take the form of traditional reports for sharing with other professionals and, in the case of children, to meet education requirements, but can be supplemented by other formats or information. These supplementary formats include video footage and a "A Book About Me," which presents relevant assessment information within an attractive, engaging book, created specifically to quickly pass information to people who may interact with an individual with ASD but may be unfamiliar with that person.

the provision of pragmatic intervention in which the functional use of preverbal and verbal communication skills are enhanced in natural and semistructured interactions. Interventions incorporate multimodal AAC systems that allow a child to use strengths in visuospatial processing.

Within SCERTS and the more general assessment model proposed by Kublin et al. (1998), the Communication and Symbolic Behavior Scales™ (CSBS™; Wetherby & Prizant, 2002a) are used to develop a profile of the child's communication and related abilities. The CSBS evolved from early studies (e.g., Wetherby et al., 1989) in which opportunities for sampling communicative behaviors were created using structured activities that resembled natural child–adult interactions (Wetherby & Prizant, 1992). The CSBS toolkit includes materials to encourage routine activities with a caregiver, such as construction and symbolic play, and structured communication sampling activities (Wetherby & Prizant, 2002a). In this way, a continuum from unstructured to structured activities is used to sample behaviors. These behaviors are analyzed using standard procedures to develop a profile of communicative functions, means (gestural and vocal), reciprocity, social-affective signaling, and verbal and nonverbal symbolic behavior. Wetherby and Prizant (1992) presented results for children with various forms of disabilities, including ASD, demonstrating differences in profiles that assist in both diagnoses and intervention planning.

By incorporating semistructured sampling activities, the CSBS provides opportunities to try visual supports, such as graphic symbols, as a means of scaffolding symbolic development. As an example, the provision of a graphic symbol or a sign for HELP can be provided to a child who shows frustration when handed a deactivated windup toy. When the child hands the symbol to the adult or attempts a sign or gesture, the adult activates the toy. Such AAC strategies can be coupled with other strategies, such as intersected eye gaze (the adult moves between the object of interest and the child, intersecting the child's line of sight to the object, and then responds as soon as the child's gaze meets the adult's eyes) (Warren, 1995), as a way of enhancing reciprocity.

Such structured assessment tasks can be supplemented by informant reports, ranging from in-depth interviews to checklists. In-depth interviews provide caregivers the opportunity to identify concerns and describe the home situation, and allow the clinician to explore attitudes toward AAC modalities (e.g., Goldbart & Marshall, 2004) and cultural influences (e.g., Shannon & Soto, 2004). Caregiver checklists can be used to supplement information obtained through direct observation of the child. An example is the Communication and Symbolic Behavior Scales Developmental Profile (CSBS DP™) Infant/Toddler Checklist (Wetherby & Prizant, 2002b), designed to gather information about predictors of language development, including emotion and use of eye gaze; use of gestures, sounds and words; understanding words; and use of objects. Also, the MacArthur-Bates Communicative Development Inventories (CDI; Fenson et al., 2006) are parent checklists that provide information on the use of gestures, single words, and word combinations. The CDI for infants has been found to be valid for children with developmental delays (Rescorla, 1993), Down syndrome (Miller, Sedey, & Miolo, 1995) and ASD (Charman, Drew, Baird, & Baird, 2003).

Later Childhood   For older children who do not develop functional speech, structured observations remain relevant as a means of obtaining information on the continued use of nonverbal communication. Materials, such as the CSBS™ toykit, may be substituted for more age-appropriate materials (e.g., a flashlight with the batteries removed). Also, for children who are using speech, representative language samples provide information about spontaneous expressive language skills, receptive language ability, and the proportion and function of echolalia. Roberts (1999), for example, obtained language samples for 23 young children with ASDs annually over 3 years. These samples were analyzed for the percentages of echolalia and mitigated echolalia and compared with expressive and receptive language measures using a standardized test. Roberts found that proportions of echolalic speech decreased over time while mitigated speech increased, with concomitant increases in receptive language. Extending this approach to include dynamic assessment could include the introduction of augmented input to test if it resulted in reduced echolalia, increased spontaneous language, or mitigated echolalia.

As in the studies by Roberts (1989; 1999), formal testing can provide a means of determining receptive language skills. Formal tests can also be used to develop profiles of reading and reading-related skills. Iacono and Cupples (2001, 2004) have developed protocols that include phonemic awareness, word recognition and word attack, and reading comprehension suitable for children and adults with disabilities, including those with complex communication needs.

Both children with and without spoken communication skills require functional analysis of speech and other behaviors. Given that echolalia can serve both interactive and noninteractive functions (Prizant & Duchan, 1981), functional analysis of echolalic utterances is warranted. Data gathered using communication sampling procedures can be analyzed using functional protocols, such as those described by Prizant and Duchan (1981). Functional analysis of other behaviors that are problematic, such as ritualistic behavior, aggression, and self-injury, are also critical in informing interventions that may incorporate the use of functional communication training (Mirenda, 1997). Data obtained by indirect assessments using interviews and checklists, systematic observations, and hypothesis testing provide the basis for functional analysis of behaviors (see Sigafoos et al., 2003). Determination of the functions of problem behaviors facilitates the development of AAC interventions that can enable their replacement with conventional and readily recognized signals (e.g., use of a graphic symbol to indicate the desire to end an activity; see Chapter 12).

Adolescents and Adults   The apparent neglect of adults with ASDs in the assessment literature may reflect 1) a lack of access to communication intervention services for this group or 2) the disappearance of adults with ASDs and complex communication needs as an identifiable group within the research literature. Research on the communication of adults with ASDs can be found within that addressing intellectual disabilities in general (e.g., Iacono et al., 2005), including the AAC intervention literature (e.g., Hamilton & Snell, 1993; Romski & Sevcik, 1996).

There are some assessments designed for people with intellectual disabilities—or more generally, those who use or could benefit from AAC—that may be useful for people who also have ASDs. One such assessment tool is the Triple C: Checklist of Communicative Competencies (Bloomberg & West, 1999), designed to be completed by support workers as a means of sensitizing them to potentially communicative behaviors demonstrated by their adult clients who lack linguistics skills (i.e., clients whose communication skills range from unintentional to early symbolic; see Iacono et al., 2005). The Triple C checklist provides a basis for collaborative planning of multimodal communication supports (see Chapter 16).

Another tool that offers potential for profiling the communication of adolescents and adults with ASD is the Social Networks inventory, even though it was developed more generally for people with complex communication needs (Blackstone & Hunt Berg, 2003). This inventory provides a systematic strategy for collecting information about how a person communicates with individuals across five circles of communication partners, moving from close family to people encountered regularly in community settings. Where possible, the individual with complex communication needs is interviewed directly; informants, such as a parent/advocate or key support person, are also interviewed. Information is gathered about modalities used with people in each circle of communication partners, their effectiveness (i.e., results in the desired effect) and efficiency (i.e., is recognizable to the communication partner), people who play key roles in supporting the individual's communication, and strategies they use to support interaction.

Research into the use of the Social Networks inventory is limited. A recent study by Iacono et al. (2004) indicated that the inventory proved useful in profiling the communication skills, modality preferences, and learning styles of three adults with developmental disabilities, including two with ASD. An unanticipated outcome was the finding that the structured interview format allowed the informants—parents and key support workers—to discuss their concerns, attitudes, and roles in supporting these adults.

Other tools that are appropriate for use with adolescents or adults with intellectual disability are the Pragmatics Profile of Everyday Communication Skills—Adults (Dewart and Summers, n.d.) and the Pre-Verbal Communication Schedule (Kiernan & Reid, 1987), although the latter may only be suitable for students because of the terminology used. The extent to which any of these checklists or interview schedules are suitable for people with ASDs, or whether they enable a profile of skills that identifies characteristics of ASD to support their valid use with this group, has not been explored in the research literature.

The use of communication sampling procedures, as used in the CSBS with children, has also been found to be useful in assessing the current communication skills of adults with intellectual disabilities. McLean, Brady, McLean, and Behrens (1999) used a structured series of interactive routines with adults with severe intellectual disability. Each activity included something that was unexpected, such as offering a sealed jar containing a food item. These sampling strategies allowed the researchers to determine the participants' level of intentionality and communicative functions expressed through nonsymbolic and symbolic communicative acts. Such direct assessments supplement the information provided through informant reports, while also allowing the opportunity to test various AAC modalities and strategies, as previously described for children.

Functional behavior analysis remains integral to AAC assessments for adolescents and adults with ASDs because of their high incidence of behavior problems (Howlin, 1997), which is a likely impetus for seeking support services. Such functional assessment needs to be part of a dynamic and transactional assessment of the adolescent or adult, within his or her daily or regular environments.

CLINICAL ILLUSTRATION: STEVE

In this section, a clinical case illustrates the implementation of principles of the lifespan model of assessment with Steve, a 40-year-old man with ASD. Steve lives in supported accommodation in the community with four other adults. He was diagnosed with autism when he was 4 years of age. A year later, he was also diagnosed as having moderate intellectual disability and epilepsy. Until 12 years ago, he lived with his parents. Steve has demonstrated behavior problems since early childhood, which were cited as the reason by a local regular school for excluding him. Instead he attended a school for children with intellectual disabilities. He was referred for a communication assessment because his continued behavior problems, including aggression, property destruction, and of greatest concern, self-injurious behaviors such as banging his head on the floor, wall, or any hard surface and, more recently, pressing his eyes with his fingers and banging his head with the closed fist of his right hand.

The communication assessment team included a speech-language pathologist, Steve's mother, two support workers from his home, and a support worker from his day service. Although Steve's mother was able to provide information about Steve's development and past experiences, she was suffering from health problems and could take only a limited role in a dynamic assessment process and intervention. Steve's father did not participate because of advanced dementia. In contrast, Steve's support workers, particularly those from his home, were motivated to be active members of the team and thus maintain Steve's place in the day service and reduce his episodes of self-injurious behavior and aggression, which had resulted in staff injuries.

The assessment comprised gathering previous records, including school reports, in-depth interviews with Steve's mother and support workers using the Social Networks inventory, administration of the Triple C checklist, dynamic assessment conducted by the support workers, structured observations by the speech pathologist, and a functional behavior assessment conducted using an informant checklist and observations to test hypotheses developed from the checklist information.

Previous Learning History

According to Steve's school reports and his mother's recollections, in the early years at school Steve developed a few phrases, such as "Go away," "Not now," and a few single words for preferred and motivating activities, including "bubbles" and "water." He also was able to vocalize along to favorite nursery rhymes and, when given time, could fill in the word to complete the phrase. Steve was reported to be fascinated by shiny objects, running water, and music, particularly familiar nursery rhymes. If his teacher or teacher's aide sang, "Twinkle, twinkle little…" and waited, Steve could, after a pause, say, "star." However, Steve did not engage in social-affective signaling; instead, he used adults to achieve goals, such as handing over an object he needed help with and waiting, or leading the adult by the hand to a door to request to go outside. The school tried a variety of AAC systems, both aided and unaided, although little information was available on how they were used or the extent to which they assisted Steve in receptive or expressive communication. School staff reported that although he knew the classroom routine, he would insist upon engaging in activities that he preferred and became exceptionally distressed if told "no" or if he was redirected to another unfamiliar activity.

It was during his school years that Steve's behavior problems worsened. Around the time of puberty, a referral to a child psychiatrist resulted in the trial of medications to address apparent anxiety and depression. At the time of the communication assessment, Steve was on medication for epilepsy and had not had a seizure for many years. His mother noted that he had not had a medication review for a number of years; she was concerned that it might have contributed to the apparent bouts of anxiety that resulted in self-injury or aggression.

Current Assessments

The Triple C checklist was completed by Steve's three support workers (home and day service) and then discussed with the speech-language pathologist. The information from the checklist indicated that Steve was an intentional/informal communicator, using informal strategies of gestures, vocalizations, and facial expressions, as well as problem behaviors to communicate intentionally. This level of communication was confirmed by the speech-language pathologist's observations of Steve during a mealtime routine and structured communication sampling. In addition, completion of the Social Networks inventory indicated that Steve tended to use gestures at home and with family, but rarely with people in the community. In fact, the support workers and Steve's mother felt that he preferred not to go out into the community, as this was where he was likely to demonstrate aggression and sometime self-injury. An exception was the local bakery, which was familiar to Steve because he went there routinely and was served by the same person.

The functional behavior checklist led to the development of hypotheses that Steve tended to be aggressive when something he had not anticipated occurred. Also, it was felt that self-injury was most likely to occur when Steve was in unfamiliar places, with unfamiliar people, or when he was stopped from participating in a preferred routine activity. However, there were times when his behaviors did not appear to be related to environmental factors or communication frustration.

Hypothesis Testing and Use of AAC Scaffolds

Water restrictions because of drought led to a natural testing of one of the hypotheses regarding Steve's aggression and self-injurious behaviors. Previously, Steve had watered the garden daily, but this had been reduced to two days a week to comply with city regulations. On days when Steve was not allowed to water the garden, he was stopped by staff and episodes of self-injury and aggression occurred. On these days, the support workers provided an opportunity for Steve to spend time hand washing small items of clothes and also assisted him in cleaning the grill. When reviewing incident reports of aggression, the group hypothesized that their attempts to provide physical prompts to complete activities had initiated aggression because support workers had approached Steve from behind without providing a verbal explanation. They changed this strategy so that they now approached him from the front and provided an explanation of what they were about to do. They also decided to pair these explanations with a physical object and a gesture to signify the activity (e.g., showing Steve a small bucket containing a few clothes requiring washing and pointing to the laundry room).

In addition, support staff organized a review of Steve's medication by his general practitioner. His medication was changed and support workers reported that Steve seemed calmer. Daily charts of behavior indicated that Steve's problem behaviors reduced substantially; during a 3-month period, there was only one incidence report.

Support staff, with the help of the speech-language pathologist, gathered information about the use of AAC to aid in Steve's understanding and social communication. By observing Steve's responses to objects in routine activities, they learned that Steve associated certain activities with particular objects (e.g., the large scrubbing brush with cleaning the grill). In thinking about Steve's daily environment, they decided to consistently use objects to cue Steve into a change in his routine, but also to accompany them with spoken information. They also implemented a trial of showing Steve options for drinks, both hot and cold, to see if he would indicate a preference by touching the container, a skill that his mother reported that he used at home.

Consensus Building

Two meetings were attended by all members of the assessment team. Objectives for intervention and also for further assessment were developed based on the information that had been gathered. Three objectives were agreed upon for intervention: 1) to create a personal communication dictionary (i.e., a record of Steve's informal modes of communication, signs, and their meanings) to enable all staff to share the same information and respond to Steve consistently; 2) to pair real objects with an activity to enhance Steve's understanding of changes in routine and anticipation of new experiences through the consistent use of the same real objects; and 3) to use keyword signs and natural gestures when interacting with Steve to provide consistent visual cues to accompany speech and real objects. In addition, an objective was set for continued assessment whereby staff would add to the personal communication dictionary if they observed any new behavior or communication through gesture, sign, or vocalization and record if and how these additions changed interactions with Steve. Staff believed that it was possible to achieve these aims by the next review of Steve's service plan in 6 months and were actively engaged in the process.

Documenting Assessment Outcomes

The speech-language pathologist summarized the outcomes of the assessment in a two-page report. Then, with the input of the support workers, strategies that were found to enhance Steve's communication were documented in the personal communication dictionary, using pictures to demonstrate AAC strategies wherever possible. The report was structured according to Steve's current communication skills and modalities, his preferred communication partners, and opportunities that were currently available in his home, in the day service, and in the community. The report also listed further strategies that would be attempted to determine the extent to which Steve's communication partners could be extended (e.g., attending new places in the community) and how to prepare Steve for new places and people through the use of a real objects and keyword signs (e.g., *change, different, okay, relax/calm down, doesn't matter, good work*). Sample dialog or scripts for staff were provided, with the keyword signs selected and illustrated.

RESEARCH IMPLICATIONS

The lifespan model of assessment for people with ASDs has been drawn from extant literature in the fields of AAC and ASD. This literature is based on notions of current best practice, which, in turn, has been based to varying extents on empirical support. The extent to which this model addresses the needs of people with ASDs across the lifespan warrants investigation. Drawing on existing research, there is a need for empirical exploration of how best to incorporate AAC modalities and strategies into dynamic assessment. Further investigation is also needed on the perspectives of caregivers and other support people in terms of their roles in an assessment team, as well as culturally appropriate strategies for professionals to use when developing collaborations and building consensus. Research to date has incorporated qualitative procedures that allow an in-depth exploration of family and support person perspectives (e.g., Goldbart & Marshall, 2004; Shannon & Soto, 2004). Such methods may be appropriate for expanding the research base on family- and person-centered approaches to assessment.

A need exists for the development and testing of assessment protocols that allow for the systematic collection of information about a person's learning style and preferences, especially in relation to AAC. Such approaches may best incorporate observations in both familiar and unfamiliar settings that vary from structured to unstructured, as well as informant reports. These protocols may incorporate existing tools, such as the Triple C and the Social Networks Inventory, to determine the extent to which they profile the skills and learner characteristics of people with ASDs. In addition, there is a need for further development of assessment tools designed to highlight such profiles of adolescents and adults, in the manner of the CSBS™ for children. Such development will allow ASDs to become apparent in adults with intellectual disabilities who have never been diagnosed with ASDs. Determining how such tools inform intervention, particularly the development of AAC and its use across contexts to support social communication, would be the next step.

CONCLUSION

The convergence of principles, strategies, and tools relating to ASDs, AAC, and intellectual disabilities provides direction for the assessment of people with ASDs and planning interventions based on or incorporating AAC. This convergence has been articulated in the lifespan model of assessment in an attempt to enhance the social communication of people with ASDs and complex communication needs through access to AAC systems that meet their current and future needs, desires, and preferences. Variation in the extent to which such needs have been addressed in the literature points to the need for research to test the empirical basis for the model and its clinical and educational utility.

REFERENCES

Abbeduto, L., & Boudreau, D. (2004). Theoretical influences on research on language development and intervention in individuals with mental retardation. *Mental Retardation and Developmental Disabilities Research Reviews, 10,* 184–192.

Akhtar, N., Dunham, F., & Dunham, P. (1991). Directive interactions and early vocabulary development: The role of joint attentional focus. *Journal of Child Language, 18,* 41–49.

American Speech-Language-Hearing Association. (2006). Guidelines for speech-language pathologists in diagnosis, assessment, and treatment of autism spectrum disorders across the life span. Retrieved November 10, 2006, from http://www.asha.org/members/deskref-journal/deskref/default

Atkin, K., & Perlman Lorch, M. (2006). Hyperlexia in a 4-year-old boy with autism spectrum disorder. *Journal of Neurolinguistics, 19,* 253–269.

Ballaban-Gil, K., Rapin, I., Tuchman, R., & Shinnar, S. (1996). Longitudinal examination of the behavioral, language, and social changes in a population of adolescents and young adults with autistic disorder. *Pediatric Neurology, 15,* 877–900.

Baranek, G., Parham, L.D., & Bodfish, J. (2005). Sensory and motor features in autism: Assessment and intervention. In F. Volkmar, R. Paul, A. Klin, & D. Cohen (Eds.), *Handbook of autism and pervasive developmental disorders,Vol. 2. Assessment, interventions and policy* (3rd ed., pp. 831–857). New York: John Wiley & Sons.

Beukelman, D.R., & Mirenda, P. (2005). *Augmentative and alternative communication: Supporting children and adults with complex communication needs* (3rd ed.). Baltimore: Paul H. Brookes Publishing Co.

Blackstone, S., & Hunt Berg, M. (2003). *Social networks: A communication inventory for individuals with complex communication needs and their communication partners: Manual.* Monterey, CA: Augmentative Communication.

Bloomberg, K., & West, D. (1999). *Triple C: Checklist of Communicative Competencies.* Melbourne: Scope.

Bloomberg, K., West, D., & Iacono, T. (2003). PICTURE IT: An evaluation of a training program for carers of adults with severe and multiple disabilities. *Journal of Intellectual and Developmental Disability, 28,* 260–282.

Carpenter, M., & Tomasello, M. (2000). Joint attention, cultural learning, and language acquisition. In S.F. Warren & J. Reichle (Series Eds.) & A.M. Wetherby & B.M. Prizant (Vol. Eds.), *Communication and language intervention series: Vol. 9. Autism spectrum disorders: A transactional developmental perspective* (pp. 31–54). Baltimore: Paul H. Brookes Publishing Co.

Charman, T., Drew, A., Baird, C., & Baird, G. (2003). Measuring early language development in preschool children with autism spectrum disorder using the MacArthur Communicative Development Inventory (Infant Form). *Journal of Child Language, 30,* 213–236.

Crais, E., & Calculator, S. (1998). Role of caregivers in the assessment process. In S.F. Warren & J. Reichle (Series Eds.) & A.M. Wetherby, S.F. Warren, & J. Reichle (Vol. Eds.), *Communication and language intervention series: Vol. 7.Transitions in prelinguistic communication* (pp. 261–283). Baltimore: Paul H. Brookes Publishing Co.

Dewart, H. & Summers, S. (n.d.). *The Pragmatics Profile of Everyday Communication Skills in Adults.* Retrieved April 3, 2007, from http://wwwedit.wmin. ac.uk/psychology/pp/

Dunst, C., Johanson, C., Trivette, C., & Hamby, D. (1991). Family-oriented early intervention policies and practice: Family-centered or not? *Exceptional Children, 58,* 115–134.

Fenson, L., Marchman, V.A., Thal, D., Dale, P.S., Reznick, J.S., & Bates, E. (2006). *The MacArthur-Bates Communicative Development Inventories (CDIs)* (2nd ed.). Baltimore: Paul H. Brookes Publishing Co.

Forster, S., & Iacono, T. (2007). Perceptions of communication before and after a speech pathology intervention for an adult with intellectual disability. *Journal of Intellectual and Developmental Disabilities, 32,* 302–314.

Goldbart, J., & Marshall, J. (2004). "Pushes and pulls" on the parents of children who use AAC. *Augmentative and Alternative Communication, 20,* 194–208.

Greenspan, S., & Wieder, S. (1997). Developmental patterns and outcomes in infants and children with disorders in relating and communicating: A chart review of 200 cases of children with autistic spectrum diagnoses. *Journal of Developmental and Learning Disorders, 1,* 87–184.

Hamilton, B., & Snell, M. (1993). Using the milieu approach to increase spontaneous communication book use across environments by an adolescent with autism. *Augmentative and Alternative Communication, 9,* 259–272.

Howlin, P. (1997). Prognosis in autism: Do specialist treatments affect long-term outcome? *European Child & Adolescent Psychiatry, 6,* 55–72.

Howlin, P. (2004). *Autism and Asperger syndrome.* London: Routledge.

Howlin, P., Goode, S., Hutton, J., & Rutter, M. (2004). Adult outcome for children with autism. *Journal of Child Psychology and Psychiatry, 45,* 212–229.

Iacono, T., Bloomberg, K., & West, D. (2005). A preliminary investigation into the internal consistency and construct validity of the Triple C: Checklist of communicative competencies. *Journal of Intellectual and Developmental Disability, 30,* 139–145.

Iacono, T., & Cupples, L. (2001). Assessment of phonological awareness and reading. Retrieved April 5, 2005, from http://www.cddh.org.au/accessability

Iacono, T., & Cupples, L. (2004). Assessment of phonemic awareness and word reading skills of people with complex communication needs. *Journal of Speech, Language, and Hearing Research, 47,* 437–449.

Iacono, T., Forster, S., Bryce, R., & Bloomberg, K. (2004, October). *Perspectives on communication in adults with severe intellectual disability according to a social networks inventory.* Paper presented at the International Society for Augmentative and Alternative Communication biennial conference, Natal, Brazil.

Kiernan, C., & Reid, B. (1987). *Pre-verbal communication schedule.* London: NFER-Nelson.

Kublin, K., Wetherby, A.M., Crais, E., & Prizant, B.M. (1998). Prelinguistic dynamic assessment: A transactional perspective. In S.F. Warren & J. Reichle (Series Eds.) & A.M. Wetherby, S.F. Warren, & J. Reichle (Vol. Eds.), *Communication and language intervention series: Vol. 7.Transitions in prelinguistic communication* (pp. 285–312). Baltimore: Paul H. Brookes Publishing Co.

Light, J., Roberts, B., Dimarco, R., & Greiner, N. (1998). Augmentative and alternative communication to support receptive and expressive communication for people with autism. *Journal of Communication Disorders, 31,* 153–180.

Lord, C., & Paul, R. (1997). Language and communication in autism. In D. Cohen & F. Volkmar (Eds.), *Handbook of autism and pervasive developmental disorders* (2nd ed., pp. 195–224). New York: John Wiley & Sons.

Lord, C., & Risi, S. (2000). Diagnosis of autism spectrum disorders in young children. In S.F. Warren & J. Reichle (Series Eds.) & A.M. Wetherby & B.M. Prizant (Vol. Eds.), *Communication and language intervention series: Vol. 9. Autism spectrum disorders: A transactional developmental perspective* (pp. 11–30). Baltimore: Paul H. Brookes Publishing Co.

Lynch, E., & Hanson, M. (Eds.). (2004). *Developing cross-cultural competence: A guide for working with young children and their families* (3rd ed.). Baltimore: Paul H. Brookes Publishing Co.

McCathren, R., Warren, S., & Yoder, P. (1996). Prelinguistic predictors of later language development. In S.F. Warren & J. Reichle (Series Eds.) & K.N. Cole, P.S. Dale, & D.J. Thal (Vol. Eds.), *Communication and language intervention series: Vol. 6. Assessment of communication and language* (pp. 57–75). Baltimore: Paul H. Brookes Publishing Co.

McEvoy, R., Loveland, K., & Landry, S. (1988). The functions of immediate echolalia in autistic children: A developmental perspective. *Journal of Autism and Developmental Disorders, 18,* 657–668.

McLean, J., & Snyder-McLean, L. (1978). *A transactional approach to early language training.* Columbus, OH: Charles E. Merrill.

McLean, L., Brady, N., McLean, J., & Behrens, G.A. (1999). Communication forms and functions of children and adults with severe mental retardation in community institutional settings. *Journal of Speech, Language, and Hearing Research, 42,* 231–240.

Miller, J., Sedey, A., & Miolo, G. (1995). Validity of parent report measures of vocabulary development for children with Down syndrome. *Journal of Speech and Hearing Research, 38,* 1037–1044.

Mirenda, P. (1997). Supporting individuals with challenging behavior through functional communication training and AAC: Research review. *Augmentative and Alternative Communication, 13,* 207–225.

Mirenda, P. (2001). Autism, augmentative communication and assistive technology: What to we really know? *Focus on Autism and Other Developmental Disabilities, 16,* 141–151.

Mirenda, P., & Schuler, A. (1988). Augmenting communication for persons with autism: Issues and strategies. *Topics in Language Disorders, 9,* 24–43.

Mundy, P., & Sigman, M. (1989). Specifying the nature of social impairment in autism. In G. Dawson (Ed.), *Autism: Nature, diagnosis and treatment* (pp. 3–21). New York: Guilford Press.

Mundy, P., Sigman, M., & Kasari, C. (1990). A longitudinal study of joint attention and language development in autistic children. *Journal of Autism and Developmental Disability, 20,* 115–128.

Mundy, P., Sigman, M., Ungerer, J., & Sherman, T. (1987). Nonverbal communication and play correlates of language development of autistic children. *Journal of Autism and Developmental Disorders, 17,* 349–364.

Nation, K., Clarke, P., Wright, B., & Williams, C. (2006). Patterns of reading ability in children with autism spectrum disorders. *Journal of Autism and Developmental Disorders, 36,* 911–919.

Nigam, R. (2001). Dynamic assessment of graphic symbol combinations by children with autism. *Focus on Autism and Other Developmental Disabilities, 16,* 190–197.

O'Brien, C., & O'Brien, J. (2002). The origins of person-centered planning: A community of practice perspective. In S. Holburn & P. Vietze (Eds.), *Person-centered planning: Research, practice and future directions* (pp. 3–28). Baltimore: Paul H. Brookes Publishing Co.

Paul, R. (2005). Assessing communication in autism spectrum disorders. In F. Volkmar, R. Paul, A. Klin & D. Cohen (Eds.), *Handbook of autism and pervasive developmental disorders:Vol. 2. Assessment, interventions & policy* (3rd ed., pp. 799–816). New York: John Wiley & Sons.

Prizant, B. (1983). Language acquisition and communicative behavior: Towards an understanding of the "whole" of it. *Journal of Speech and Hearing Disorders, 48,* 296–307.

Prizant, B., & Duchan, J. (1981). The functions of immediate echolalia in autistic children. *Journal of Speech and Hearing Disorders, 46,* 241–249.

Prizant, B.M., Wetherby, A.M., Rubin, E., Laurent, A.C., & Rydell, P.J. (2005). *The SCERTS® Model: A comprehensive educational approach for children with autism spectrum disorders. Vol. 1: Assessment.* Baltimore: Paul H. Brookes Publishing Co.

Prizant, B.M., Wetherby, A.M., & Rydell, P. (2000). Communication intervention issues for children with autism spectrum disorder. In S.F. Warren & J. Reichle (Series Eds.) & A.M. Wetherby & B.M. Prizant (Vol. Eds.), *Communication and language intervention series: Vol. 9. Autism spectrum disorders: A transactional developmental perspective* (pp. 193–224). Baltimore: Paul H. Brookes Publishing Co.

Rescorla, L. (1993). Use of parental report in the identification of communicatively delayed toddlers. *Seminars in Speech and Language, 14,* 264–277.

Roberts, J. (1989). Echolalia and comprehension in autistic children. *Journal of Autism and Developmental Disorders, 19,* 271–281.

Roberts, J. (1999). *A comparison of the development of language skills in young children with autism and young children with developmental language disability.* Unpublished doctoral dissertation. Macquarie University, Sydney.

Rogers, S., Cook, I., & Meryl, A. (2005). Imitation and play in autism. In F. Volkmar, R. Paul, A. Klin & D. Cohen (Eds.), *Handbook of autism and pervasive developmental disorders:Vol. 1. Diagnosis, development, neurobiology, and behavior* (3rd ed., pp. 382–405). New York: John Wiley & Sons.

Romski, M., & Sevcik, R. (1996). *Breaking the speech barrier: Language development through augmented means.* Baltimore: Paul H. Brookes Publishing Co.

Rydell, P., & Mirenda, P. (1994). Effects of high and low constraint utterances on the production of immediate and delayed echolalia in young children with autism. *Journal of Autism and Developmental Disorders, 24,* 719–735.

Sanderson, H. (2000). Person-centred planning: Key features and approaches. Retrieved 5th March, 2007, from http://www.doh.gov.uk/vpst/pcp.htm

Shannon, M.S., & Soto, G. (2004). Perceptions of AAC: An ethnographic investigation of Mexican-American families. *Augmentative and Alternative Communication, 20,* 209–227.

Sigafoos, J., Arthur, M., & O'Reilly, M. (2003). *Challenging behaviour and developmental disability.* London: Whurr.

Snowling, M., & Frith, U. (1986). Comprehension in "hyperlexic" readers. *Journal of Experimental Child Psychology, 42,* 392–415.

Tager-Flusberg, H. (1997). Perspectives on language and communication in autism. In D. Cohen & F. Volkmar (Eds.), *Handbook of autism and pervasive developmental disorders* (2nd ed., pp. 894–899). New York: John Wiley & Sons.

Tager-Flusberg, H., Calkins, S., Nolin, T., Baumberger, T., Anderson, M., & Chadwick-Dias, A. (1990). A longitudinal study of language acquisition in autistic and Down syndrome children. *Journal of Autism and Developmental Disorders, 20,* 1–21.

Warren, S. (1995). *Early language intervention.* Seminar presented to Macquarie University Special Education Centre, Sydney.

Westby, C. (1999). Assessing and facilitating text comprehension problems. In H. Catts & A. Kamhi (Eds.), *Language and reading disabilities* (pp. 154–219). Boston: Allyn & Bacon.

Wetherby, A.M., & Prizant, B.M. (1992). Profiling young children's communicative competence. In S.F. Warren & J. Reichle (Series & Vol. Eds.), *Communication and language intervention series: Vol. 1. Causes and effects in communication and language intervention* (pp. 217–254). Baltimore: Paul H. Brookes Publishing Co.

Wetherby, A.M., & Prizant, B.M. (2002a). *Communication and Symbolic Behavior Scales™ (CSBS™).* Baltimore: Paul H. Brookes Publishing Co.

Wetherby, A.M., & Prizant, B.M. (2002b). *CSBS DP™ Infant-Toddler Checklist and Easy-Score Software.* Baltimore: Paul H. Brookes Publishing Co.

Wetherby, A.M., Prizant, B.M., & Hutchinson, T. (1998). Communicative, social/affective, and symbolic profiles of young children with autism and pervasive developmental disorders. *American Journal of Speech-Language Pathology, 7,* 79–91.

Wetherby, A.M., Prizant, B.M., & Schuler, A. (2000). Understanding the nature of communication and language impairments. In S.F. Warren & J. Reichle (Series Eds.) & A.M. Wetherby & B.M. Prizant (Vol. Eds.), *Communication and language intervention series: Vol. 9. Autism spectrum disorders: A transactional developmental perspective* (pp. 109–141). Baltimore: Paul H. Brookes Publishing Co.

Wetherby, A.M., Schuler, A., & Prizant, B.M. (1997). Enhancing language and communication development: Theoretical foundations. In D. Cohen & F. Volkmar (Eds.), *Handbook of autism and pervasive developmental disorders* (2nd ed., pp. 513–538). New York: John Wiley & Sons.

Wetherby, A., Yonclas, D., & Bryan, A. (1989). Communicative profiles of preschool children with handicaps: Implications for early identification. *Journal of Speech and Hearing Disorders, 54,* 148–158.

World Health Organization. (2001). *The international classification of functioning, disability and health—ICF.* Albany, NY: World Health Organization.

II

Communication Modalities

3

Presymbolic Communicators with Autism Spectrum Disorders

CHARITY M. ROWLAND

Presymbolic behavior[1] is important to the discussion of communication in autism spectrum disorders (ASDs) because many individuals with these disorders lack meaningful speech. Estimates are that approximately one third to one half of individuals with ASDs do not use speech as a primary communication mode (Bryson, 1996; Lord & Paul, 1997; Luyster et al., 2005; National Research Council, 2001; Prizant, 1996). Furthermore, approximately 20%–30% of individuals with ASDs who initially acquire speech on a typical developmental schedule subsequently lose speech (either permanently or temporarily), generally between the first and third year (Prizant, 1996). Of course, lacking speech does not necessarily mean lacking symbolic communication skills; however, we have no definitive data on the number of individuals with ASDs who use AAC systems that involve symbols. This chapter describes evidence on the development of presymbolic communicative behaviors in individuals with ASDs and reviews intervention strategies and models currently available for these presymbolic communicators.

---

[1]The terms *presymbolic, preverbal, nonverbal,* and *nonspeaking* are used inconsistently in the developmental and AAC literatures. In this chapter, I use *presymbolic* to describe communication that does not involve any sort of symbolic system. I use *symbolic* to describe communication involving any sort of symbolic system, whether it involves speech or an AAC system such as Blissymbolics or tangible symbols (two- or three-dimensional symbols). However, where I have reported on the research or intervention programs of other authors, I have used the terms that the authors used to describe their work.

PRESYMBOLIC COMMUNICATION
AND THE DEVELOPMENT OF LANGUAGE

In the 1970s, Elizabeth Bates and her colleagues published longitudinal studies that suggested the importance of presymbolic communication to the development of language (Bates, Benigni, Bretherton, Camaioni, & Volterra, 1979; Bates, Camaioni, & Volterra, 1975). They documented the development of intentional communication in typically developing children, realized initially through gestural and vocal "performatives" and later through early speech. That seminal research (since elaborated by Camaioni, Aureli, Bellagamba, & Fogel, 2003) documented parallel developments in gestural and vocal modalities, with each modality becoming increasingly decontextualized as communication undergoes the transition from deictic (interpretable only in context) to representational (interpretable independent of context).

Gestures versus Symbols

It is important to understand the essential difference between presymbolic communicative behaviors and symbols. Nonspeech vocalizations and gestures are generally quite effective, are fairly universally understood (at least within a given culture), and are versatile—one can point to anything, whine about anything, and tug anybody's arm. Because they can refer to anything, none of these gestures by themselves mean anything in particular; in fact, their power lies in the very fact that they do not have specific meanings. Their limitation—and it is a serious one—is that they can refer only to things that are physically present (i.e., things that can be pointed toward, looked at, or touched). Thus, presymbolic communication limits communicators to the "here and now." In contrast, most symbols have a direct correspondence with a specific referent. Since a symbol refers to one thing and one thing only, its meaning is generally clear, even if its referent is physically or temporally distant (Rowland & Schweigert, 2000a, 2000b). A number of studies have suggested that the timing and size of an early gestural repertoire is predictive of eventual language acquisition (McCathren, Warren, & Yoder, 1996; Morford & Goldin-Meadow, 1992) and that the use and understanding of gestures are appropriate language intervention goals for a variety of language-impaired populations (Capone & McGregor, 2004).

Why Bother?

One may question the wisdom of teaching someone without speech to use presymbolic behaviors, given that symbols are so much more powerful (especially if the learner is an older child or an adult). There are two good reasons to do so. First, an individual who cannot communicate using any sort of symbolic system needs to be able to communicate *right now* about whatever is important to him or her. If symbolic communication is not a viable option at the moment, then it makes sense to concentrate on presymbolic means of communication. Second, presymbolic communication lays the foundation for symbolic communication in individuals with disabilities, as well as in typically developing children. Research on communication intervention for individuals experiencing a wide range of severe and multiple impairments has shown that those who do not have presymbolic means of communication are less successful in acquiring any sort of symbolic means. For example, Rowland and Schweigert (2000a) conducted a 3-year intervention study that involved 41 presymbolic children with developmental disabilities (including 9 with ASDs) to examine the use of tangible symbol systems (two- and three-dimensional symbols) as a means of symbolic communication. All of the students who began the study with intentional presymbolic communication, whether nonconventional or conventional in nature, learned to use some form of tangible symbol; 10 students subsequently learned to use some form of abstract symbol. The 16 students who began the study without any intentional communication initially received instruction on the use of presymbolic communicative behaviors. Subsequent to this instruction, 10 students learned to use some form of tangible symbol, although none learned to use abstract symbols during the study. This research showed that, once individuals learn to communicate presymbolically, it is a fairly straightforward matter to teach them to use some sort of symbolic system to communicate, assuming that the targeted symbol system is one that makes sense to them.

Developmental Foundations of Presymbolic Communication

Communicating presymbolically requires many of the same skills that speech requires, but the cognitive and motor demands are less taxing than are those required for speech. The generic ability to communicate, realized initially through presymbolic communication, is based on certain basic social and cognitive milestones (Rowland & Schweigert, 2003a) that tend to be compromised in individuals with ASDs.

Social Foundations   As infants develop socially, they must first figure out that they are somehow separate from everything else in the world. They must then learn to differentiate between the people and objects that they encounter in the environment, and finally must grasp the fact that people (but *not* objects) can serve as social agents. The establishment of social bonds, social orienting, and social approach form a basic foundation for communication skill development; however, these areas are notably impaired in individuals with ASDs (Dawson et al., 2004; Landa, Holman, & Garrett-Mayer, 2007; Siegel, 1996; Wetherby & Prizant, 2000). It is much easier to teach communication skills to someone who appears to enjoy the attention of other people than to someone who seems to prefer objects to people. Nonetheless, a lack of social attachment does not mean that it is impossible to teach an individual to communicate. Rowland and Schweigert (2004) provided explicit instructions for working around an apparent disinterest in other people to teach presymbolic communication skills by making access to desired nonsocial items dependent on behavior directed to the person who controls such access. As an example, they described the experience of a young boy who first learned to tolerate the presence of another person while he interacted with his favorite toy, then learned to tolerate interaction with another person preceding access to the toy, and finally learned to touch another person to request access to the toy.

Cognitive Foundations The most important cognitive skills related to the development of presymbolic communication are social contingency awareness, communicative intent, and memory (Rowland & Schweigert, 2003a). Memory is not typically an impediment for individuals with ASDs. From a presymbolic perspective, this is good; a few gestures stored in long-term memory can go a long way because they can be used over and over again in different contexts. However, social contingency awareness and communicative intent are of concern. Contingency awareness involves understanding the predictable relationships between events (e.g., hitting a light switch will cause a light to come on). Awareness of social contingencies, or causal relationships between people, is the foundation for communicative intent. Individuals with ASDs may have difficulty attending to and understanding social contingencies (Siegel, 1996). Communicative intent distinguishes a purposeful communicative behavior or act from one that only appears to be communicative because someone (mis)interprets it as being produced with meaning. Communicative intent evolves at the point that interactions with other people take on dual orientation (i.e., a simultaneous orientation to both a communication partner and a topic or referent). A lack of dual orientation, or joint attention, is a core characteristic of individuals with ASDs and will be described in the following section. Still, individuals with ASD may be taught to use specific presymbolic behaviors to establish joint attention, as demonstrated by Kasari, Freeman, and Paparella (2006).

PRESYMBOLIC COMMUNICATION SKILLS OF INDIVIDUALS WITH ASD

Many authors have examined the use of sociocommunicative behaviors by individuals with ASDs. Presymbolic behaviors, such as pointing and hand guiding, deliver specific messages (*look at that, get that for me*). More general sociocommunicative behaviors, such as social orientation and joint attention, help to deliver the messages implied by such behaviors. Joint attention is sometimes viewed as a constellation of specific behaviors contributing to shared meaning, the ideal outcome of intentional communication. Initiating joint attention is distinct from responding to joint attention, and many believe that only initiating joint attention rises to the level of purely socially motivated behavior (Jones & Carr, 2004). In the presymbolic individual, joint attention is typically accomplished by alternating one's gaze between a partner and an object of interest or by pointing, giving, or showing an object to another person. In this regard, pointing has been studied more than any other specific gesture. Many studies distinguish between imperative pointing (which is used to regulate behavior) and declarative pointing (which is used to direct attention).

The research reviewed in this section is restricted to studies involving young children, for whom a presymbolic repertoire is less likely to have been affected by therapeutic interventions. These studies are categorized as either retrospective (i.e., involving reflection on the prior skills of children who are later identified as experiencing ASDs), concurrent or cross sectional (i.e., measuring the relationships between different skills that are recorded at the same time in groups distinguished by disability or by age), longitudinal (i.e., tracking skill development forward at repeated intervals over a significant period of time), or prospective (i.e., measuring skills as they develop in children who are initially undiagnosed, some of whom eventually develop ASDs and some of whom do not).

Retrospective Studies

Retrospective studies of young children with ASDs have revealed anomalies in presymbolic communication from an early age. Studies of home movies or videotapes provide extremely selective glimpses of the behavior of young children. For instance, Adrien et al. (1993) found that five behaviors related to socialization, communication, and attention differentiated children with ASDs from typically developing children prior to 1 year of age. After 1 year of age, eight additional behaviors, including some related to environmental adaptation and emotion, discriminated between the two groups. Baranek (1999), using similar techniques, found a pattern of depressed response to name, poor visual attention to nonsocial stimuli, aversion to touch, and excessive mouthing of objects in 9- to 12-month-old children with ASDs as compared to children with developmental disabilities or typically developing children. Maestro et al. (2002) examined movies of children with ASDs and typically developing children that were made during the first 6 months of life and found depressed levels of five behaviors related to social attending, but no differences in nonsocial attending.

Deficits in dyadic (i.e., person–person) and triadic (i.e., person–object–person) social engagement were described by parents retrospectively in the first 2 years of life in children referred for sociocommunicative disorders who were later diagnosed with ASDs (Wimpory, Hobson, Williams, & Nash, 2000). Parents retrospectively reported that specific presymbolic skills, including eye contact, babbling, and responsiveness to name and to smiles were lost prior to age 2 years, both by children who experienced word loss (speech regression) and by those who experienced regression without word loss (Luyster et al., 2005). Disconcertingly, children who experienced word loss were reported to have had more nonverbal communicative behaviors prior to word loss than did those who did not experience word loss. These data are unsettling because they cast doubt that the presence of early communication skills protects against subsequent regression.

Concurrent and Cross-Sectional Studies

Many concurrent and cross-sectional studies use scale scores from standardized assessments as dependent measures, whereas others catalogue the use of specific communicative behaviors produced during elicitation tasks or naturalistic observations. Stone, Ousley, Yoder, Hogan, and Hepburn (1997) found a lower rate and number of communicative acts; less commenting, pointing, showing, and eye gaze; and more leading the partner by the hand in 2- to 3-year-old children with ASDs than in children with developmental delays or language impairments who were matched on chronological age, mental age, and expressive vocabulary. Wetherby, Prizant and Hutchinson (1998) found smaller repertoires of conventional and distal gestures and less coordination of gestures with vocalizations in 1- to 5-year old children with pervasive developmental disorders (PDDs) as compared with children with developmental language delays matched on expressive language. Carpenter, Pennington, and Rogers (2002) found greater individual differences in the order of skill acquisition in 12 children with ASDs between the ages of 3 and 4 years as compared with children with developmental delays, as well as a tendency to show imitative learning and referential language prior to joint attention and attention sharing. They suggested that imitation may be a "detour" to learning language, which circumvents the more social means used by other children. Charman, Drew, Baird, and Baird (2003) used the MacArthur-Bates Communicative Development Inventories (CDIs) to assess 134 children with ASDs between the ages of 1 and 7 years (Fenson et al., 2006). They found greater delays of "late gestures" than of "early" ones in comparison with the normative sample for the instrument. As they noted, the early gestures (as defined by the CDIs) all require social referencing, whereas the later ones involve objects, do not need to be produced in a social context, and may be learned through imitation. Dawson et al. (2004) found impairments in social attention, joint attention, and attention to adults' distress in 3- to 4-year-old children with ASDs relative to children with developmental disabilities who were matched for mental age and typically developing children. Joint attention was the single best predictor both of group membership and of concurrent language ability. Warreyn, Roeyers, Van Wetswinkel, and De Groote (2007) elicited declarative initiation of joint attention, declarative response to joint attention, and imperative initiation of joint attention in 2- to 5-year-old children with ASDs and PDD-not otherwise specified and in a control group matched for mental age, chronological age, and language. They found that the children with ASDs made less eye contact with their mothers; were slower to follow adult points; were less able to shift gaze smoothly between their mothers and an object of interest; and had a tendency to gaze at their mother's finger, hand, or arm rather than the item to which she was pointing.

Longitudinal Studies

Longitudinal studies shed light on the trajectory of communication skill development and associations between different behaviors over time. Camaioni, Perrucchini, Muratori, and Milone (1997) found earlier comprehension and production of imperative pointing as compared with declarative pointing in three 2- to 4-year-old children with ASDs over the course of 2 years. Sigman and Ruskin (1999) found concurrent associations between language skills and initiating joint attention, responding to joint attention, and responding to social interaction for 54 children with autism between the ages of 2 and 6 years. They found predictive associations for language measured 1 year later for those same skills and for initiating social interaction. Finally, responding to joint attention predicted gains in expressive language at a 10- to 13-year follow-up.

Camaioni, Perrucchini, Muratori, Parrini, and Cesari (2003) followed five 3- to 5-year-old children with ASDs for 15–20 months, all of whom developed imperative pointing during this time. Only one child developed declarative pointing. Of the four children who comprehended pointing, three did so before they used pointing themselves. Drew, Baird, Taylor, Milne, and Charman (2007) studied children with ASDs and PDDs at 21 and 42 months of age; they found an association between the frequency of social acts and comments and later language scores.

Toth, Munson, Meltzoff, and Dawson (2006) calculated the contribution of joint attention, imitation, and symbolic play to early and concurrent language in 60 preschoolers with ASDs; they found that protodeclarative initiation of joint attention and immediate imitation were most strongly related to concurrent language ability, whereas toy play and deferred imitation were most strongly related to the rate of language development between 4 and 6.5 years of age. They suggested that the first set of skills (initiation of joint attention and symbolic play) are "starter skills" that set the stage for communicative exchanges, whereas the second set (toy play and deferred imitation) promote expansion of communication skills over succeeding years. Thurm, Lord, Lee, and Newschaffer (2007) followed 118 children with ASDs, PDDs, or other developmental disabilities at ages 2, 3, 4, and 5 years; they found that imitation of sounds at age 2 years was a strong predictor of expressive language, while response to joint attention was predictive of receptive language at 5 years.

Prospective Studies

Because they begin prior to a diagnosis of ASD or other disability, prospective studies provide the most convincing data related to the diagnostic value of various early skills. A prospective study of 150 high-risk siblings of children with ASDs followed from 6–24 months (Zwaigenbaum et al., 2005) found anomalies in eye contact, visual behavior (tracking and disengagement), orienting to name, smiling, affect, passivity, extreme distress, and fewer early and late gestures (as defined by the MacArthur-Bates CDIs) at 12 months of age in children who were diagnosed with ASDs at 24 months of age, as compared with other high-risk children and to low-risk children matched for chronological age. Eighteen-month assessments showed that the children's low levels of both early and late gestures persisted (Mitchell et al., 2006). The most recent case series report on nine children in this group (Bryson et al., 2007) documented few communicative gestures at either 12 or 18 months of age in a subset of participants who demonstrated an early decline in IQ (occurring between 12 and 24 months of age). Another large-scale prospective study of 125 children at high and low risk of ASD (related to the diagnosis of ASD in older siblings) from 14 to 24 months of age revealed impairments in joint attention and decreases over time in the diversity of both nonverbal and verbal forms of communication (Landa, Holman, & Garrett-Mayer, 2007). Children with an early diagnosis of ASD showed unconventional forms of communication that were difficult to interpret.

Summary

Overall, young children with ASDs seem to have smaller gestural repertoires than peers without ASDs who are matched on various demographics. Furthermore, these gestural repertoires may actually diminish over time. Wetherby (2006) noted that, unlike children with other language impairments, children with ASDs do not seem to use gestures to compensate for a lack of speech. Rather, they often resort to inappropriate actions to regulate the behavior of others instead of using conventional gestures. She suggested that the high-contact gestures that typically precede the development of conventional gestures serve to reenact aspects of a situation that the user wishes to reinstate and that, like echolalic speech, these reenactments only later acquire symbolic meaning.

Joint attention (especially initiation of joint attention) also seems to be compromised in children with ASDs. Pointing is often used only for imperative rather than declarative purposes. Some evidence suggests that joint attention is a strong predictor of language development. Yoder and McDuffie (2006) consider joint attention to be a social behavior that elicits language by increasing the likelihood that social partners will provide the appropriate language stimulation. Given the reliable anomalies documented in the presymbolic communication skills of children with ASDs and the fact that many do not acquire speech, it is appropriate to consider intervention strategies that target presymbolic communication. In some cases, improved presymbolic skills may allow individuals with ASDs to better communicate their needs and desires. In other cases, such skills may serve as a bridge to symbolic forms of communication.

EDUCATIONAL INTERVENTIONS FOR PRESYMBOLIC COMMUNICATORS WITH ASD

Interventions targeting presymbolic communication range from single strategies that target isolated skills to comprehensive models that address the full range of communication development. In this section, some common intervention strategies are described and comprehensive intervention models are reviewed.

Specific Strategies

Intervention strategies that have been studied in the quest to promote presymbolic communication in individuals with ASDs include those used to promote symbolic communication. However, because it is more likely that presymbolic communication will be targeted in young children than in older children or adults, the most popular approaches are likely to have a strong developmental foundation that is especially appropriate to the child-centered contexts of early childhood settings. These approaches are less likely to be behavioral in nature and are more likely to emphasize the use of natural contexts and contingencies. Four different strategies are described below.

Social-Interactive and Naturalistic Strategies

Social-interactive and naturalistic strategies typically include contingent imitation, naturally occurring reinforcement, time delay, and environmental arrangement applied in natural contexts. Hwang and Hughes (2000a) reviewed social-interactive interventions for preschool and elementary children. They found that few of the 16 qualifying studies involved preschoolers who were nonverbal and few targeted early social-communicative skills. A number of studies suggested that contingent imitation was associated with increases in preverbal behaviors, but overall the authors suggested that verbal behaviors were more responsive to social-interactive interventions than were preverbal social/emotional behaviors. Their own intervention study (Hwang & Hughes, 2000b) used a social-interactive package of strategies to teach eye contact, initiation of joint attention (alternating gaze, pointing, and showing), and motor imitation to three nonverbal 3-year-old children with ASDs. Rates of targeted behaviors increased from baseline to training, but increases were less for initiation of joint attention. Generalization probes showed virtually no maintenance for initiation of joint attention.

Rowland and Schweigert (2000a, 2000b, 2001) used social-interactive and naturalistic strategies to teach children with ASDs to use tangible symbols (i.e., objects or pictures that bear a concrete relationship to the referents that they represent). Tangible symbols are manipulable, making it possible to conduct a literal exchange of information; they are created for the individual user based on his or her experience with the referent. Instruction was delivered in a naturalistic and spontaneous manner in the midst of activities that the learners thoroughly enjoyed. Of the 41 participants, nine were children with ASD ages

3–9 years. Eight children learned to use tangible symbols; two of these children first learned to use three-dimensional symbols and subsequently learned to use two-dimensional symbols, whereas the others were able to start with two-dimensional symbols. Four students began to use speech after learning to use tangible symbols; two of these children were using speech as their primary mode of communication at the last contact.

Peer-Mediated Interventions   Interactions between peers, a natural context for social skill attainment for most children, has been embraced as a logical context for intervention for children with ASDs. However, mere immersion in peer activities without intervention has proven ineffective in terms of promoting interaction between peers (DiSalvo & Oswald, 2002). A variety of peer-mediated approaches have been examined, including those that promote group or dyadic interaction (e.g., Wolfberg, 2003; Wolfberg & Schuler, 1993), those that focus on the skill training of typically developing peers (e.g., Garfinkle & Schwartz, 2002; Koegel & Koegel, 2006; Roeyers, 1996), those that focus on the skill training of children with ASDs (e.g., Zanolli, Daggett, & Adams, 1996), and combinations of these approaches (e.g., Gonzalez-Lopez & Kamps, 1997). As a rule, these approaches involve peers who are cognitively, verbally, and socially adept enough to understand and implement training that is delivered verbally. These approaches are likely to target children with symbolic communication skills and are less likely to target presymbolic communicators.

Behavioral Techniques   Although all instructional strategies target behavior change and involve some level of behavioral analysis, those labeled as "behavioral" tend to involve the instruction of isolated skills over repeated trials using extrinsic reinforcement to control responses. Sometimes the targeted behaviors, although communicative in form, are reproduced without communicative function. For example, Martins and Harris (2006) used behavioral techniques and a multiple baseline design to teach three 3- to 4-year-old children with ASDs to respond to bids for joint attention by head turning and gazing at an object at which an adult was looking. All participants had some verbal ability but did not demonstrate joint attention. Although skill acquisition was demonstrated (as measured in vivo by adults who conducted the training), follow-up was not extensive and it was not clear how long the behavior would have been maintained in the absence of extrinsic reinforcement.

Whalen and Schreibman (2003) explicitly targeted response to joint attention (gazing and pointing), initiation of joint attention (pointing), and coordinated joint attention (gaze shifting) in 4-year-old children with ASDs, using a combination of discrete trial training and Pivotal Response Treatments (PRT; Koegel & Koegel, 2006). For four of five participants, gains in response to joint attention (RJA) far outstripped gains in initiation of joint attention (IJA). In unstructured follow-up probes with an experimenter, three participants maintained posttraining rates of response to joint attention, while only one maintained posttraining rates of initiation of joint attention. However, because training for response to joint attention always occurred first, more practice may have been provided for this training by follow-up, if one assumes that IJA training would naturally afford opportunities for both RJA and IJA.

Using the Physical Environment to Scaffold Presymbolic Communication
Another instructional strategy involves harnessing naturally reinforcing aspects of the physical environment to encourage communication. This approach capitalizes on an apparent affinity for nonsocial stimulation that is seen in many individuals with ASDs. Reichle (1991) described mechanisms for teaching communicative behavior to learners who do not seem to enjoy social interaction. For instance, he paired the elicitation of response to joint attention with a powerful nonsocial reinforcer to scaffold the use of nonverbal joint attention. The goal of such techniques, in Reichle's words, is "to establish people as things that one should want to approach" (p. 142).

Rowland and Schweigert (2007) also described such an approach, based on an analysis of object interaction skills in young children with PDDs. Parents assessed the object interaction skills of 2- to 5-year-old children with PDDs and their typically developing classmates using the *Hands-On Learning at Home* assessment (Rowland & Schweigert, 2003b). This is a checklist of early object-interaction skills that are needed to negotiate the physical and social environments. The checklist includes four strands: obtaining objects, practical uses of objects, representational uses of objects, and social uses of objects. Children with PDDs scored significantly lower than their typically developing age mates on all four strands of the instrument, with greater discrepancies for representational and social uses of objects. Despite these significant delays in object-interaction skills, these skills remain a relative strength for the population, at least as compared with communication skills. In the intervention component of this research, another group of young children with PDDs was taught to use objects for social purposes, targeting skills from the social uses strand of the *Hands-On Learning at Home* assessment and using instructional procedures described in Rowland and Schweigert (2003c). All of the individuals learned new social skills over the course of intervention, suggesting that the relatively strong object-interaction skills of individuals with

PDDs may be used to scaffold the acquisition of social communication skills (Rowland & Schweigert, 2003c).

Intervention Programs

A number of comprehensive instructional approaches have been developed over the past two decades that are appropriate for individuals with ASDs who are operating at the presymbolic level. Some of these programs specifically target the development of presymbolic means of communication, whereas others target more general social interaction skills. Most of them were developed for young children, but some were developed to address the needs of older individuals operating at a presymbolic level. Notably, none of these programs involve massed/discrete trial training or the delivery of extrinsic reinforcement. Most of these programs are supported by web sites through which instructional materials may be purchased; in some cases, regular training opportunities are also offered. Table 3.1 summarizes the major features of these programs.

Child's Talk   Child's Talk (Aldred, 2002; http://bramhallsalt. org/childstalk.asp) is a parental intervention program based on typical parent–infant interactions. The manual is under development and is expected to be available in 2009. The approach is almost exclusively prelinguistic, is emphatically focused on the promotion of early stages of communication, and eschews any demands on the child to use speech or sign language. The program involves parent workshops and monthly videotapes of parent–child interactions that serve as the basis for facilitated discussions of strategies for parents to use at home to promote shared attention and social engagement. Parents are expected to work one to one with their child for 30 minutes a day. Child-focused techniques unfold in six stages, beginning with mirroring the child's behavior. A pilot randomized controlled trial (RCT) comparing Child's Talk to routine care (Aldred, Green, & Adams, 2004) showed increases in both parents' synchronous communication (i.e., comments, acknowledgements, or social interactions) and children's communicative acts, and decreases in parents' asynchronous communication (i.e., directing, controlling, or demanding), as coded from video recordings of parent–child interactions. Participants excluded children who showed "no evidence of any desire to interact with adults" (p. 1423). An RCT in the United Kingdom, the Preschool Autism Communication Trial, is underway to compare Child's Talk to routine clinical care (investigators: Green, Aldred, Pickles, Macdonald, Le Couteur, McConachie, Charman, Byford, Howlin, and Slonims).

Table 3.1. Overview of instructional models for presymbolic communicators with an autism spectrum disorder (ASD)

Model	Developed specifically for learners with ASD?	Targeted level of communication	Targeted skills	Intervention agent
Child's Talk	Yes	Presymbolic communicators	Prelinguistic behaviors	Parents
Design to Learn products	Yes (Design to Learn and Hands-On Learning materials); No (First Things First and Tangible Symbol Systems)	Presymbolic communicators	Presymbolic communication (First Things First); object interaction skills (Hands-On Learning); tangible symbols (Tangible Symbol Systems)	Educators
Developmental, Individual-Difference, Relationship-Based model	Yes	Presymbolic and symbolic communicators	Shared attention/regulation; engagement/relating; problem solving; two-way intentional communication; creating symbols/ideas; logical thinking	Educators, with parent involvement
Early Start Denver model	Yes (toddlers)	Presymbolic communicators	Receptive communication, expressive communication, social interaction, imitation; cognitive skills; play; fine motor skills; gross motor skills; independence/behavior; joint attention	Educators, with strong parent involvement
The Hanen Program: More than Words	Yes (5 years of age and younger)	Nonverbal and verbal communicators	Presymbolic communication skills	Parents
Intensive interaction	No	Prespeech communicators	Holistic interaction	Caregivers

InterAACtion	No: adolescents and adults with severe/profound disabilities	Unintentional and intentional communicators	Nonverbal communication skills	Educators
Joint attention mediated learning	Yes (toddlers)	Presymbolic communicators	Focusing on faces; turn taking; responding to joint attention; initiating joint attention	Parents
Responsive teaching	Yes (included with children who have developmental delays)	Presymbolic and symbolic communicators	Cognition; communication; socio-emotional functioning; motivation	Parents
Responsivity education and prelinguistic milieu teaching	No	Low-frequency communicators (presymbolic or symbolic)	For learners: nonverbal communication (verbal communication is targeted after prelinguistic criteria met); for parents: responsivity	Educators and parents
SCERTS® Model	Yes	Presymbolic and symbolic communicators	Joint attention; symbol use; self and mutual regulation/dysregulation; transactional support	Educators and parents

Design to Learn Products   A number of products have been developed by Rowland and Schweigert that address communication skills in individuals of any age who experience severe or multiple disabilities (www.designtolearn.com). *First Things First* (Rowland & Schweigert, 2004) is a manual describing strategies for teaching presymbolic communication skills to individuals with severe communication disorders, including autism. It focuses on the three most basic communicative intents: requesting *more,* gaining attention, and making choices. The approach emphasizes how to harness an individual's intrinsic motivations and establish logical intervention targets based on close progress monitoring. A section addressing learners who are uninterested in interacting with other people is especially pertinent to individuals with ASDs.

Design to Learn, an environmental inventory developed especially for children with PDDs (Rowland & Schweigert, 2003d), is designed to track opportunities to learn communication and object interaction skills that are provided in classroom activities for a specific student. *A Teacher's Guide to Hands-On Learning* and the accompanying *Hands-On Learning at Home* and *Hands-On Learning at School* assessments (Rowland & Schweigert, 2000b, 2003c, 2003e) also were developed specifically for children with PDDs. These materials address a range of object interaction skills, including those related to representational skills and social interactions. *Tangible Symbol Systems*, a manual (Rowland & Schweigert, 2000b) and DVD (Rowland & Schweigert, 2005), provide detailed information about teaching individuals who have mastered a basic level of presymbolic communication skills to use two- and three-dimensional symbols to communicate. The study described earlier that involved nine children with ASDs demonstrated the bridging function of tangible symbol systems (Rowland & Schweigert, 2000a).

All *Design to Learn* materials are meant to be used in an integrated approach. The *First Things First* and *Tangible Symbol Systems* materials in particular are designed to promote a seamless transition from presymbolic communication to symbolic communication. The *Design to Learn* products were developed over a long series of research and demonstration projects that employed a variety of methods to validate the instructional approaches and materials in real-world settings, including single subject and group pre/post designs.

Developmental, Individual-Difference, Relationship-Based Model   Greenspan and Wieder (1998, 2006) harnessed insights from many years of clinical experience with individuals with ASDs into an organizational framework to guide assessment and relationship-focused intervention. The Developmental, Individual-Difference, Relationship-Based (DIR) model was developed for children and is family focused, although guidelines are provided for applying the techniques to adolescents and adults as well (Greenspan & Wieder, 2006; www.playworks.cc/DIRmodel.html and www.floortime.org).

This model rejects the notion of isolated developmental domains in favor of learning through interactive processes based on affective relationships that are sensitive to the sensory and motor processing skills of the individual. Attention is paid to identifying the strengths and weaknesses of family members; the model plays to the strengths of family members to bring out the best in the target child. The framework involves six core levels of emotional development: regulation and interest in the world; engaging and relating; intentionality and two-way communication; social problem solving, mood regulation and sense of self; creating symbols and using words and ideas; and emotional thinking, logic, and sense of reality. These six stages lay the foundation for three more advanced stages of relatively abstract thought and reflection that receive less attention. Floor time, a widely used technique that is included as one component of the model (but that is often erroneously considered to constitute the entire model), involves frequent, intensive, one-to-one interactive sessions dictated by the child's own interests. The authors have used retrospective chart reviews to track the outcomes in a large group of children with ASDs for whom they recommended interventions that lasted from 2 to 8 years (Greenspan & Wieder, 1997). They have also revisited the progress of 16 children, selected from a subgroup representing the most successful 20 of the original 200 children, at 10–15 years after the start of treatment (Wieder & Greenspan, 2005). These children received a wide array of interventions, including the Greenspan/Wieder approach. No experimental studies of the effectiveness of this approach have been completed to date.

Early Start Denver Model   The Early Start Denver Model (Smith, Rogers, & Dawson, 2007) is a comprehensive early intervention approach for children with ASDs as young as 12 months, which was adapted from the Denver Model developed for preschoolers with ASDs (Rogers, Hall, Osaki, Reaven, & Herbison, 2000). It is based on Stern's (1985) model of the infant's interpersonal, intersubjective development. There is a strong emphasis on imitation as well as emotional sharing, joint attention, and social motivation. The Early Start Denver Model combines principles of applied behavior analysis, PRT, and relationship-focused intervention and requires heavy parent involvement.

Domains covered by the curriculum include receptive communication, expressive communication, social interaction, imitation, cognitive skills, play skills, fine motor skills, gross motor skills, independence/behavior, and joint attention—all of which are taught at four developmental levels. Spontaneous communication is an area of focus and nonverbal communication is emphasized initially. The model involves home-based intensive therapy (25–30 hours per week) provided by trained therapists, plus parent-provided intervention (up to 10 hours per week). This model is the focus of an RCT that will compare use of the Promoting First Relationships program (Kelly, Zuckerman, Sandoval, & Buehlman, 2003) at 8 months of age followed by use of the Early Start Denver Model at 12 months of age to community-based interventions (investigators: Dawson and Rogers).

The Hanen Program   The Hanen Centre in Toronto provides parent training on an interactive language intervention program based on Sussman's (1999) *More Than Words* book and is supported by posters and a forthcoming DVD (www.hanen.org). This is an expansion of another parent program based on the *It Takes Two to Talk* book (Pepper & Weitzman, 2004) that addresses the needs of children with language delays. *More Than Words* was designed specifically for parents of children with ASDs under the age of 5 years (*Talkability,* also by Sussman [2006], addresses the needs of verbal children with ASDs). The program reflects a social-pragmatic perspective and targets young children with ASDs who are either nonverbal or verbal. Both child-led and parent-led (i.e., prompted) interactions are targeted, along with language modeling. Topics include recognizing communication; how parents affect children's communication; setting goals; following the child's lead; taking turns; playing games; receptive communication; the use of visual supports, music, books, and toys; and encouraging play with peers.

This is a popular program that has been used to train many parents in North America. Research on the effectiveness of the program includes one study involving a delayed control group (McConachie, Randle, & Le Couteur, 2005) that focused on the verbal behavior of participants and a multiple case study involving three families (Girolametto, Weitzman, & Sussman, 2006). Two RCTs are currently underway to investigate the efficacy of the Hanen program, one in Canada (investigator: Fombonne) and one in the United States (investigators: Carter, Tager-Flusberg, Stone, and Messinger).

Intensive Interaction   The Intensive Interaction program (www.intensiveinteraction.co.uk), described in Kellett and Nind

(2003), Nind and Hewett (2001, 2005), and Caldwell (2006), specifically targets prespeech individuals who have significant learning challenges and/or autism. Nind and Hewett (2005) described Intensive Interaction as "for those people whose signals we do not understand and whom we may have difficulty perceiving as being social and communicative" (p. 11). Intensive Interaction has been used primarily with adults. It originates in the clinical work of Ephraim (1986), which was originally called "augmented mothering" and was based on the principles of mother–child interactions.

The Intensive Interaction approach stresses intuitive responding and structured reflection, enjoining caregivers to engage in playful interactions based on what their clients want to do. The model emphatically rejects the teaching of specific tasks and targeted outcomes in favor of a holistic, interactive approach implemented in an atmosphere of "tasklessness." It is one of a number of interactive approaches developed in the United Kingdom, seemingly in a backlash against rigidly prescriptive and mechanistic approaches. Notably, caregivers are encouraged to attribute intentionality to potentially communicative behaviors, striving to break into the "inner language" of the individual. Involuntary actions (such as sounds and breathing patterns), inner-directed nonverbal utterances, and both gestures and imitations on the part of the client are all considered communicative. Copying the client's sounds and motions is seen as a major avenue toward engagement. Progress is documented through narratives and discussions rather than charts and checklists. Case studies of the program's impact have been published (Hewett & Nind, 1998; Nind, 1996), but there is no experimental evidence of the effectiveness of this program (see Chapter 16 for additional information about this approach).

InterAACtion   The InterAACtion model (Bloomberg, West, & Johnson, 2004) evolved from the Triple C Checklist of Communication Competencies (Bloomberg & West, 1998), a communication skill assessment designed for adolescents and adults with severe/profound disabilities that has been subjected to construct validity studies (Iacono, Blomberg, & West, 2005). The InterAACtion package (http://www. scopevic.org.au/therapy_crc_r&p.html) includes a manual and videotape/DVD (Bloomberg, 2002), as well as handouts for communication partners that describe specific communication strategies. The model specifically targets unintentional and intentional communicators who are adults and as such is unique among the programs described here. The complete kit includes software for making communication aids such as time tables, chore charts, and community request cards. This program is described more fully in Chapter 16.

Joint Attention Mediated Learning   Joint Attention Mediated Learning (JAML; Scherz & Odom, 2007) is a parent-implemented home-based intervention developed for toddlers with ASDs. The manual is yet unpublished. The relationship-based JAML program includes four phases: focusing on faces, turn taking, responding to joint attention, and initiating joint attention. Each phase has two levels: the first is driven by parent initiative and the second is driven by child initiative. The focus is on increasing the child's desire to learn and interact rather than on teaching specific skills. Significantly, parents are the designated participants; they are expected to create activities to encourage social participation, with coaching and support from professionals. A pilot study of JAML (Schertz & Odom, 2007) involved the parents of three 22- to 33-month-old toddlers who were rated as severely autistic in a single subject, multiple baseline design that showed promising results. JAML is the subject of a current study involving toddlers at risk for ASDs, which will involve both a multiple baseline component and a group experimental design (investigators: Schertz, Odom, and Baggett).

Responsive Teaching   Responsive teaching (http://www.responsiveteaching.org) is a relationship-focused, parent-implemented intervention for young children with ASDs or developmental delays that was developed by Mahoney and McDonald (2007). The curriculum is supported by software that may be used to select intervention objectives, develop instructional plans, track progress, and develop reports (Mahoney, 2007). Responsive teaching may be used by parents at home or by professionals in educational settings. Discussion topics are provided to help professionals explain the rationale for each objective to parents. The approach is predicated on the assumption that increased parental responsiveness will be associated with improved socioemotional functioning of the child.

Responsive teaching involves 16 pivotal behavioral objectives in the domains of cognition, communication, social-emotional functioning, and motivation that are characterized as developmentally critical and subject to influence by maternal responsiveness. A study of the effect of responsive teaching on 20 children with ASDs between the ages of 3 and 5 years compared measures taken before and after 8–14 months of weekly 1-hour parent training sessions (Mahoney & Perales, 2003). Significant increases in maternal response and affect and in a number of child measures of social interaction and temperament were found. Children whose mothers' responsivity improved the most showed the most improvement themselves.

Another similarly designed study (Mahoney & Perales, 2005) compared the use of responsive teaching in 12- to 54-month-old children with PDDs versus children with developmental disabilities who were matched on developmental age by language and cognitive measures. Results were similar to those reported for the study by Mahoney and Perales (2003). In addition, children with PDDs showed greater improvement overall than children with developmental disabilities. Two RCTs are currently underway. One RCT by Mahoney will compare responsive teaching to parent–child interaction therapy (Herschell, Calzada, Eyberg, & McNeil, 2002) for young children with ASDs and other developmental disabilities; the other will compare the use of responsive teaching to a control treatment (investigators: Baranek, Watson, Reznick, and Crais).

Responsivity Education and Prelinguistic Milieu Teaching

Responsivity education and prelinguistic milieu teaching (RPMT) was described by Yoder and Warren (1998, 2002) and by Warren et al. (2006), but is not yet available in the form of a curriculum or manual. The model, based on a transactional approach to parent–infant interactions (McLean & Snyder-McLean, 1978), was developed for young children who are low-frequency communicators (i.e., they show evidence of less than one spontaneous and intentional communicative act per minute). The prelinguistic milieu teaching component of the model targets nonverbal communicative acts and is designed to be implemented by professionals working one to one with the child several times a week. Key principles include arranging the environment to occasion communication, following the child's attentional lead, and building social routines. Learning is supported through prompts, models, and natural consequences.

The responsive education component provides training to parents to promote their responsivity to the nonverbal behaviors that are targeted in the prelinguistic milieu teaching component. The Hanen program is used to implement this component. A comparison study of nonverbal and low-verbal preschoolers with ASDs who were randomly assigned to either RPMT or the Picture Exchange Communication System (PECS; Frost & Bondy, 2002) showed that RPMT was more effective in terms of increasing the number of object exchange turns and initiation of joint attention for those entering with higher levels of initiating joint attention, while PECS was more effective for those entering with one instance or less of initiating joint attention (Yoder & Stone, 2006a, 2006b). PECS resulted in greater gains in the number and variety of nonimitative words than RPMT. This is a difficult pair of treatments to compare because unlike PECS, RPMT explicitly teaches presymbolic behaviors and only targets words after specific prelinguistic criteria have been met. Thus, behaviors such as gestures, alternating gaze, and vocalizations—which may have constituted more appropriate targets for some of the participants—were not among the dependent variables measured.

SCERTS®: Social Communication, Emotional Regulation, and Transactional Support   The SCERTS Model (Prizant, Wetherby, Rubin, Laurent, & Rydell, 2005a, 2005b) is a comprehensive educational approach developed specifically for individuals with ASDs (but is also applicable to other individuals with developmental disabilities) that proceeds from a social-pragmatic approach informed by the developmental sequence of symbolic skill acquisition in typically developing children (Prizant, Wetherby, Rubin, & Laurent, 2003). It is described as a lifespan approach. The approach addresses core challenges that are typical of individuals with ASDs: social communication (joint attention and symbol use), emotional regulation (self and mutual regulation/dysregulation), and transactional support (interpersonal learning, support to families, and support to professionals). Under the first two domains, specific milestones, goals, and objectives are provided for the child in three stages: the social partner stage (i.e., preverbal intentional communication); the language partner stage (i.e., emerging and early language) and the conversational partner stage (i.e., advanced language). Intervention plans are predicated on a comprehensive assessment process and are systematically identified and documented using planning and tracking forms provided. A program evaluation is also provided to rate the educational program, support to families, and support to professionals provided by the program.

The approach, although extensively documented, is implemented in a highly individualized manner. Parents are viewed as active partners but are not expected to take over as primary instructors. Contributing research has been meticulously summarized by Wetherby, Rubin, Laurent, Prizant, and Rydell (2006). An RCT is currently underway that will compare the SCERTS Model to an information/education/support model for children 18 months of age or younger (investigators: Wetherby and Lord; see Chapter 7 for additional information about this approach).

RESEARCH IMPLICATIONS AND CONCLUSIONS

Much remains to be discovered about the development of presymbolic communication in individuals with ASDs, its role in language acquisition, and effective instructional practices. Suggestions that specific communicative behaviors may be used first without meaning and that meaning may later be attached to their use (e.g. Wetherby, 2006) have important ramifications for intervention. The fact that there seem to be differences in communication development and outcomes for individuals with early- versus late-onset ASDs or for those who experience speech regression versus those who do not only add to the complexity of the work ahead. A number of avenues for future research are indicated.

Additional longitudinal studies on the natural course of presymbolic communication in children with ASDs and its ramifications for language development would be helpful. Specifically, research along the lines of that conducted by Camaioni, Aureli, Bellagamba, and Fogel (2003) would be illuminating. This elegant research involving typically developing children examined the communicative "frames" shared by mothers and infants in their second year. This approach embraces the concept that communication is best studied through the joint meaning developed between communication partners rather than through the separate contributions of each partner. A similar study of communicative frames involving young children with ASDs and their parents would contribute to our understanding of the development of shared meaning in ASDs. Studies that address the developmental course of communication in children with early-onset versus late-onset ASD, in groups of young children categorized according to their current communicative repertoires, and in groups with and without speech regression are also indicated. Additional prospective studies that probe the diagnostic value of specific presymbolic behaviors (as opposed to scores from standardized assessment instruments that provide only gross measures of early communication) also are warranted.

In terms of appropriate intervention, the research supporting the programs described above is uneven at best. Some of the programs integrate individual components that are derived from well-researched principles of child development, a few have been the topic of limited RCTs, and still others have been the topic of case studies or case reviews and are essentially unsupported by scientific evidence. To date, no single approach has been validated in a real-world setting using an experimental research design with appropriate controls for internal and external validity. The few RCTs that have been conducted compare a specific intervention program to a nontreatment control group or to a contrasting treatment. In the former case, it is very difficult to control the dose and nature of intervention that control groups receive in community-based programs, especially because families of children with ASDs are likely to seek intensive services for their children. In the latter case, contrasting intervention programs often target different outcomes, making it difficult to establish dependent variables that are appropriate across both of the compared treatments. Smith et al. (2007) suggested a number of appropriate designs for studies of psychosocial interventions for ASDs that may have some influence on future research. New scientific evidence of treatment effectiveness should be available soon, as the results of RCTs on early intervention that are now underway (many of which are funded by Autism Speaks; www.autismspeaks.org) become available.

The National Research Council (2001) asserted that "[i]ntervention research is not yet available to predict which specific intervention approaches or strategies work best with which individuals. No one approach is equally effective for all individuals, and not all individuals in outcome studies have benefited to the same degree" (p. 64). In a similar vein, Kasari (2002) concluded her review of early intervention techniques for young children with ASDs by stressing the need to identify the "active ingredients" of multifaceted programs that are associated with improvement and to identify the characteristics of individuals for whom a given strategy is helpful or not. A combination of research on the developmental course of presymbolic and symbolic communication in ASDs, the identification of different behavioral constellations among subpopulations, and the conduct of RCTs on the effectiveness of existing intervention programs will shed light on the match between specific instructional strategies and the characteristics of presymbolic individuals with ASDs who do or do not benefit from them.

REFERENCES

Adrien, J.L., Lenoir, P., Martineau, J., Perrot, A., Hameury, L., Larmande, C., & Sauvage, D. (1993). Blind ratings of early symptoms of autism based on family home movies. *Journal of the Academy of Individual and Adolescent Psychiatry, 32,* 617–626.

Aldred, C. (2002). Child's Talk: Early communication intervention for children with autism and pervasive developmental disorders. *Good Autism Practice, 3,* 44–57.

Aldred, C., Green, J., & Adams, C. (2004). A new social communication intervention for children with autism: Pilot randomized controlled treatment study suggesting effectiveness. *Journal of Child Psychology and Psychiatry, 45,* 1420–1430.

Baranek, G.T. (1999). Autism during infancy: A retrospective video analysis of sensory-motor and social behaviors at 9–12 months of age. *Journal of Autism and Developmental Disorders, 29,* 213–224.

Bates, E., Benigni, L., Bretherton, I., Camaioni, L., & Volterra, V. (1979). *The emergence of symbols: Cognition and communication in infancy.* New York: Academic Press.

Bates, E., Camaioni, L., & Volterra, V. (1975). The acquisition of performatives prior to speech. *Merrill-Palmer Quarterly, 21,* 205–226.

Bloomberg, K., (2002). *InterAACtion: Strategies for intentional and unintentional communicators* [Videotape]. Victoria, Australia: Communication Resource Centre.

Bloomberg, K., & West, D. (1998). *Triple C: Checklist of Communication Competencies*. Victoria, Australia: Communication Resource Centre.

Bloomberg, K., West, D., & Johnson, H. (2004). *InterAACtion: Strategies for intentional and unintentional communicators*. Victoria, Australia: Communication Resource Centre.

Bryson, S. (1996). Brief report: Epidemiology of autism. *Journal of Autism and Developmental Disorders, 26,* 165–167.

Bryson, S., Zwaigenbaum, L., Brian, J., Roberts, W., Szatmari, P., Rombough, V., et al. (2007). A prospective case series of high-risk infants who developed autism. *Journal of Autism and Developmental Disorders, 37,* 12–24.

Caldwell, P. (2006). *Finding you, finding me*. London: Atheneum Press.

Camaioni, L., Aureli, T., Bellagamba, F., & Fogel, A. (2003). A longitudinal examination of the transition to symbolic communication in the second year of life. *Infant and Child Development, 12,* 1–26.

Camaioni, L., Perucchini, P., Muratori, F., & Milone, A. (1997). Brief report: A longitudinal examination of communicative gestures deficit in young children with autism. *Journal of Autism and Developmental Disorders, 27,* 715–725.

Camaioni L., Perucchini, P., Muratori F., Parrini, B., & Cesari, A. (2003). The communicative use of pointing in autism: Developmental profile and factors related to change. *European Psychiatry, 18,* 6–12.

Capone, N., & McGregor, K. (2004). Gesture development: A review for clinical and research practices. *Journal of Speech, Language, and Hearing Research, 47,* 173–186.

Carpenter, M., Pennington, B., & Rogers, S. (2002). Interrelations among social-cognitive skills in young children with autism. *Journal of Autism and Developmental Disorders, 32*(2), 91–106.

Charman, T., Drew, A., Baird, C., & Baird, G. (2003). Measuring early language development in preschool children with autism spectrum disorder using the MacArthur Communicative Development Inventory (Infant Form). *Journal of Child Language, 30,* 213–236.

Dawson, G., Toth, K., Abbott, R., Osterling, J., Munson, J., Estes, A., & Liaw, J. (2004). Early social attention impairments in autism: Social orienting, joint attention and attention to distress. *Developmental Psychology, 40,* 271–283.

DiSalvo, C., & Oswald, D. (2002). Peer-mediated interventions to increase the social interaction of children with autism: Consideration of peer expectancies. *Focus on Autism and Other Developmental Disabilities, 17*(4), 198–207.

Drew, A., Baird, G., Taylor, E., Milne, E., & Charman, T. (2007). The Social Communication Assessment for Toddlers with Autism (SCATA): An instrument to measure the frequency, form, and function of communication in toddlers with autism spectrum disorder. *Journal of Autism and Developmental Disorders, 37,* 648–666.

Ephraim, G. (1986). *A brief introduction to augmented mothering*. Radlett, England: Harperbury Hospital School.

Fenson, L., Marchman, V.A., Thal, D.J., Dale, P.S., Reznick, J.S., & Bates, E. (2006). *MacArthur-Bates Communication Development Inventories (CDIs)* (2nd ed.). Baltimore: Paul H. Brookes Publishing Co.

Frost, L., & Bondy, A. (2002). *Picture Exchange Communication System training manual* (2nd ed.). Newark, DE: Pyramid Education Products.

Garfinkel, A.N., & Schwartz, I.S. (2002). Peer imitation: Increasing social interactions in children with autism and other developmental disabilities in inclusive preschool classrooms. *Topics in Early Childhood Special Education, 22,* 26–38.

Girolametto, L., Weitzman, E., & Sussman, F. (2006). Using case study methods to investigate the effects of interactive intervention for individuals with autism spectrum disorders. *Journal of Communication Disorders, 40,* 470–492.

Gonzalez-Lopez, A., & Kamps, D.M. (1997). Social skills training to increase social interactions between children with autism and their typical peers. *Focus on Autism & Other Developmental Disabilities, 12,* 2–14.

Greenspan, S., & Wieder, S. (1997). Developmental patterns and outcomes in infants and individuals with disorders in relating and communicating: A chart review of 200 cases of individuals with autism spectrum diagnoses. *Journal of Developmental and Learning Disorders, 1,* 87–141.

Greenspan, S., & Wieder, S. (1998). *The individual with special needs: Encouraging intellectual and emotional growth.* Reading, MA: Addison-Wesley.

Greenspan, S., & Wieder, S. (2006). *Engaging autism.* Cambridge, MA: DaCapo Press.

Herschell, A.D., Calzada, E.J., Eyberg, S.M., & McNeil, C.B. (2002). Parent–Child Interaction Therapy: New directions for research. *Cognitive and Behavioral Practice, 9,* 9–16.

Hewett, D., & Nind, M. (1998). *Interaction in action: Reflections on the use of Intensive Interaction.* London: David Fulton.

Hwang, B., & Hughes, C. (2000a). The effects of social interactive training on early social communicative skills of children with autism. *Journal of Autism and Developmental Disorders, 30,* 331–343.

Hwang, B., & Hughes, C. (2000b). Increasing early social-communicative skills of preverbal preschool children with autism through social interactive training. *Journal of the Association for Persons with Severe Handicaps, 25,* 18–28.

Iacono, T., Bloomberg, K., & West, D. (2005). A preliminary investigation into the internal consistency and construct validity of the Triple C: Checklist of Communicative Competencies. *Journal of Intellectual and Developmental Disabilities, 130,* 127-138.

Jones, E., & Carr, E. (2004). Joint attention in children with autism: Theory and intervention. *Focus on Autism and Other Developmental Disabilities, 19,* 13–26.

Kasari, C. (2002). Assessing change in early intervention programs for children with autism. *Journal of Autism and Developmental Disorders, 32,* 447–461.

Kasari, C., Freeman, S., & Paparella T. (2006). Joint attention and symbolic play in young individuals with autism: A randomized controlled intervention study. *Journal of Individual Psychology & Psychiatry, 47,* 611–620.

Kellet, M., & Nind, M. (2003). *Implementing Intensive Interaction in schools: Guidance for practitioners, managers and coordinators.* London: David Fulton.

Kelly, J.F., Zuckerman, T., Sandoval, D., & Beuhlman, K. (2003). *Promoting First Relationships: A curriculum for service providers to help parents and other caregivers meet young children's social and emotional needs.* Seattle: NCAST-AVENUW Publications.

Koegel, R.L., & Koegel, L.K. (2006). *Pivotal response treatments for autism: Communication, social, and academic development.* Baltimore: Paul H. Brookes Publishing Co.

Landa, R.J., Holman, K.C., & Garret-Mayer, E. (2007). Social and communication development in toddlers with early and later diagnosis of autism spectrum disorders. *Archives of General Psychiatry, 64,* 853–864.

Lord, C., & Paul, R. (1997). Language and communication in autism. In D. Cohen & F. Volkmar (Eds.), *Handbook of autism and pervasive developmental disorders* (pp. 195–225). New York: John Wiley & Sons.

Luyster, R., Richler, J., Risi, S., Hsu, W., Dawson, G., Bernier, R., et al. (2005). Early regression in social communication in autism spectrum disorders: A CPEA study. *Developmental Neuropsychology, 27,* 311–336.

Maestro, S., Muratori, F., Cavallaro, M.C., Pei, F., Stern, D., Golse, B., & Palacio-Espasa, F. (2002). Attentional skills during the first 6 months of age in autism spectrum disorder. *Journal of the Academy of Child and Adolescent Psychiatry, 41,* 1239–1245.

Mahoney, G. (2007). *Autism and developmental delays in young children.* Austin, TX: PRO-ED.

Mahoney, G., & McDonald, J.D. (2007). *Autism and developmental delays: The Responsive Teaching curriculum for parents and professionals.* Austin, TX: PRO-ED.

Mahoney, G., & Perales, F. (2003). Using relationship-focused intervention to enhance the social-emotional functioning of young children with autism spectrum disorders. *Topics in Early Childhood Special Education, 23,* 77–89.

Mahoney, G., & Perales, F. (2005). Relationship-focused early intervention with children with pervasive developmental disorders and other disabilities: A comparative study. *Developmental and Behavioral Pediatrics, 26,* 77–85.

Martins, M., & Harris, S. (2006). Teaching children with autism to respond to joint attention initiations. *Child and Family Behavior Therapy, 28,* 51–69.

McCathren R.B., Warren, S.F., & Yoder, P.J. (1996). Prelinguistic predictors of later language development. In S.F. Warren & J. Reichle (Series Eds.) & K.N. Cole, P.S. Dale, & D.J. Thal (Vol. Eds.), *Communication and language intervention series: Vol. 6. Assessment of communication and language* (pp. 57–76). Baltimore: Paul H. Brookes Publishing Co.

McConachie, H. Randle, V., & Le Couteur, A. (2005). A controlled trial of a training course for parents of individuals with suspected autism spectrum disorder. *Journal of Pediatrics, 147,* 335–340.

McLean, J.E., & Snyder-McLean, L. (1978). *A transactional approach to early language training.* Columbus: OH: Charles E. Merrill.

Mitchell, S., Brian, J., Zwaigenbaum, L., Roberts, W., Szatmari, P., Smith, I., et al. (2006). Early language and communication development of infants later diagnosed with autism spectrum disorder. *Developmental and Behavioral Pediatrics, 27,* 69–78.

Morford, M., & Goldin-Meadow, S. (1992). Comprehension and production of gesture in combination with speech in one-word speakers. *Journal of Child Language, 19,* 559–580.

National Research Council. (2001). *Educating children with autism.* Committee on Educational Interventions for Children with Autism, Division of Behavioral and Social Sciences and Education. Washington, DC: National Academies Press.

Nind, M. (1996). Efficacy of Intensive Interaction: Developing sociability and communication in people with severe and complex learning difficulties using an approach based on caregiver–infant interaction. *European Journal of Special Needs Education, 11,* 48–66.

Nind, M., & Hewett, D. (2001). *A practical guide to Intensive Interaction.* Kidderminster, England: British Institute of Learning Disabilities.

Nind, M., & Hewett, D. (2005). *Access to communication: Developing the basics of communication with people with severe learning difficulties through Intensive Interaction* (2nd ed.). London: David Fulton.

Pepper, J., & Weitzman, E. (2004). *It takes two to talk: A practical guide for parents of individuals with language delays.* Toronto: The Hanen Centre.

Prizant, B. (1996). Brief report: Communication, language, social and emotional development. *Journal of Autism and Developmental Disorders, 20,* 173–178.

Prizant, B., Wetherby, A., Rubin, E., & Laurent, A. (2003). The SCERTS® Model: A transactional, family-centered approach to enhancing communication and socio-emotional abilities of individuals with autism spectrum disorder. *Journal of Infants and Young Individuals, 16,* 296–316.

Prizant, B.M., Wetherby, A.M., Rubin, E., Laurent, A.C., & Rydell, P.J. (2005a). *The SCERTS® Model: A comprehensive educational approach for children with autism spectrum disorders. Vol. I: Assessment.* Baltimore: Paul H. Brookes Publishing Co.

Prizant, B.M., Wetherby, A.M., Rubin, E., Laurent, A.C., & Rydell, P.J. (2005b). *The SCERTS® Model: A comprehensive educational approach for children with autism spectrum disorders. Vol. II: Intervention.* Baltimore: Paul H. Brookes Publishing Co.

Reichle, J. (1991). Developing communicative exchanges. In J. Reichle, J. York, & J. Sigafoos (Eds.), *Implementing augmentative and alternative communication: Strategies for learners with severe disabilities* (pp. 133–156). Baltimore: Paul H. Brookes Publishing Co.

Roeyers, H. (1996). The influence of nonhandicapped peers on the social interactions of children with a pervasive developmental disorder. *Journal of Autism and Developmental Disorders, 26,* 303–320.

Rogers, S., Hall, T., Osaki, D., Reaven, J., & Herbison, J. (2000). The Denver Model: A comprehensive, integrated approach to young children with autism and their families. In S. Harris & J. Handleman (Eds.), *Preschool education programs for children with autism* (2nd ed., pp. 95–134). Austin, TX: PRO-ED.

Rowland, C., & Schweigert, P. (2000a). Tangible symbols, tangible outcomes. *Augmentative and Alternative Communication, 16,* 61–78.

Rowland, C., & Schweigert, P. (2000b). *Tangible Symbol Systems.* Portland, OR: Oregon Health & Science University.

Rowland, C., & Schweigert, P. (2001). A concrete bridge to abstract communication for children with autism. *Proceedings of the Autism Society of America Millennium of Hope National Conference on Autism.* Arlington, TX: Future Horizons.

Rowland, C., & Schweigert, P. (2003a). Cognitive skills and AAC. In D.R. Beukelman & J. Reichle (Series Eds.) & J.C. Light, D.R. Beukelman, & J. Reichle (Vol. Eds.), *Augmentative and alternative communication series. Communicative competence for individuals who use AAC: From research to effective practice* (pp. 241–275). Baltimore: Paul H. Brookes Publishing Co.

Rowland, C., & Schweigert, P. (2003b). *Hands-On Learning at Home.* Portland, OR: Oregon Health & Science University.

Rowland, C., & Schweigert, P. (2003c). *Teacher's guide to Hands-On Learning.* Portland, OR: Oregon Health & Science University.

Rowland, C., & Schweigert, P. (2003d). *Design to Learn.* Portland, OR: Oregon Health & Science University.

Rowland, C., & Schweigert, P. (2003e). *Hands-On Learning at School.* Portland, OR: Oregon Health & Science University.

Rowland, C., & Schweigert, P. (2004). *First Things First.* Portland, OR: Oregon Health & Science University.

Rowland, C., & Schweigert, P. (2005). *Tangible Symbol Systems* [DVD]. Portland, OR: Oregon Health & Science University.

Rowland, C., & Schweigert, P. (2007). *Object lessons: How children with pervasive developmental disorder use objects to interact with the physical and social environments.* Manuscript submitted for publication.

Schertz, H., & Odom, S. (2007). Promoting joint attention in toddlers with autism: A parent-mediated developmental model. *Journal of Autism and Developmental Disorders, 37,* 1562–1575.

Siegel, B. (1996). *The world of the autistic individual: Understanding and treating autistic spectrum disorders.* New York: Oxford University Press.

Sigman, M., & Ruskin, E. (1999). Continuity and change in the social competence of children with autism, Down syndrome and developmental delays. *Monographs of the Society for Research in Child Development, 64,* 256.

Smith, C.M., Rogers, S., & Dawson, G. (2007). The Early Start Denver Model: A comprehensive early intervention approach for toddlers with autism. In J.S. Handleman & S.L. Harris (Eds.), *Preschool education programs for children with autism* (3rd ed., pp. 65–101). Austin, TX: PRO-ED.

Smith, T., Scahill, L., Dawson, G., Guthrie, D., Lord, C., Odom, S., et al. (2007). Designing research studies on psychosocial interventions in autism. *Journal of Autism and Developmental Disorders, 37,* 354–366.

Stern, D.N. (1985). *The interpersonal world of the human infant.* New York: Basic Books.

Stone, W., Ousley, O., Yoder, P., Hogan, K., & Hepburn, S. (1997). Nonverbal communication in two- and three-year-old individuals with autism. *Journal of Autism and Developmental Disorders, 27,* 677–695.

Sussman, F. (1999). *More than words.* Toronto: The Hanen Centre.

Sussman, F. (2006). *Talkability.* Toronto: The Hanen Centre.

Thurm, A., Lord, C., Lee, L., & Newschaffer, C. (2007). Predictors of language acquisition in preschool children with autism spectrum disorders. *Journal of Autism and Developmental Disorders, 37,* 1721–1734.

Toth, K., Munson, J., Meltzhoff, A., & Dawson, G. (2006). Early predictors of communication development in young children with autism spectrum disorder: Joint attention, imitation, and toy play. *Journal of Autism and Developmental Disorders, 36,* 993–1005.

Warren, S.F., Bredin-Oja, S.L., Fairchild, M., Finestack, L.H., Fey, M.E., & Brady, N.C. (2006). Responsivity education/prelinguistic milieu training. In S.F. Warren & M.E. Fey (Series Eds.) & R.J. McCauley & M.E. Fey (Vol. Eds.), *Communication and language intervention series: Treatment of language disorders in children* (pp. 47–75). Baltimore: Paul H. Brookes Publishing Co.

Warreyn, P., Roeyers, H., Van Wetswinkel, U., & De Groote, I. (2007). Temporal coordination of joint attention behavior in preschoolers with autism spectrum disorder. *Journal of Autism and Developmental Disorders, 37,* 501–512.

Wetherby, A.M. (2006). Understanding and measuring social communication in children with autism spectrum disorders. In T. Charman & W. Stone (Eds.), *Social and communication development in autism spectrum disorders* (pp. 3–34). New York: Guilford Press.

Wetherby, A.M., & Prizant, B.M. (Vol. Eds.). (2000). *Autism spectrum disorders: A transactional developmental perspective.* In S.F. Warren & J. Reichle (Series Eds.), *Communication and language intervention series: Vol. 9.* Baltimore: Paul H. Brookes Publishing Co.

Wetherby, A.M., Prizant, B.M., & Hutchinson, T.A. (1998). Communicative, social/affective, and symbolic profiles of young children with autism and pervasive developmental disorders. *American Journal of Speech-Language Pathology, 7,* 79–91.

Wetherby, A.M., Rubin, E., Laurent, A.C., Prizant, B.M., & Rydell, P J. (2006). *Summary of research supporting the SCERTS® Model.* Retrieved November 5, 2007, from http://scerts.com/ResearchSupportingtheSCERTSModel10-7-06.pdf

Whalen, C., & Schreibman, L. (2003). Joint attention training for children with autism using behavior modification procedures. *Journal of Psychology and Psychiatry, 44,* 456–468.

Wieder, S., & Greenspan, S. (2005). Can individuals with autism master the core deficits and become empathetic, creative, and reflective? A ten to fifteen year follow-up of a subgroup of individuals with autism spectrum disorders (ASD) who received a comprehensive developmental, individual-difference, relationship-based (DIR) approach. Retrieved November 5, 2007 from http://www.playworks.cc/articles/DIRstudy—10yearfollowup.pdf

Wimpory, D., Hobson, R., Williams, J., & Nash, S. (2000). Are infants with autism socially engaged? A study of recent retrospective parental reports. *Journal of Autism and Developmental Disorders, 30,* 525–536.

Wolfberg, P. (2003). *Peer play and the autism spectrum: The art of guiding individuals' socialization and imagination.* Shawnee Mission, KS: Autism Asperger Publishing Company.

Wolfberg, P., & Schuler, A. (1993). Integrated play groups: A model for promoting the social and cognitive dimensions of play in individuals with autism. *Journal of Autism and Developmental Disorders, 23,* 467–489.

Yoder, P.J., & McDuffie, A. (2006). Treatment of responding to and initiating joint attention. In T. Charman & W. Stone (Eds.), *Social and communication development in autism spectrum disorders: Early identification, diagnosis, & intervention* (pp. 117–142). New York: Guilford Press.

Yoder, P., & Stone, W. (2006a). A randomized comparison of the effect of two prelinguistic communication interventions on the acquisition of spoken communication in preschoolers with ASD. *Journal of Speech, Language, and Hearing Research, 49,* 698–711.

Yoder, P., & Stone, W. (2006b). Randomized comparison of two communication interventions for preschoolers with autism spectrum disorders. *Journal of Consulting and Clinical Psychology, 74,* 426–435.

Yoder, P.J., & Warren, S.F. (1998). Maternal responsivity predicts the extent to which prelinguistic intervention facilitates generalized intentional communication. *Journal of Speech, Language and Hearing Research, 41,* 1207–1219.

Yoder, P.J., & Warren, S.F. (2002). Effects of prelinguistic milieu teaching and parent responsivity education on dyads involving children with intellectual disabilities. *Journal of Speech, Language and Hearing Research, 45,* 1158–1174.

Zanolli, K., Daggett, J., & Adams, T. (1996). Teaching preschool age autistic children to make spontaneous initiations to peers using priming. *Journal of Autism and Related Disorders, 26,* 407–422.

Zwaigenbaum, L., Bryson, S., Rogers, S., Roberts, W., Brian, J., & Szatmari, P. (2005). Behavioral manifestations of autism in the first year of life. *International Journal of Developmental Neuroscience, 23,* 143–152.

4

Research on the Use of Manual Signs and Graphic Symbols in Autism Spectrum Disorders

A Systematic Review

OLIVER WENDT

According to recent estimates, approximately 14%–25% of children diagnosed with an autism spectrum disorder (ASD) present with little or no functional speech (Lord & Bailey, 2002; Lord, Risi, & Pickles, 2004; Volkmar, Lord, Bailey, Schultz, & Klin, 2004). These individuals rely on augmentative and alternative communication (AAC) to meet their daily communication needs. AAC refers to an area of educational and clinical practice that aims to supplement or replace an individual's natural speech and/or handwriting through aided or unaided communication approaches. Aided communication requires an aid or device external to the body to represent, select, or transmit messages. Examples of aided communication are pictographic symbols sets and systems or electronic systems with speech generation. Unaided

The research presented in this chapter was supported by grants from the American Speech-Language-Hearing Association, the Purdue Clifford Kinley Trust, the Purdue Research Foundation, and a Sigma Xi Grant-in-Aid of Research. The author wishes to thank the following graduate and undergraduate students for their valuable assistance with many phases of this work: Katie Angermeier, Megan Clark, Krista Davidson, Johanna Hassink, Jill Lievense, Sam Mathew, and Nicole Smith. The author is also grateful to Lyle Lloyd and Ralf W. Schlosser for their input on earlier versions of this manuscript.

communication does not rely on any external aid or device and involves using only the individual's own body as the mode of communication. Examples of unaided communication are body language and fingerspelling (Lloyd, Fuller, & Arvidson, 1997).

For many years, AAC interventions for individuals with ASDs focused primarily on the use of unaided communication strategies and manual signing in particular (e.g., Schaeffer, Kollinzas, Musil, & McDowell, 1978). After professionals realized the apparent visuoperceptual strengths that many children with ASDs demonstrate, increasing attention was paid to the application of aided strategies, such as pictographic symbol sets and other graphic symbol sets/systems (Mirenda & Schuler, 1989). These developments were further advanced by a need to justify the use of AAC over traditional speech therapy for individuals with severe communication impairments. Once practitioners, families, and funding agencies started to recognize the benefits of using AAC with this population, AAC was used more and more frequently for children on the autism spectrum with no functional speech. In the early 1990s, the controversial approach of facilitated communication was widely explored in the ASD field, but was largely abandoned because of a lack of scientific evidence for the validity of the technique (for systematic reviews, see Biermann, 1999; Nußbeck, 1999; Probst, 2005).

Subsequently, a debate evolved about the characteristics of individuals with ASDs in relation to AAC modalities. At the center of this debate, questions focused on the most appropriate AAC option for individuals with ASDs: an unaided AAC approach, such as manual signs and gestures, or an aided AAC approach, such as graphic symbol sets/systems (Mirenda, 2001, 2003).

This discussion emerged at a time when clinical psychology promoted the idea of "empirically supported interventions" (Lonigan, Elbert, & Johnson, 1998, p. 139) and several other fields in allied health care and education started to embrace the principles of evidence-based practice (EBP) as a major paradigm for service delivery (Schlosser, 2003; Straus, Richardson, Glasziou, & Haynes, 2005). EBP involves the integration of the best and current research evidence with clinical/educational expertise and stakeholder perspectives during clinical or educational decision making (Schlosser & Raghavendra, 2004). For this purpose, the practitioner 1) asks a well-built question concerning a child with an ASD, 2) searches for research evidence, 3) appraises the evidence, 4) applies the evidence by integrating it with his or her clinical expertise and relevant stakeholder perspectives to arrive at a decision, and 5) evaluates whether the decision resulted in desired outcomes.

The primary purpose of this chapter is to provide practitioners and other stakeholders with a summary of appraised research evidence related to the use of manual signs and graphic symbols for individuals with ASDs. To give an overview on the currently existing research base, the author located research studies that met the inclusion criteria for several recently conducted systematic reviews and meta-analyses on AAC for individuals with ASDs. These references were updated through an additional literature search. Studies that focused on manual signs, gestures, and selection-based graphic symbol sets/systems were extracted for review in this chapter. Exchange-based graphic symbol systems, such as the Picture Exchange Communication System (PECS), were excluded because related research on PECS is covered in Chapter 10 of this book. Although manual signs and graphic symbols are often used in studies investigating the effects of functional communication training on the reduction of problem behavior, this body of research was also excluded because it is addressed in Chapter 12 and has been the topic of several reviews (e.g., Bopp, Brown, & Mirenda, 2004; Mancil, 2006).

All of the reviewed studies provide the EBP practitioner with evidence that can be characterized as "prefiltered." Such evidence is generated when one or several experts on a subject area have reviewed and presented the methodologically strongest data in the field (Guyatt & Rennie, 2002). Prefiltered evidence established through a systematic review substantially reduces the time and expertise required for practitioners to locate and appraise individual studies (Schlosser, Wendt, & Sigafoos, 2007). Time pressure and missing resources are documented barriers to EBP implementation that can be overcome by applying prefiltered evidence (Zipoli & Kennedy, 2005). It is hoped that the prefiltered evidence presented in this chapter will assist practitioners and other stakeholders in clinical decision making. Therefore, the sections on manual signs and graphic symbols conclude with implications for clinical practice in light of the research evidence. An additional purpose for this chapter is to identify gaps in the current research base and derive plausible directions for future research—research that intends to further promote EBP implementation when using manual signs or graphic symbols with individuals with ASDs.

DESIGN OF THE REVIEW

In this section, procedures for retrieving and appraising the studies will be described, along with methods for estimating effect size.

Retrieval and Appraisal of Studies

Reviewed studies were retrieved from previously conducted systematic reviews and meta-analyses of the larger body of AAC research related to ASDs. Fortunately, an increasing number of systematic reviews have synthesized the research base in this area (e.g., Schlosser & Wendt, 2008a, 2008b; Wendt, 2007). Systematic reviews (if well conducted) provide an excellent, comprehensive source of research evidence and therefore rank highly on EBP hierarchies of evidence (e.g., Schlosser & Rhagavendra, 2004). Their value lies in the systematic application of procedures to minimize bias while locating, appraising, and synthesizing evidence (Petticrew & Roberts, 2006). For example, transparency and objectivity of the review process are implemented through a well-documented and comprehensive literature search strategy, which minimizes the danger of subjective inclusion or oversight of relevant studies.

To supplement and update the body of research literature obtained from previous reviews, an additional literature search was conducted using the keywords and search procedures employed in the meta-analysis by Wendt (2007) that were relevant to retrieve studies on manual signs and/or graphic symbols. The temporal cutoff for this search was set to December 2007. Obtained documents were evaluated by two independent raters using the identical inclusion criteria and coding procedures that were established in the Wendt review. All previously and newly retrieved documents that met the inclusion criteria underwent an assessment of study quality. This assessment was accomplished by applying the certainty framework that was originally proposed by Simeonsson and Bailey (1991) and subsequently adapted and used by several authors (Granlund & Olsson, 1999; Millar, Light, & Schlosser, 2006; Schlosser & Sigafoos, 2002, 2006). This framework classifies the certainty of evidence into four groupings from conclusive to preponderant and from suggestive to inconclusive, based on three dimensions: research design, interobserver agreement of the dependent variable, and treatment integrity.

Conclusive evidence establishes that the outcomes are undoubtedly the results of the intervention based on a sound design and adequate or better interobserver agreement and treatment integrity. Preponderant evidence ascertains that the outcomes are not only plausible but they are also more likely to have occurred than not, despite minor design flaws and with adequate or better interobserver agreement and treatment integrity. Suggestive evidence establishes that the outcomes are plausible and within the realm of possibility due to a strong design but inadequate interobserver agreement and/or treatment integrity, or due to minor design flaws and inadequate interobserver agreement and/or treatment integrity. Inconclusive evidence ascertains that the outcomes are not plausible due to fatal flaws in design.

The studies were grouped into tables in terms of the certainty of evidence categories (see Appendixes 4A and 4B). Studies were sequenced from the best available evidence first, followed by less convincing evidence (e.g., suggestive evidence). Within each level of evidence, studies were sequenced alphabetically by author. Only evidence evaluated as being suggestive or better is discussed in terms of implications for practice. Studies that were deemed inconclusive are not appropriate for informing practice due to their fatal design flaws. They may be considered only in terms of directions for future research. Studies of this type have been listed last in each appendix.

Estimating Effect Size

Based on the research design of a study, different effect size metrics were applied to aggregate study outcomes and derive a quantitative measure for the extent of treatment or experimental effect caused by the intervention or independent variable. It should be noted that there are currently no meta-analytic techniques that permit meaningful aggregation or averaging of single-subject design with group design effectiveness measures (Allison & Gorman, 1993). Thus, effect size estimates for group experiments were calculated and interpreted separately from that of single-subject experiments. A direct comparison of both types of outcome measures is not permissible. Effect size estimates are presented in Appendixes 4A and 4B in a separate column labeled with the applied effect size metrics.

Group Design Effect Size Indices and Their Interpretation

When a group design was present, one of two different effect size indices were chosen that are based on the standard mean difference: Cohen's d or Hedges' g. Cohen's d was derived by calculating the difference between the two group means (i.e., the control group and the experimental group) divided by the standard deviation for those means (Cohen, 1988). When group studies had small samples sizes ($N < 20$), Hedges' g was used instead of Cohen's d to avoid small sample bias (Lipsey & Wilson, 2001). Hedges' g is a simple correction of d based on the pooled standard deviation. It was computed by using the square root of the mean square error from the analysis of variance testing for differences between the two groups. Standard mean difference effect sizes such d and g can range from -3.00 to $+3.00$. Cohen (1988) provided a widely used convention to interpret the magnitude of the effect size: an effect size less than 0.20 is considered small, 0.20–0.50 is medium, 0.50–0.80 is important, and greater than 0.80 is large.

***Single-Subject Experimental Design Effect Size Indices
and Their Interpretation***   Single-subject experimental designs
study the effect of treatment in terms of either increases or decreases in
specific target behaviors. Based on the intended direction of the
observed behavior, one of two nonparametric techniques was chosen
to aggregate the outcomes of single-subject experimental designs
and determine the magnitude of an effect. For studies aimed at
increasing target behavior, the percentage of nonoverlapping data
(PND) was applied (Scruggs, Mastropieri, & Casto, 1987). The PND
method requires the calculation of nonoverlap between baseline and
successive intervention (or generalization) phases by identifying the
highest data point in baseline and determining the percentage of data
points during intervention (or generalization or maintenance) exceeding this level.

PND scores can range from 0% to 100% and can be interpreted
using the conventions set by Scruggs, Mastropieri, Cook, and Escobar
(1986). A PND score greater than 90% is considered highly effective,
70%–90% is fairly effective, 50%–70% is questionably effective, and less
than 50% reflects unreliable or ineffective treatments. When PND
scores were summarized across participants or outcome variables, the
median PND score (rather than the mean) was taken as a measure of
overall effectiveness, because PND scores are usually not distributed
normally and the median is less affected by outliers than the mean
(Scruggs et al., 1986).

For studies intending to decrease behavior, the mean baseline
reduction (MBR) procedure was used (Kahng, Iwata, & Lewin, 2002).
The MBR measure is calculated by 1) subtracting the mean of the last
three intervention points from the last three baseline points, 2) dividing
the result by the mean of the last three baseline points, and 3) multiply-
ing by 100. This reveals a mean percent reduction from baseline (Olive
& Smith, 2005). MBR scores also fall in the range of 0% to 100%, with the
MBR reflecting the behavior reduction percentage. A reduction of 100%
represents total elimination of the target behavior based on comparison
of the specified treatment data points, whereas a reduction of 0% indicates no change compared with baseline (Kahng et al., 2002).

RESEARCH SYNTHESIS: MANUAL SIGNS AND GESTURES

Manual signs were one of the first forms of AAC taught to individuals
with ASDs without functional speech (e.g., Carr, Binkoff, Kologinsky, &
Eddy, 1978). The approach was introduced in the 1970s and has been
used successfully with this population for more than 30 years. The
term *manual sign* can refer to a natural sign language (e.g., American

Sign Language) or to the production of manual signs as a code for a spoken language (Blischak, Lloyd, & Fuller, 1997).

Originally, the rationale for introducing manual sign communication instead of speech was based on four major assumptions (Sundberg, 1993; Sundberg & Partington, 1998). First, learning manual signs or gestures has specific advantages over learning speech. It may be an easier option than speech because many individuals with ASDs struggle when confronted with the task of imitating sounds, but are able to imitate at least a few fine or gross motor movements that are demonstrated by their communication partners (Sundberg & Partington, 1998). Second, if an individual does not possess a strong motor or vocal imitative repertoire, then it might be less difficult to teach him or her to imitate motor movements than to teach word imitation (Sundberg, 1993). Motor imitation is an easier behavior to teach because an instructor can make use of physical prompting and fading procedures (Sundberg & Partington, 1998); that is, it is easier to provide a physical prompt for a motor behavior such as a hand movement than it is to prompt a vocalization or speech sound. Third, because manual signs are less transient than words, manual sign learning may be less demanding of verbal memory and abstract understanding (Fulwiler & Fouts, 1976). Fourth, using manual signs may help to overcome a negative emotional history with speech that many individuals with autism experience as a result of prolonged lack of progress (Sundberg & Partington, 1998). Introducing manual signs eliminates this problem by creating an alternative mode for functional communication.

By the mid-1980s, manual signs were often taught in combination with speech. This approach was referred to as *total communication* or *simultaneous communication* (Mirenda & Erickson, 2000). Total communication was originally developed in the field of deafness in the 1960s to emphasize the importance of communication (as well as language development) apart from specific communication modes or methods (Lloyd et al., 1997). Thus, total communication stressed the use of the most appropriate communication strategy for each individual. As a communication method, pairing manual signs and speech was the preferred AAC approach during the 1980s for people labeled as "severely handicapped" (including those with autism) in the United States, the United Kingdom, and Australia (Mirenda & Erickson, 2000). This enthusiasm started to fade as research revealed a generalized imitation deficit in learners with ASDs (Dawson & Adams, 1984; Smith & Bryson, 1994), which challenged the promise of total communication as a successful intervention approach for this population.

Gestures are body movements or sequences of coordinated body movements to represent an object, idea, action, or relationship without the linguistic features of manual signs (Lloyd et al., 1997). Examples of gestures include pointing or yes-no headshakes. In general, gestural communication is one of the earliest developing nonlinguistic forms of unaided communication (see Chapter 3). Before linguistic development starts, young children typically use gestures when communicating and interacting with people in the environment (Loncke & Bos, 1997); thus, the use of gestures serves as a precursor to later development of language skills (Morford & Goldin-Meadow, 1992). However, individuals with ASDs rarely use gestures for communicative purposes, even if they have difficulty speaking (Loveland, Landry, Hughes, Hall, & McEvoy, 1988). Because gestural development is often targeted as an important focus of early communication intervention (Rogers, 1999; Rogers, Hepburn, Stackhouse, & Wehner, 2003), research on gestures is included in this review, along with research on manual signs.

Review and Appraisal

A total of 21 experimental studies on the application of manual signs or gestures met the inclusion criteria for this review. All participants in these studies were diagnosed with autism. The experiments, which include 18 single-subject experimental designs and three group designs, are summarized in Appendix 4A. Following the study appraisal format for this review, the focus of Appendix 4A is on evidence ranked better than inconclusive, beginning with conclusive evidence and followed by preponderant and suggestive evidence. Two group studies and two single-subject experimental designs were ranked as inconclusive; their results are provided last in Appendix 4A, but are not discussed in further detail. The remaining studies targeted three different outcome variables: 14 focused on teaching manual signs or gestures and primarily monitored symbol acquisition as an outcome variable, 2 compared the effects of simultaneous communication versus sign alone and/or speech training, and 1 examined the effects of manual signing relative to variations of manual sign instructions. Results are reported according to these major groups.

Results for the Acquisition and Production of Manual Signs and Gestures   Studies in this category varied in terms of the conditions under which sign language or gestures were taught. They also varied in the specific behaviors that were observed to indicate that the symbol had been acquired.

Among the conclusive evidence, one study by Anderson (2001) monitored the acquisition of sign items for six participants as part of an experiment comparing acquisition and use of manual signs versus

PECS. Although the overall results indicated PECS to be superior to manual signs for item requesting, the study demonstrated that the six participants were very successful in acquiring manual signs, with all PNDs equal to 100%. Another study (Buffington, Krantz, McClannahan, & Poulson, 1998) taught gestures in combination with oral speech (e.g., saying *"look"*) for indicating tasks and measured the frequency of correctly produced gestural and verbal responses. This intervention yielded PND scores in the range of highly effective for all four participants.

Among the preponderant evidence, Ingersoll, Lewis, and Kroman (2007) investigated the use of a naturalistic imitation intervention called reciprocal imitation training to teach descriptive gestures. Reciprocal imitation training led to a substantial increase in gesture imitation among all five participants, three of whom achieved PND scores in the range of fairly or highly effective. Reciprocal imitation training was less effective in increasing the spontaneous use of gestures; under this condition, only two individuals showed PNDs in the fairly effective range. Participants with less developed language skills were generally more likely to demonstrate spontaneous gesture use than those who had some verbal fluency. Tincani (2004) conducted an experiment comparing manual signing with PECS relative to effects on requesting and speech production. For requesting, manual signing was fairly effective for two participants, but not as effective as PECS. For speech production, another two participants were highly successful in increasing their vocalizations after manual signing was introduced, as demonstrated by PNDs equal to 100%. In this case, manual signing appeared to be superior to PECS.

The majority of studies provided suggestive evidence, including an early study by Carr, Binkoff, Kologinsky, and Eddy (1978) that evaluated the impact of a training procedure using prompting, fading, and stimulus rotation on a sign production task. The procedure yielded highly effective expressive sign labeling, with PNDs equal to 100% for all four participants. Carr and Kemp (1989) conducted an experiment to determine whether leading (i.e., taking an adult by the hand to a desired item) could be replaced with a pointing gesture as a means of requesting. Again, the intervention led to highly effective use of pointing for requests in all four participants.

A study by Carr and Kologinsky (1983; experiment 1) evaluated whether a combination of prompting, fading, differential reinforcement, and incidental teaching affected the acquisition of spontaneous sign requests and generalization of requests across communication partners. All three participants in this study were very successful in acquiring spontaneous requesting and generalizing those requests across partners, with PNDs consistently equal to 100%. In a related study, Carr and Kologinsky (1983; experiment 2) investigated whether targeted prompting and reinforcement would result in increased signed requesting, with generalization across adults and settings. In terms of sign acquisition, the procedure was highly effective for three participants. It also proved to be highly effective for all participants when generalization across settings was examined. Slightly different results were obtained for generalization across partners; the procedure was highly effective for one participant and fairly effective for another. Finally, as a follow-up to the 1983 study, Carr, Kologinsky, and Leff-Simon (1987) examined the effects of prompting, fading, stimulus rotation, and differential reinforcement on descriptive signing of action-object phrases. PND scores revealed that this teaching procedure was highly effective for the three participants in this study. All of them acquired signed action–object phrases and were able to generalize those phrases to new situations.

Keogh, Whitman, Beeman, Halligan, and Starzynski (1987) evaluated the effects of a treatment package that included verbal prompts, modeling, physical guidance, positive reinforcement, fading, and chaining procedures to teach one participant an interactive signing dialogue within a naturalistic snack time routine. The intervention was highly effective in increasing the participant's sign repertoire, but led to a PND indicating ineffectiveness when it came to generalizing signed communication to new partners. In a related experiment (Sommer, Whitman, & Keogh, 1988), the same participant was taught a behavioral script to sign interactively with other children in a play situation. PND scores indicated questionable effectiveness of this intervention for sign acquisition, as well as for generalizing signed communication to another play situation.

Schepis et al. (1982) investigated the effects of modified incidental teaching strategies on manual sign acquisition in four participants. When expressive signing was observed, PND scores indicated the teaching program to be highly effective for one participant, fairly effective for another, questionably effective for a third, and ineffective for the last participant. Finally, Sundberg, Endicott, and Eigenheer (2000) compared the efficacy of two procedures for the acquisition of signed tacts (i.e., object labels) by two participants. The standard procedure of using a general verbal prompt (e.g., "*What is that?*") yielded PND scores ranging from questionable to highly effective across acquisition and maintenance phases. This procedure was found to be less effective than using a specific intraverbal prompt (e.g., "*Sign* [spoken word]"), which consistently produced PNDs in the highly effective range during both acquisition and maintenance.

Results for Targeting Receptive Speech   In the only study in this category, Carr and Dores (1981) provided simultaneous communication training to three participants and measured their correct responses on a receptive language discrimination task. PND scores indicated a highly effective intervention for all participants.

Results for Studies Comparing Simultaneous Communication, Sign-Alone Instruction, and Oral Instruction   Studies in this group compared the effects of simultaneous communication versus sign-alone training and/or oral training. Barrera, Lobato-Barrera, and Sulzer-Azaroff (1980) taught expressive language skills to one participant using three different instructional models: simultaneous sign training, nonverbal sign-alone training, and oral training. Increases in expressive language skills were noted as the number of words successfully produced either through expressive signing or oral speech. Whereas sign-alone and oral training resulted in PND scores of questionable effectiveness, simultaneous communication led to a PND score considered to be fairly effective. Remington and Clarke (1983) compared simultaneous communication versus sign-alone training in two participants and monitored the effects on expressive sign labeling and speech comprehension. For both participants, PND scores revealed no difference between treatment conditions, both of which were highly effective in increasing sign production as well as speech comprehension.

Yoder and Layton (1988) conducted a randomized controlled trial with 60 participants with limited speech skills to examine the interaction effects of pretreatment verbal imitation abilities and sign or speech training conditions on speech production. When adjusted for sample size, the effect sizes were small ($g < 0.20$) and were not significantly different across four treatment conditions: speech-alone training, sign-alone training, simultaneous communication, and alternating presentation of speech and sign training. Regardless of the treatment condition, pretreatment speech imitation skills proved to be a strong predictor of later speech production.

Implications for Practice

The available body of research on manual signs and gestures for children with ASDs reveals strong intervention effectiveness scores for symbol acquisition and production, as well as for related outcomes such as speech comprehension and production. These results suggest that manual signing and gestures are very effective communication options for individuals with ASDs. In addition to the proposed advantages of manual signs that were described earlier, this success can be due to a number of reasons. First, when compared with spoken language, manual signs provide a more iconic form of representation—that is, many manual signs strongly resemble their referents (Loncke & Bos, 1997). For example, the sign for DRINK is produced by moving a hand close to the mouth and turning it slightly back and forth as if holding a cup and drinking from it. The strong resemblance between the sign and the object or action it represents may help people with ASDs to learn sign language quite rapidly. Oral speech, on the other hand, is not iconic—except for onomatopoeic words that imitate, echo, or otherwise suggest the concept they describe (e.g., *beep* or *click*).

In addition, manual signs have a particular advantage in that they are unaided and therefore free from the need for access to external equipment. Because of this independence from environmental support, manual signs—like speech—are highly portable, cannot be lost or left behind, and enable individuals who sign to communicate under virtually all circumstances (Anderson, 2001; Sundberg, 1993; Sundberg & Partington, 1998). In addition, manual signs allow trained communication partners (e.g., parents, caregivers, siblings) to understand communicative messages quickly and easily.

However, one of the primary drawbacks of communicating through manual signs and gestures relates to the demands these techniques place on communication partners. Communication partners who are not skilled in manual signing and/or gestural communication will have great difficulty understanding individuals with ASDs who use these modes of communication (Mirenda & Erickson, 2000). Unfamiliar communication partners might understand some of the more iconic signs and gestures, but are likely to struggle with more abstract and idiosyncratic symbols and thus require an interpreter to act as an intermediary. The learning demands for family members, teachers, classmates, and community members who need to communicate with an individual with ASDs via manual signs or gestures are quite arduous if independence from an interpreter is desired (Mirenda & Erickson, 2000). Nonetheless, manual signs and/or gestures can play a significant role as one component of a multimodal communication system that works across different communication environments and that includes partners both with and without experience in using these techniques.

Implications for Future Research

Whereas the majority of studies on manual signing and gestures documented successful acquisition and, in some cases, generalization of these communication modes, only a few studies compared manual signing or gestures against an aided mode of communication such as graphic symbols (e.g., Anderson, 2001; Tincani, 2004). More comparative efficacy studies are needed to clarify whether learners with ASD are likely to benefit from one of these communication modalities more than another (Mirenda, 2003). As is evident from this review, some studies have investigated the effect of manual signs and gestures on speech production and reception, but these studies are small in number and some have methodological limitations. Future research is needed to further explore these potential outcomes using methodologically sound designs. Finally, when examining the number of studies based on manual signs versus those based on gestures, it appears that gestures are underrepresented and are not well researched in this population. This is surprising because gestural communication is positively correlated with vocal (i.e., speech) development in both typically developing children and in those with ASDs (Mundy & Gomes, 1998; Mundy, Sigman, & Kasari, 1990). More research investigating the effects of gestural communication is needed to clarify the potential of this unaided communication mode.

RESEARCH SYNTHESIS: GRAPHIC SYMBOLS

Compared with manual signs, graphic symbols have been employed in AAC interventions for individuals with ASDs more recently; as a result, the research base in this area is less well developed. In the early 1980s, clinicians discovered the relatively strong visuospatial strengths of individuals with ASDs and pointed out the potential benefits of visuospatial graphic symbols due to their nontransient nature (e.g., Schuler & Baldwin, 1981).

One of the earliest published research reports in this area was by Lancioni (1983), who investigated the application of pictorial symbols (i.e., line drawings) to facilitate symbol comprehension. Two children with autism were taught to follow pictorial directions printed on cards. Instruction started with simple object discriminations (e.g., touching a pictured object) and ended with activities involving a peer partner (e.g., bringing an object to a typical peer using a certain sequence of steps). Both participants succeeded in following a large number of pictorial directions correctly and were able to generalize the skill to new line drawings. This report was one of the first to provide empirical evidence for the use of graphic symbols for comprehension. Some commonly used applications of graphic symbols for individuals with ASDs that are not part of an electronic communication aid or an exchange-based communication system are discussed in the following section.

Visual Schedules

A widely used augmented visual input approach involves the use of pictorial or written schedules to assist individuals with ASDs in understanding and following predictable activity sequences in the classroom or at home (e.g., Mirenda, 2001; Quill, 1997; Wood, Lasker, Siegel-Causey, Beukelman, & Ball, 1998). Applications in this area are twofold: 1) individuals with ASDs or their caregivers can be instructed to use within-task pictorial schedules to help with completion of specific activities in school and home environments (e.g., Hall, McClannahan, & Krantz, 1995; Pierce & Schreibman, 1994) and 2) individuals can be given between-task schedules to retrieve information about what will happen next as they switch from one activity to another (e.g., Flannery & Horner, 1994; Krantz, MacDuff, & McClannahan, 1993; MacDuff, Krantz, & McClannahan, 1993). Reports indicate that pictorial or written schedules can lead to improvement in independent self-management skills; in some cases, problem behaviors can be diminished or eliminated when these supports are given (e.g., Mirenda, MacGregor, & Kelly-Keough, 2002). Chapter 11 in this volume provides a narrative review of visual schedule research for individuals with ASDs.

Visual Supports to Facilitate Choice Making

Visual supports based on graphic symbols can also enhance choice making for individuals with ASDs (e.g., Peterson, Bondy, Vincent, & Finnegan, 1995). Such strategies seem particularly useful for individuals who benefit from additional input for language comprehension. For example, Vaughn and Horner (1995) demonstrated that the disruptive and aggressive behavior of a young man with an ASD was reduced when he was provided with verbal plus photographic choices for food items; concurrently, his acceptance rates for food choices increased. Choice-making interventions that incorporate AAC are discussed further in Chapter 12.

Graphic Symbols for Expressive Communication

Graphic symbols can enhance the expressive communication skills of individuals with ASDs when they are used to compose messages on communication boards or communication wallets. A relatively large number of studies have targeted expressive communication as an outcome; in some cases, these studies examine different aspects of instruction related to graphic symbol acquisition (e.g., milieu teaching techniques or discrete trial training; Hamilton & Snell, 1993; Spillane, 1999).

Augmented Input and Aided Language Stimulation

Augmented input (also known as augmented communicative input) refers to a variety of strategies in which communication partners combine the use of AAC (usually in the form of graphic symbols) with natural speech. These strategies serve the purpose of augmenting spoken input to facilitate an AAC user's comprehension, while at the same time providing models of symbol use (Lloyd et al., 1997). One augmented input approach that uses graphic symbols with individuals with ASDs is aided language stimulation (AiLS). AiLS was introduced by Goossens' and Elder as a technique for augmenting both the input and the output of a person using AAC (Elder & Goossens', 1994; Goossens', Crain, & Elder, 1992). The aim of AiLS is to teach individuals how to understand and apply visual-graphic symbols for communication. The role of the communication partner in AiLS is to "highlight symbols on the user's communication display as he or she interacts and communicates verbally with the user" (Goossens' et al., 1992, p. 101). Additional forms of augmented input, including the System for Augmenting Language (Romski & Sevcik, 1996), are reviewed in Chapter 8 of this volume.

Review and Appraisal

A total of 15 experimental studies on the application of graphic symbols displayed sufficient quality to meet the inclusion criteria for this review. To be included, studies had to concentrate on the application of graphic symbols as part of a nonelectronic, selection-based communication set or system. Studies that employed graphic symbols in conjunction with PECS or other exchange-based approaches or as part of an intervention that used speech-generating devices (SGDs) were not included. (For in-depth reviews of SGD and PECS research, respectively, see Chapters 5 and 10 in this volume.)

The majority of participants in the retrieved studies were diagnosed with autism, although some presented with secondary conditions (e.g., hypotonia or severe intellectual disability) and others had a diagnosis of pervasive developmental disorder, pervasive developmental disorder-not otherwise specified, or Rett syndrome. All of the included studies used single-subject experimental designs and are summarized in Appendix 4B, in which conclusive evidence is presented first, followed by preponderant and suggestive evidence. Six single-subject experimental designs were ranked as inconclusive; their summaries are presented last in Appendix 4B without further discussion. The remaining studies investigated a variety of graphic symbols drawn from the following sets and systems: colored photographs, line drawings, Picture Communication Symbols (PCS), Premack symbols (all sets); Blissymbols, orthography, and Rebus (all systems). Several outcome variables were targeted, including requesting and transitioning skills, identifying orthography, labeling under different instructional procedures, and spontaneous picture card use.

Results for Teaching Requesting Skills   The majority of studies focused on the teaching of requesting skills. One study by Johnston, Nelson, Evans, and Palazolo (2003) provided conclusive evidence. The three children in this experiment used PCS to request entrance into a play group. Instructional procedures involved a naturalistic intervention that included creating communicative opportunities, modeling desired behavior, least-to-most prompting, and time delay. PND scores for symbol acquisition indicated high effectiveness for one participant and questionable effectiveness for the other two participants. Over time, however, the intervention proved highly effective in maintenance for all three children.

Among the studies with suggestive evidence, Kozleski (1991) compared the effectiveness and efficiency of request training using five different graphic symbol sets and systems: Blissymbols, colored photographs, orthography, Premack, and Rebus. Each of the graphic symbol sets/systems produced a perfect PND of 100% across all four participants, suggesting that all were equally effective. Regarding efficiency, Kozleski (1991) noted that sets/systems displaying a high degree of iconicity (e.g., photographs and Rebuses) appeared to be acquired more readily than less iconic sets/systems. However, a priori ratings of iconicity for the different graphic symbols were not obtained. Thus, the conclusion related to learning efficiency is difficult to sustain because the sets/systems differed considerably in a number of ways, including iconicity (Schlosser & Sigafoos, 2002).

In another study by Reichle et al. (2005), an adult with an ASD was taught to use a PCS to request assistance and to engage independently in a vocational assembly task. The intervention resulted in a PND score of questionable effectiveness for the requesting task, but was highly effective for completion of the assembly task. Sigafoos (1998) explored the effects of differential reinforcement to teach the conditional use of requesting and reaching. The participant was instructed to point to a line drawing of the _want_ symbol to request items that were placed out of reach and to reach directly for items within close proximity. PND scores revealed the intervention to be fairly effective for both conditions. Taken together, these studies indicate that there is suggestive to conclusive evidence that teaching the use of graphic symbols is effective in promoting the acquisition of requesting behavior in individuals with ASDs.

Results for Targeting Transitioning Skills

Two included studies focused on the application of graphic symbols as visual supports for transitioning activities. One study (Bryan & Gast, 2000) provided preponderant evidence that visual activity schedules increase on-task and on-schedule behavior. The four participants in this experiment increased their performance during literacy-based activities when an individualized picture activity schedule containing line-drawn pictures of academic tasks was available. Performance dropped when the schedule was missing. The intervention was also successful in decreasing undesirable off-task behaviors with irrelevant materials and inappropriate behaviors, such as refusals and tantrums. PND scores indicated the picture activity schedule to be highly effective across all four participants; identical scores were yielded for generalizing performance to novel activity schedules.

Another study by Dettmer, Simpson, Smith Myles, and Ganz (2000) presented suggestive evidence that visual supports may be highly effective in decreasing the latency between an instructional cue and the start of new activities. The two participants in this study were taught to follow a photo album and a visual schedule filled with line drawings when transitioning between different types of community and educational activities. These visual supports were highly effective (PNDs of 100%) for both children in decreasing the amount of time needed to move from one activity to another.

Results for Identifying Orthography

A study by Hetzroni and Shalem (2005) provided preponderant evidence that children with autism can learn to match orthographic symbols to corresponding logos in an effective manner. The authors combined orthographic symbols from the Hebrew alphabet with food item logos in a computer-based intervention to teach six participants the symbol meanings. The computer-based fading procedure gradually decreased the presence of the logos until participants recognized the orthographic symbols standing alone. Mixed results were obtained for this strategy. PND scores were in the range of fairly effective for three participants, but indicated questionable effectiveness for the other three. It is important to note that the scope of this study was restricted to matching orthographic symbols to corresponding food item logos. Successful mastery of such a matching task does not indicate the participants' ability to use the same orthographic symbols for functional communication purposes.

Results for Instructional Strategies   In the only study in this category, Spillane (1999) investigated the effects of different instructional strategies on PCS acquisition by comparing discrete trial training versus incidental teaching. Ranked as suggestive evidence, the experiment was limited to only one child with autism who showed very low acquisition rates when asked to label preferred items by selecting the corresponding symbol. The study found no difference in the effectiveness of the two teaching strategies; PND scores indicated unreliable treatment for both conditions. The study is limited by its restriction to one participant with autism and inappropriate replication using a participant without autism; thus, no definite conclusion can be made on the relative efficacy of one instructional strategy compared with another.

Results for Spontaneous Picture Card Use   Stiebel (1999) studied the effects of a parent-oriented problem-solving intervention on the spontaneous use of picture communication cards with three participants. The communication cards contained colored photographs and were used by the children for a variety of communicative functions, including asking for assistance, choice making, and requesting. Card instruction included a fading technique to teach the communicative function. Spontaneous use of the cards was recorded whenever the child pointed to the symbol and handed or attempted to hand it to the communication partner. This intervention yielded mixed results. PND scores were highly effective for one participant, fairly effective for another, and questionably effective for the third. A similar pattern was observed for intervention follow-up phases.

Implications for Practice

Currently, the use of graphic symbols for teaching requesting offers the most solid empirical evidence. Children and adults in these studies were successfully taught requesting for various purposes, including access to play activities, receiving assistance, and obtaining desired items. However, research in this area has not yet reached the critical mass that is required to productively inform choices about the selection of one graphic symbol set/system over another.

Practitioners may refer to symbol iconicity as one guiding factor in selecting an initial graphic symbol set/system, based on the results of Kozleski (1991), but with the limitations of that study in mind. Thus, preference may be given to highly iconic symbol set/systems in accordance with the iconicity hypothesis (i.e., a symbol that has a strong resemblance to its referent tends to be learned more readily than a symbol that has a weak visual relationship; Fristoe & Lloyd, 1979).

A study by Mirenda and Locke (1989) provided further support for such an approach. The authors investigated the role of symbol transparency by comparing real objects, photos, line drawings, Blissymbols, and written words in a match-to-sample task that was administered to individuals with autism, intellectual disability, or multiple disabilities. For these learners, symbol transparency (i.e., the degree to which the symbol was readily understood without further cues) decreased as the symbols looked less and less like the objects they represented, with the exception of miniature objects. The results of this study provided support for the following hierarchy of symbol transparency from easiest to most difficult for individuals with developmental disabilities in general: objects, color photographs, black-and-white photographs, miniature objects, line drawings, Blissymbols, and written words.

At the same time, it seems imperative to be mindful of the unique information processing and learning styles of individuals with ASDs, which might result in idiosyncratic patterns of symbol recognition and acquisition. For example, individuals with ASDs present with varying degrees of cognitive impairment; as a result, some might be more limited in their overall symbol recognition abilities than others. Subsequently, an individual may be able to use a particular symbol set/system to respond to questions, but may be unable to use the same set/system to request desired items or to engage in other communicative acts that require initiation. All of these are important aspects for the clinician to consider when making a choice among different graphic symbol sets/systems.

Graphic symbols may also be useful in interventions targeting transitions within or between educational, home, or community activities. Transitions are difficult to handle for individuals with ASDs (Cohen & Volkmar, 1997). Although limited in scope, current research provides relatively strong evidence that visual activity schedules are effective in helping individuals to independently transition from one activity to another. Such visual schedules provide a structured teaching environment, make expectations clear, and lessen the need for continuous adult prompting (Schopler, Mesibov, & Hearsey, 1995). Because school-age children with ASDs often experience new learning environments and lack consistent routines in school settings (Cohen & Volkmar, 1997), visual activity schedules may help them to stay focused on appropriate task-related behaviors with minimal adult assistance and reinforcement.

The currently available evidence is insufficient for informing clinical practice regarding the most effective instructional approaches for introducing graphic symbol sets/systems to individuals with ASDs. The extant research literature indicates the potential effectiveness of naturalistic teaching strategies (e.g., Johnston et al., 2003). However, there are currently no sound comparisons of one instructional approach against another. Practitioners will have to rely primarily on their clinical experience when choosing an appropriate instructional format.

Implications for Future Research

As evident from this review, research on graphic symbols for individuals with ASDs has not yet been extended beyond the point of teaching functional communication and closely related skills (i.e., requesting and transitioning). Future research is required and should focus on outcomes more directly related to developing natural speech, social, and language skills (e.g., increasing vocalizations, teaching action–object phrases, expanding word utterances). Such a research base is currently emerging for PECS, a structured behavioral intervention program to teach the use of visual-graphic symbols for communication (Bondy & Frost, 1994). PECS typically uses PCS to teach exchanged-based requesting skills, but recent studies have explored innovations to the PECS protocol, such as substituting PECS with Blissymbols to investigate the role of iconicity (Angermeier, Schlosser, Luiselli, Harrington, & Carter, 2008). The effect of PECS on facilitating natural speech development is also being explored (e.g., Anderson, 2001; Tincani, 2004; Tincani, Crozier, & Alazetta, 2006). These research efforts should be replicated using a variety of graphic symbol sets/systems with intervention approaches other than PECS.

As graphic symbol research continues to evolve, it would also be prudent to study variations of the independent variable (e.g., varying levels of graphic symbol iconicity or complexity) while keeping the instructional method constant. In a second step, research is needed to examine how specific participant characteristics such as the level of cognitive functioning, type of ASD, and pretreatment speech and language skills correlate with graphic symbol characteristics and related intervention outcomes. The use of randomized controlled trials and growth curve analyses, such as the techniques used in two recent treatment efficacy studies comparing PECS with responsive education and prelinguistic milieu teaching (Yoder & Stone, 2006a, 2006b), provide exemplary models for conducting such urgently needed research.

In addition to teaching the communicative function of requesting, evidence is emerging in support of using graphic symbols in visual schedules for transitions. This evidence is currently limited to only two studies that met the criteria for this review, neither of which was ranked as conclusive. The scarcity of research in this area is surprising, given that visual schedules are applied in almost every classroom containing individuals with ASDs, at least in the United States (H. Shane, personal communication, March 14, 2008). Substantiation of the effectiveness of visual schedules for facilitating transitions would provide a welcome addition to an empirical-based repertoire for teaching children with ASDs to use graphic symbols for receptive goals in addition to expressive purposes.

Children with ASDs seem to be able to match graphic symbols to orthographic symbols, as demonstrated by Hetzroni and Shalem (2005). These results are promising, but the issue of whether this matching could lead to enhanced communication has yet to be examined. Future research needs to replicate and validate these findings, while investigating the potential of orthographic symbols for more elaborated communicative functions beyond matching. Research has shown that, among the various graphic symbol sets/systems used by children who require AAC, orthographic symbols are the most difficult to acquire (Fuller, Lloyd, & Stratton, 1997). Nevertheless, traditional orthography is a very powerful graphic symbol system because it is directly related to emergent literacy and can provide opportunities for learners to interact with written words. Exploring the potential of orthography for individuals with ASDs may lead to providing more acceptable and age-appropriate communication options for this population.

CONSIDERATIONS FOR SELECTING MANUAL SIGNS AND GESTURES VERSUS GRAPHIC SYMBOLS

Many children with ASDs who have limited or no functional speech are likely to benefit from AAC interventions based on manual signs and/or graphic symbols. However, as is evident from this review, the research base for these two approaches has not yet grown to a point where it can reliably inform clinical decision making. Empirical support is emerging for certain outcomes (e.g., requesting, sign production), but is still scarce or lacking for others (e.g., gesture acquisition, transitioning). There have been very few attempts to compare the relative efficacy of manual signs and gestures to graphic symbols. In addition, despite published reports suggesting positive results for specific skill areas, there is no evidence indicating that any one AAC approach is superior to any other in yielding higher rates of spontaneous and generative communication, or in optimizing generalization (Howlin, 2006).

Under these circumstances, practitioners must supplement research evidence with additional considerations for the selection of a suitable intervention approach. In one of the few comparative efficacy studies investigating aided versus unaided AAC modes (in this case, PECS versus manual signs), Anderson (2001) noted four levels of consideration: inherent advantages and disadvantages of each modality, universal benefits, individual preference, and caregiver/ supporter preference. In the following sections, these considerations are applied to the selection of manual signs and gestures versus graphic symbols.

Advantages and Disadvantages of Manual Signs versus Graphic Symbols

Theoretical arguments have been proposed for each of these approaches; some were discussed previously in this chapter. One of the key arguments promoting the use of manual signs is that it involves an easier discrimination than does the use of graphic symbols (Michael, 1985; Sundberg & Michael, 2001; Sundberg & Partington, 1998). Graphic symbols demand conditional (i.e., multiple stimuli) discriminations, whereas manual signs depend only on unconditional (i.e., single stimulus) discriminations.

To illustrate this difference, Sundberg and Partington (1998) demonstrated that for a child to request a cup via a graphic symbol display, both the child's motivation for a cup (the first stimulus) and the presence of a symbol for cup (the second stimulus) are necessary. When manual signs are used, the motivational factor is the only necessary stimulus because the manual sign for cup does not occur in spatial form and therefore does not need to be present. Sundberg and Partington also stated that an unconditional discrimination is easier to acquire than a conditional form because it involves only a single stimulus and a single response.

Similarly, it has been argued that manual signs are easier to acquire because they need only a single rather than a multicomponent motor response (i.e., the child has only to generate the sign, rather than examine an array of graphic symbols until a specific choice is found and selected; Michael, 1985; Potter & Brown, 1997).

In opposition to these arguments, other researchers have noted that it is not reasonable to assume that individuals with ASDs have less difficulty in learning manual signs than graphic symbols, as their visual-spatial learning is usually intact (Koul, Schlosser, & Sancibrian, 2001; Mirenda & Erickson, 2000). Another advantage of graphic symbols may be that memory demands are not as high as for signs (Mirenda, 2003). Further limitations of manual signs include the fact that communication partners must be able to produce and understand them (as previously noted) and that, in some individuals, motor impairments may prevent the acquisition of manual communication (e.g., Minshew, Goldstein, &

Siegel, 1997). Recent research also indicates that learning manual signs may depend not only on children's motor abilities, but also on their functioning in domains such as symbolic processing, social skills (Bonvillian & Blackburn, 1991), and executive functioning (Seal & Bonvillian, 1997).

From a practical perspective, graphic symbols (especially when highly iconic) seem to present several potential advantages over manual signs or abstract symbols: 1) demands on memory and cognitive skill may be lower, 2) there is very little demand regarding motor ability, and 3) graphic symbols are more easily understood by unfamiliar communication partners and are easier to prompt (Howlin, 2006). Nevertheless, the disadvantages of graphic symbols should not be overlooked. In particular, the communication rate when using graphic symbols can be very low, which makes it difficult to communicate at a conversational pace. Whereas proficient oral language speakers communicate at a rate of 150–250 words per minute, selection of graphic symbols typically occurs at a rate of 2–8 words per minute (Howlin, 2006). In addition, turn taking may be restricted; syntactic or semantic relations are also difficult to transmit in the graphic symbol modality.

Successful learning of graphic symbols can occur at varying, unpredictable rates. Although some individuals with developmental disabilities are relatively fast in acquiring an initial symbol vocabulary, others progress rather slowly (Abrahamsen, Romski, & Sevcik, 1989). Furthermore, teaching graphic symbols to individuals with ASDs can present certain challenges, as reported by Konstantareas (1987) and Kiernan (1983). Their findings indicate that unprompted, spontaneous use rarely occurs, that graphic symbols are more frequently used for requesting purposes rather than for initiating social contact, and that generalization to unfamiliar contexts is particularly difficult.

From the perspective of the practitioner, it is important to consider the specific attributes of each type of AAC system, the difficulties that can be addressed instructionally, and the potential for individual benefit (Anderson, 2001). For example, manual signs might be indicated for an individual who has good hand motor skills and access to daily communication partners who are fluent in manual signing. In contrast, graphic symbols might be indicated for an individual who is a strong visual learner, presents with motor coordination and imitation difficulties, and has access primarily to communication partners who are unfamiliar with manual signs. There are, of course, a myriad of other assessment considerations required when making AAC modality decisions (see Chapter 2); all such decisions must be made on an individual basis.

Universal Benefits

The second level of consideration focuses on the universal benefits of each approach. These are the advantages inherent in each modality for all individuals, regardless of variations in their characteristics. For example, two universal benefits of manual signs include their portability and the potential for access to unlimited vocabulary. Two universal benefits of graphic symbols include their nontransient nature and the fact that they are readily understood by most communication partners.

Given the high training demands placed on communication partners by manual signs and their relatively high fine motor (hand) requirements, manual signs might best be included as one component of a multimodal communication system that also includes graphic symbols, SGDs, and an individual's extant communication modalities (e.g., gestures, vocalizations, facial expressions). If this occurred, individuals who acquire manual signs quite readily can benefit from this AAC modality while at the same time learning to use additional AAC techniques, which may have broader contextual and partner applicability. However, further research on effective strategies for teaching the conditional use of manual signs is needed to support such a multimodal approach.

To date, only a few studies have contrasted manual sign or gesture use with other modes of communication. In one such study, Sigafoos (1998) taught a child to use an SGD when it was available and a gesture (i.e., reaching) when it was not. Similarly, Sigafoos and Drasgow (2001) contrasted manual sign and SGD use in a child with developmental disabilities who did not have a confirmed diagnosis of autism. Thus, it is clear that more research is warranted into strategies for teaching the conditional use of manual signs and gestures, especially in comparison with graphic symbols.

Individual Preference

Individual preference for one modality over the other may affect correct use and maintenance after treatment. Whatever communication modality is chosen, it appears critical that the approach is fully aligned with the individual's specific interests or needs. In addition, this approach should be directly relevant to each of the person's regular environments. Using a preferred modality will also maximize success and motivation. This is especially important when communication training occurs during early intervention, when neural plasticity is high and behavioral changes can be more easily induced (Chugani, Phelps, & Mazziotta, 1987). Refined assessment procedures are required to determine response and preference patterns in very young children with ASDs. See Chapter 16 for a discussion of preference assessment in adults with ASDs.

Caregiver/Supporter Preferences

Caregivers and other supporters of individuals with ASDs also need to feel comfortable with the selected AAC approach. Consistent reinforcement across a wide range of settings and contexts is needed for an approach to be effective. The evidence-based practice process emphasizes the integration of caregivers' perspectives with research evidence and clinical expertise as an essential component of clinical decision making (Schlosser & Raghavendra, 2004). If caregivers and other supporters are not comfortable with the specific modalities employed, they will most likely fail to encourage usage at home and in the community. Thus, an individually tailored AAC system that is used only during school or work hours is of little value if an individual's caregivers are reluctant to use it or have it available at home.

As Howlin (2006) noted, typically developing children acquire natural speech and language because they are exposed to speech and language starting at birth. It is not realistic to expect individuals with severe communication disorders, such as those with ASDs, to develop effective communication skills if they are using their AAC systems only for short periods of time during the day. There is an urgent need to educate caregivers and other supporters about the benefits of AAC and to improve attitudes and practices that encourage consistent use across school, work, community, and home settings.

SUMMARY

This chapter provided an evidence-based review of two prominent AAC approaches—manual signs and graphic symbols. The primary purpose was to supply the practitioner and other relevant stakeholders with prefiltered evidence that can inform clinical and educational decision making. Therefore, numerous implications for practice were provided in light of the evidence. In this regard, it is important to acknowledge that research evidence itself cannot and should not be used to make decisions. In fact, practitioners still need to integrate any course of action gleaned from appraised research evidence with their own clinical or educational expertise, as well as with client and caretaker preferences. Thus, it is critical that practitioners conduct in-depth, individualized assessments and elicit the perspectives of caregivers and other relevant stakeholders about the research evidence and assessment results.

In terms of the research evidence itself, it is apparent that general descriptions of the characteristics of individuals with ASDs and general statements about successful or unsuccessful interventions are of little value for guiding the selection of AAC approaches for a specific person. Individuals with ASDs constitute a very heterogeneous group; evidence is emerging to indicate that the selection of an AAC approach must be made relative to specific task demands and individual characteristics, rather than on the basis of general predictive and prescriptive indicators. The research of Yoder and Stone (2006a, 2006b), which explored pretreatment object exploration or joint attention skills in relation to treatment outcomes, is an excellent example of such an individualized approach.

Research on manual sign and graphic symbols has advanced significantly over the past three decades; however, there is much more to accomplish. In general, it is noteworthy that the majority of studies on both manual signs/gestures and graphic symbols were ranked at the level of suggestive evidence. Close examination of the evidence base indicates that a failure to report treatment integrity data caused this less-than-ideal rating in most cases (Schlosser, 2002). While regrettable, the fact is that many of the studies were conducted before the importance of treatment integrity was emphasized in the field of behavioral science (e.g., Peterson, Homer, & Wonderlich, 1982). Consequently, it may be advisable to replicate some of these studies with measures of treatment integrity included, to ensure that the results are indeed the outcomes of the intended treatments.

In this review, recommendations for clinical practice and future research varied across the different aided and unaided approaches, depending on the respective status of research. Several studies (e.g., Hetzroni & Shalem, 2005; Ingersoll et al., 2007) have provided preponderant evidence that treatment produces effects under ideal conditions (i.e., efficacy [Robey, 2004] or effectiveness under ideal conditions [Schlosser, 2003]). These existing efficacy studies need to be replicated under less-than-ideal conditions to demonstrate that the interventions produce similar effects under more typical circumstances (i.e., effectiveness [Robey, 2004] or effectiveness under typical conditions [Schlosser, 2003]).

For lower-ranked evidence, researchers still need to establish that proposed treatments work under ideal conditions before progressing to more typical conditions. As the AAC field continues to move toward the adoption of evidence-based practice, such research efforts are critical to develop and refine the extant research base on manual signs and graphic symbols, toward the final goal of facilitating evidence-informed clinical decision making.

REFERENCES

Note: References marked with an asterisk (*) indicate primary research studies from systematic reviews.

Abrahamsen, A.A., Romski, M.A., & Sevcik, R.A. (1989). Concomitants of success in acquiring an augmentative communication system: Changes in attention, communication, and sociability. *American Journal on Mental Retardation, 93,* 475–496.

Allison, D.B., & Gorman, B.S. (1993). Calculating effect sizes for meta-analysis: The case of the single case. *Behaviour Research and Therapy, 31,* 621–631.

*Anderson, A.E. (2001). *Augmentative communication and autism: A comparison of sign language and the Picture Exchange Communication System.* Unpublished doctoral dissertation, University of California, San Diego.

Angermeier, K., Schlosser, R.W., Luiselli, J.K., Harrington, C., & Carter, B. (2008). Effects of iconicity on requesting with the Picture Exchange Communication System in children with autism spectrum disorder. *Research in Autism Spectrum Disorders, 2*(3), 430–446.

*Barrera, R.D., Lobato-Barrera, D., & Sulzer-Azaroff, B. (1980). A simultaneous treatment comparison of three expressive language training programs with a mute autistic child. *Journal of Autism and Developmental Disorders, 10,* 21–37.

Biermann, A. (1999). *Gestützte Kommunikation im Widerstreit.* [Facilitated Communication in Antagonism]. Berlin: Edition Marhold im Wissenschaftsverlag Volker Spiess GmbH.

Blischak, D.M., Lloyd, L.L., & Fuller, D.R. (1997). Terminology issues. In L.L. Lloyd, D.R. Fuller, & H.H. Arvidson (Eds.), *Augmentative and alternative communication: A handbook of principles and practices* (pp. 38–42). Boston: Allyn & Bacon.

Bondy, A.S., & Frost, L.A. (1994). The Picture Exchange Communication System. *Focus on Autistic Behavior, 9,* 1–19.

Bonvillian, J.D., & Blackburn, D.W. (1991). Manual communication and autism: Factors relating to sign language acquisition. In P. Siple & S.D. Fischer (Eds.), *Theoretical issues in sign language research* (pp. 255–300). Chicago: University of Chicago Press.

Bopp, K.D., Brown, K.E., & Mirenda, P. (2004). Speech-language pathologists' role in the delivery of positive behavior support for individuals with developmental disabilities. *American Journal of Speech-Language Pathology, 13,* 5–19.

*Brady, D.O., & Smouse, A.D. (1978). A simultaneous comparison of three methods for language training with an autistic child: An experimental single case analysis. *Journal of Autism and Childhood Schizophrenia, 8,* 271–279.

*Bryan, L.C., & Gast, D.L. (2000). Teaching on-task and on-schedule behaviors to high-functioning children with autism via picture activity schedules. *Journal of Autism and Developmental Disorders, 30,* 553–567.

*Buffington, D.M., Krantz, P.J., McClannahan, L.E., & Poulson, C.L. (1998). Procedures for teaching appropriate gestural communication skills to children with autism. *Journal of Autism and Developmental Disorders, 28,* 535–545.

*Carr, E.G., Binkoff, J.A., Kologinsky, E., & Eddy, M. (1978). Acquisition of sign language by autistic children. I: Expressive labeling. *Journal of Applied Behavior Analysis, 11*, 489–501.

*Carr, E.G., & Dores, P. (1981). Patterns of language acquisition following simultaneous communication with autistic children. *Analysis and Intervention in Developmental Disabilities, 1*, 347–361.

*Carr, E.G., & Kemp, D.C. (1989). Functional equivalence of autistic leading and communicative pointing: Analysis and treatment. *Journal of Autism and Developmental Disorders, 19*, 561–578.

*Carr, E.G., & Kologinsky, E. (1983). Acquisition of sign language by autistic children II: Spontaneity and generalization effects. *Journal of Applied Behavior Analysis, 16*, 297–314.

*Carr, E.G., Kologinsky, E., & Leff-Simon, S. (1987). Acquisition of sign language by autistic children III: Generalized descriptive phrases. *Journal of Autism and Developmental Disorders, 17*, 217–229.

Chugani, H., Phelps, M., & Mazziotta, J. (1987). Positron emission tomography study of human brain functional development. *Annals of Neurology, 22*, 487–497.

Cohen, D.J., & Volkmar, F.R. (1997). *Handbook of autism and pervasive developmental disorders* (2nd ed.). New York: John Wiley & Sons.

Cohen, J. (1988). *Statistical power analysis for the behavioral sciences* (2nd ed.). Mahwah, NJ: Lawrence Erlbaum Associates.

Dawson, G., & Adams, A. (1984). Imitation and social responsiveness in autistic children. *Journal of Abnormal Child Psychology, 12*, 209–225.

*Dettmer, S., Simpson, R.L., Smith Myles, B., & Ganz, J. (2000). The use of visual supports to facilitate transitions of students with autism. *Focus on Autism and Other Developmental Disabilities, 15*, 163–169.

*Dexter, M.E. (1998). *The effects of aided language stimulation upon verbal output and augmentative communication during storybook reading for children with pervasive developmental disabilities.* Unpublished doctoral dissertation, The Johns Hopkins University, Baltimore.

Elder, P., & Goossens', C. (1994). *Engineering training environments for interactive augmentative communication: Strategies for adolescents and adults who are moderately/severely developmentally delayed.* Birmingham, AL: Southeast Augmentative Communication Conference Publications.

Flannery, K.B., & Horner, R. (1994). The relationship between predictability and problem behavior for students with severe disabilities. *Journal of Behavioral Education, 4*, 157–176.

Fristoe, M., & Lloyd, L.L. (1979). Nonspeech communication. In N.R. Ellis (Ed.), *Handbook of mental deficiency: Psychological theory and research* (2nd ed., pp. 401–430). Mahwah, NJ: Lawrence Erlbaum Associates.

Fuller, D.R., Lloyd, L.L., & Stratton, M.M. (1997). Aided AAC symbols. In L.L. Lloyd, D.R. Fuller, & H.H. Arvidson (Eds.), *Augmentative and alternative communication: A handbook of principles and practices* (pp. 48–79). Boston: Allyn & Bacon.

Fulwiler, R.L., & Fouts, R.S. (1976). Acquisition of American sign language by a noncommunicating autistic child. *Journal of Childhood Autism and Childhood Schizophrenia, 6*, 43–51.

Goossens', C., Crain, S., & Elder, P. (1992). *Engineering the preschool environment for interactive, symbolic communication.* Birmingham, AL: Southeast Augmentative Communication Conference Publications.

Granlund, M., & Olsson, C. (1999). Efficacy of communication intervention for presymbolic communicators. *Augmentative and Alternative Communication, 15,* 25–37.

Guyatt, G., & Rennie, D. (2002). *Users' guide to the medical literature: Essentials of evidence-based clinical practice.* Chicago: AMA Press.

Hall, L., McClannahan, L., & Krantz, P. (1995). Promoting independence in integrated classrooms by teaching aides to use activity schedules and decreased prompts. *Education and Training in Mental Retardation and Developmental Disabilities, 30,* 208–217.

*Hamilton, B.L., & Snell, M.E. (1993). Using the milieu approach to increase spontaneous communication book use across environments by an adolescent with autism. *Augmentative and Alternative Communication, 9,* 259–272.

*Hetzroni, O.E., & Shalem, U. (2005). From logos to orthographic symbols: A multilevel fading computer program for teaching nonverbal children with autism. *Focus on Autism and Other Developmental Disabilities, 20,* 201–212.

Howlin, P. (2006). Augmentative and alternative communication systems for children with autism. In T. Charman & W. Stone (Eds.), *Social & communication development in autism spectrum disorders* (pp. 236–266). New York: Guilford Press.

*Hundert, J. (1981). Stimulus generalization after training an autistic deaf boy in manual signs. *Education and Treatment of Children, 4,* 329–337.

*Ingersoll, B., Lewis, E., & Kroman, E. (2007). Teaching the imitation and spontaneous use of descriptive gestures in young children with autism using a naturalistic behavioral intervention. *Journal of Autism and Developmental Disorders, 37,* 1446–1456.

*Johnston, S., Nelson, C., Evans, J., & Palazolo, K. (2003). The use of visual supports in teaching young children with autism spectrum disorder to initiate interactions. *Augmentative and Alternative Communication, 19,* 86–103.

Kahng, S., Iwata, B.A., & Lewin, A.B. (2002). Behavioral treatment of self-injury, 1964 to 2000. *American Journal on Mental Retardation, 107,* 212–221.

*Keogh, D., Whitman, T., Beeman, D., Halligan, K., & Starzynski, T. (1987). Teaching interactive signing in a dialogue situation to mentally retarded individuals. *Research in Developmental Disabilities, 8,* 39–53.

Kiernan, C. (1983). The use of nonvocal communication techniques with autistic individuals. *Journal of Child Psychology and Psychiatry, 24,* 339–375.

Konstantareas, M. (1987). Autistic children exposed to simultaneous communication training: A follow-up. *Journal of Autism and Developmental Disorders, 17,* 115–132.

Koul, R., Schlosser, R., & Sancibrian, S. (2001). Effects of symbol, referent, and instructional variables on the acquisition of aided and unaided symbols by individuals with autism spectrum disorders. *Focus on Autism and Other Developmental Disabilities, 16,* 162–169.

*Kozleski, E. (1991). Visual symbol acquisition by students with autism. *Exceptionality, 2,* 173–194.

Krantz, P.J., MacDuff, M.T., & McClannahan, L.E. (1993). Programming participation in family activities for children with autism: Parents' use of photographic activity schedules. *Journal of Applied Behavior Analysis, 26,* 137–138.

Lancioni, G. (1983). Using pictorial representation as communication means with low-functioning children. *Journal of Autism and Developmental Disorders, 13,* 87–105.

Lipsey, M.W., & Wilson, D.B. (2001). *Practical meta-analysis.* Thousand Oaks, CA: Sage Publications.

Lloyd, L.L., Fuller, D.R., & Arvidson, H.H. (Eds.). (1997). *Augmentative and alternative communication: A handbook of principles and practices.* Boston: Allyn & Bacon.

Loncke, F., & Bos, H. (1997). Unaided AAC symbols. In L.L. Lloyd, D.R. Fuller, & H.H. Arvidson (Eds.), *Augmentative and alternative communication: A handbook of principles and practices* (pp. 80–106). Boston: Allyn & Bacon.

Lonigan, C., Elbert, J., & Johnson, S. (1998). Empirically supported psychosocial interventions for children: An overview. *Journal of Clinical Child Psychology, 27,* 138–145.

Lord, C., & Bailey, A. (2002). Autism spectrum disorders. In M. Rutter & E. Taylor (Eds.), *Child and adolescent psychiatry* (4th ed., pp. 664–681). Oxford: Blackwell Scientific.

Lord, C., Risi, S., & Pickles, A. (2004). Trajectory of language development in autistic spectrum disorders. In M.L. Rice & S.F. Warren (Eds.), *Developmental language disorders: From phenotypes to etiologies* (pp. 7–29). Mahwah, NJ: Lawrence Erlbaum Associates.

Loveland, K.A., Landry, S.H., Hughes, S.O., Hall, S.K., & McEvoy R.E. (1988). Speech acts and the pragmatic deficits of autism. *Journal of Speech and Hearing Research, 31,* 593–604.

MacDuff, G.S., Krantz, P.J., & McClannahan, L.E. (1993). Teaching children with autism to use photographic activity schedules: Maintenance and generalization of complex response chains. *Journal of Applied Behavior Analysis, 26,* 89–97.

Mancil, G.R. (2006). Functional communication training: A review of the literature related to children with autism. *Education and Training in Developmental Disabilities, 41,* 213–224.

Michael, J. (1985). Two kinds of verbal behavior plus a possible third. *The Analysis of Verbal Behavior, 3,* 1–4.

Millar, D., Light, J.C., & Schlosser, R.W. (2006). The impact of augmentative and alternative communication intervention on the speech production of individuals with developmental disabilities: A research review. *Journal of Speech, Language, and Hearing Research, 49,* 248–264.

Minshew, N.J., Goldstein, G., & Siegel, D.J. (1997). Neuropsychologic functioning in autism: Profile of a complex information processing disorder. *Journal of the International Neuropsychological Society, 3,* 303–316.

Mirenda, P. (2001). Autism, augmentative communication, and assistive technology: What do we really know? *Focus on Autism and Other Developmental Disabilities, 16,* 141–151.

Mirenda, P. (2003). Toward functional augmentative and alternative communication for students with autism: Manual signs, graphic symbols, and voice output communication aids. *Language, Speech, and Hearing Services in Schools, 34*, 203–216.

Mirenda, P., & Erickson, K.A. (2000). Augmentative communication and literacy. In S.F. Warren & J. Reichle (Series Eds.) & A.M. Wetherby & B.M. Prizant (Vol. Eds.), *Communication and language intervention series: Vol. 9. Autism spectrum disorders: A transactional developmental perspective* (pp. 333–367). Baltimore: Paul H. Brookes Publishing Co.

Mirenda, P., & Locke, P.A. (1989). A comparison of symbol transparency in nonspeaking persons with intellectual disabilities. *Journal of Speech and Hearing Disorders, 54*, 131–140.

Mirenda, P., MacGregor, T., & Kelly-Keough, S. (2002). Teaching communication skills for behavior support in the context of family life. In J.M. Lucyshyn, G. Dunlap, & R.W. Albin (Eds.), *Families and positive behavior support: Addressing problem behaviors in family contexts* (pp. 185–208). Baltimore: Paul H. Brookes Publishing Co.

Mirenda, P., & Schuler, A.L. (1989). Augmenting communication for persons with autism: Issues and strategies. *Topics in Language Disorders, 9*, 24–43.

Morford, M., & Goldin-Meadow, S. (1992). Comprehension and production of gesture in combination with speech in one-word speakers. *Journal of Child Language, 19*, 559–580.

Mundy, P., & Gomes, A. (1998). Individual differences in joint attention skill development in the second year. *Infant Behavior & Development, 21*, 469–482.

Mundy, P., Sigman, M., & Kasari, C. (1990). A longitudinal study of joint attention and language development in autistic children. *Journal of Autism and Developmental Disorders, 20*, 115–128.

Nußbeck, S. (1999). *Gestützte Kommunikation. Ein Ausdrucksmittel für Menschen mit geistiger Behinderung?* [Facilitated Communication. A means of expression for people with mental retardation?]. Göttingen, Germany: Hogrefe-Verlag.

Olive, M.L., & Smith, B.W. (2005). Effect size calculations and single subject designs. *Educational Psychology, 25*, 313–324.

*Oxman, J., Konstantareas, M.M., & Liebovitz-Bojm, S.F. (1979). Simultaneous communication training and vocal responding in nonverbal autistic and autistic-like children. *International Journal of Rehabilitation Research, 2*, 394–396.

Peterson, L., Homer, A.L., & Wonderlich, S.A. (1982). The integrity of independent variables in behavior analysis. *Journal of Applied Behavior Analysis, 15*, 477–492.

Peterson, S.L., Bondy, A.S., Vincent, Y., & Finnegan, C.S. (1995). Effects for altering communicative input for students with autism and no speech: Two case studies. *Augmentative and Alternative Communication, 11*, 93–100.

Petticrew, M., & Roberts, H. (2006). *Systematic reviews in the social sciences: A practical guide.* Malden, MA: Blackwell Publishing.

Pierce, K., & Schreibman, L. (1994). Teaching daily living skills to children with autism in unsupervised settings through pictorial self-management. *Journal of Applied Behavior Analysis, 27,* 471–482.

Potter, B., & Brown, D. (1997). Review of the studies examining the nature of selection-based and topography-based verbal behavior. *The Analysis of Verbal Behavior, 14,* 85–104.

Probst, P. (2005). "Communication unbound—or unfound?": Ein integratives Literatur-Review zur Wirksamkeit der Gestützten Kommunikation (Facilitated Communication/FC) bei nichtsprechenden autistischen und intelligenzgeminderten Personen. *Zeitschrift für Klinische Psychologie, Psychiatrie und Psychotherapie, 53,* 93–128.

Quill, K. (1997). Instructional considerations for young children with autism: A rationale for visually cued instruction. *Journal of Autism and Developmental Disorders, 27,* 697–714.

*Reichle, J., & Brown, L. (1986). Teaching the use of a multipage direct selection communication board to an adult with autism. *Journal of the Association for Persons with Severe Handicaps, 11,* 68–73.

*Reichle, J., McComas, J., Dahl, N., Solberg, G., Pierce, S., & Smith, D. (2005). Teaching an individual with severe intellectual delay to request assistance conditionally. *Educational Psychology, 25,* 275–286.

*Reichle, J., Sigafoos, J., & Remington, B. (1991). Beginning an augmentative communication system with individuals who have severe disabilities. In B. Remington (Ed.), *The challenge of severe mental handicap: A behavior analytic approach* (pp. 189–213). New York: John Wiley & Sons.

*Remington, B., & Clarke, S. (1983). Acquisition of expressive signing by autistic children: An evaluation of the relative effects of simultaneous communication and sign-alone training. *Journal of Applied Behavior Analysis, 16,* 315–328.

Robey, R.R. (2004). A five-phase model for clinical-outcome research. *Journal of Communication Disorders, 37,* 401–411.

Rogers, S.J. (1999). An examination of the imitation deficit in autism. In J. Nadel & G. Butterworth (Eds.), *Imitation in infancy* (pp. 254–283). New York: Cambridge University Press.

Rogers, S.J., Hepburn, S.L., Stackhouse, T., & Wehner, E. (2003). Imitation performance in toddlers with autism and those with other developmental disorders. *Journal of Child Psychology and Psychiatry, 44,* 763–781.

Romski, M.A., & Sevcik, R.A. (1996). *Breaking the speech barrier: Language development through augmented means.* Baltimore: Paul H. Brookes Publishing Co.

*Saraydarian, K.A. (1994). *Simultaneous referent recognition-production training for nonverbal children with autism.* Unpublished doctoral dissertation, Columbia University Teachers College, New York.

Schaeffer, B., Kollinzas, G., Musil, A., & McDowell, P. (1978). Spontaneous verbal language for autistic children through signed speech. *Sign Language Studies, 21,* 317–352.

*Schepis, M.M., Reid, D.H., Fitzgerald, J.R., Faw, G.D., VanDenPol, R.A., & Welty, P.A. (1982). A program for increasing manual signing by autistic and profoundly retarded youth within the daily environment. *Journal of Applied Behavior Analysis, 15,* 363–379.

Schlosser, R.W. (2002). On the importance of being earnest about treatment integrity. *Augmentative and Alternative Communication, 18,* 36–44.

Schlosser, R.W. (2003). *The efficacy of augmentative and alternative communication: Toward evidence-based practice.* San Diego: Academic Press.

Schlosser, R.W., & Raghavendra, P. (2004). Evidence-based practice in augmentative and alternative communication. *Augmentative and Alternative Communication, 20,* 1–21.

Schlosser, R.W., & Sigafoos, J. (2002). Selecting graphic symbols for an initial request lexicon: Integrative review. *Augmentative and Alternative Communication, 18,* 102–123.

Schlosser, R.W., & Sigafoos, J. (2006). Augmentative and alternative communication interventions for persons with developmental disabilities: Narrative review of comparative single-subject experimental studies. *Research in Developmental Disabilities, 27,* 1–29.

Schlosser, R.W., & Wendt, O. (2008a). Augmentative and alternative communication interventions for children with autism. In J.K. Luiselli, D.C. Russo, & W.P. Christian (Eds.), *Effective practices for children with autism: Educational and behavior support interventions that work* (pp. 325–389). Oxford, England: Oxford University Press.

Schlosser, R.W., & Wendt, O. (2008b). Effects of augmentative and alternative communication intervention on speech production in children with autism: A systematic review. *American Journal of Speech-Language Pathology, 17*(3), 212–230.

Schlosser, R.W., Wendt, O., & Sigafoos, J. (2007). Not all systematic reviews are created equal: Considerations for appraisal. *Evidence-based Communication Assessment and Intervention, 1,* 138–150.

Schopler, E., Mesibov, G.B., & Hearsey, K. (1995). Structured teaching in the TEACCH system. In E. Schopler & G.B. Mesibov (Eds.), *Learning and cognition in autism* (pp. 243–267). New York: Plenum Press.

Schuler, A.L., & Baldwin, M. (1981). Nonspeech communication and childhood autism. *Language, Speech, and Hearing Services in Schools, 12,* 246–257.

Scruggs, T.E., Mastropieri, M.A., & Casto, G. (1987). The quantitative synthesis of single subject research methodology: Methodology and validation. *Remedial and Special Education, 8,* 24–33.

Scruggs, T.E., Mastropieri, M.A., Cook, S.B., & Escobar, C. (1986). Early intervention for children with conduct disorders: A quantitative synthesis of single-subject research. *Behavioral Disorders, 11,* 260–271.

Seal, B.C., & Bonvillian, J.D. (1997). Sign language and motor functioning in students with autistic disorders. *Journal of Autism and Developmental Disorders, 27,* 437–466.

*Sigafoos, J. (1998). Assessing conditional use of graphic mode requesting in a young boy with autism. *Journal of Developmental and Physical Disabilities, 10,* 133–151.

Sigafoos, J., & Drasgow, E. (2001). Conditional use of aided and unaided AAC: A review and clinical case demonstration. *Focus on Autism and Other Developmental Disabilities, 16,* 152–161.

*Sigafoos, J., Laurie, S., & Pennell, D. (1996). Teaching children with Rett syndrome to request preferred objects using aided communication:

Two preliminary studies. *Augmentative and Alternative Communication, 12,* 88–96.

Simeonsson, R., & Bailey, D. (1991). Evaluating programme impact: Levels of certainty. In D. Mitchell & R. Brown (Eds.), *Early intervention studies for young children with special needs* (pp. 280–296). London: Chapman and Hall.

Smith, I., & Bryson, S. (1994). Imitation and action in autism: A critical review. *Psychological Bulletin, 116,* 259–273.

*Sommer, K.S., Whitman, T.L., & Keogh, D.A. (1988). Teaching severely retarded persons to sign interactively through the use of a behavioral script. *Journal in Developmental Disabilities, 9,* 291–304.

*Spencer, L.G. (2002). *Comparing the effectiveness of static pictures vs. video modeling on teaching requesting skills to elementary children with autism.* Unpublished doctoral dissertation, Georgia State University, Atlanta.

*Spillane, M.M. (1999). *The effect of instructional method on symbol acquisition by students with severe disabilities.* Unpublished doctoral dissertation, The University of Nebraska, Lincoln.

*Stiebel, D. (1999). Promoting augmentative communication during daily routines. *Journal of Positive Behavior Interventions, 1,* 159–169.

Straus, S.E., Richardson, W.S., Glasziou, P., & Haynes, R.B. (2005). *Evidence-based medicine: How to practice and teach EBM* (3rd ed.). Edinburgh: Churchill Livingstone.

Sundberg, M.L. (1993). Selecting a response form for nonverbal persons: Facilitated communication, pointing systems, or sign language? *The Analysis of Verbal Behavior, 11,* 99–116.

*Sundberg, M.L., Endicott, K., & Eigenheer, P. (2000). Using intraverbal prompts to establish tacts for children with autism. *The Analysis of Verbal Behavior, 17,* 89–104.

Sundberg, M.L., & Michael, J. (2001). The benefits of Skinner's analysis of verbal behavior for children with autism. *Behavior Modification, 25,* 698–724.

Sundberg, M.L., & Partington, J. (1998). *Teaching language to children with autism or other developmental disabilities.* Pleasant Hill, CA: Behavior Analysts.

*Tincani, M. (2004). Comparing the Picture Exchange Communication System (PECS) and sign-language training for children with autism. *Focus on Autism and Other Developmental Disabilities, 19,* 152–163.

Tincani, M., Crozier, S., & Alazetta, L. (2006). The Picture Exchange Communication System: Effects on manding and speech development for school-aged children with autism. *Education and Training in Developmental Disabilities, 41,* 177–184.

Vaughn, B., & Horner, R.H. (1995). Effects of concrete versus verbal choice systems on problem behavior. *Augmentative and Alternative Communication, 11,* 89–92.

Volkmar, F.R., Lord, C., Bailey, A., Schultz, R.T., & Klin, A. (2004). Autism and pervasive developmental disorders. *Journal of Child Psychology and Psychiatry, 45,* 135–170.

Wendt, O. (2007). The effectiveness of augmentative and alternative communication for individuals with autism spectrum disorders: A systematic review and meta-analysis. Doctoral dissertation, Purdue University, 2006. *Dissertation Abstracts International: Section A: Humanities and Social Sciences, 68.*

Wood, L., Lasker, J., Siegel-Causey, E., Beukelman, D., & Ball, L. (1998). An input framework for augmentative and alternative communication. *Augmentative and Alternative Communication, 14,* 261–267.

*Yoder, P.J., & Layton, T.L. (1988). Speech following sign language training in autistic children with minimal verbal language. *Journal of Autism and Developmental Disorders, 18,* 217–229.

Yoder, P.J., & Stone, W.L. (2006a). A randomized comparison of the effect of two prelinguistic communication interventions on the acquisition of spoken communication in preschoolers with ASD. *Journal of Speech, Language, and Hearing Research, 49,* 698–711.

Yoder, P., & Stone, W.L. (2006b). Randomized comparison of two communication interventions for preschoolers with autism spectrum disorders. *Journal of Consulting and Clinical Psychology, 74,* 426–435.

Zipoli, R.P., & Kennedy, M. (2005). Evidence-based practice among speech–language pathologists: Attitudes, utilization, and barriers. *American Journal of Speech-Language Pathology, 14,* 208–220.

Overview and Appraisal of Studies Involving Manual Signs and Gestures

Study	Purpose	Participants (chronological age in years, months; functional speech)	Design	Outcomes	Effect size estimate: Percentage of nonoverlapping data or standard mean difference (Cohen's *d* and Hedges' *g*)	Appraisal
Anderson (2001)	To compare PECS with manual signing in terms of acquisition	6 children: John (2,11; few words), Cory (2,3; none), Alex (2,7; none), Maya (2,10; none), Ryan (4,11; few words), Sara (1,11; none)	Adapted alternating treatments within a multiple probes design	Sign item acquired	John, 100; Cory, 100; Alex, 100; Maya, 100; Ryan, 100; Sara, 100	Conclusive. Strong design, solid IOA and TI
Buffington, Krantz, McClannahan, & Poulson (1998)	To demonstrate the effects of modeling, prompting, and reinforcement on the acquisition of gestures	4 children: Anne (6,5), Oscar (6,4), Kevin (4,5); all with some spoken language	Multiple probe design across behaviors	1. Acquisition: pointing and saying "look" to indicate 2. Generalization across settings and stimuli	1. Acquisition: Anne, 94; Oscar, 96; Kevin, 96; Nick, 95 2. Generalization: time-series data were not provided	1. Acquisition: conclusive. Excellent design, IOA and TI. 2. Generalization: inconclusive. The generalization is unclear based on the results reported.
Ingersoll, Lewis, & Kroman (2007)	To examine whether reciprocal imitation training can successfully	5 children: Noel (3,2), Gage (4,1), Zane (3,7), Isaiah (3,7), Graham (2,10); all	Multiple baseline design across subjects	1. Total gesture imitation 2. Combined gesture imitation	(Acquisition/maintenance) 1. Total gesture imitation: Noel, 96/100; Gage,	Preponderant. Sound design, replication across 5 participants; generalization and follow-up

	Purpose	Participants	Design	Dependent variables	Outcomes	Comments
	teach immediate gesture imitation and whether increases in imitation would lead to spontaneous use of gestures	with some spoken language but deficits in gesture imitation		3. Total spontaneous gesture use 4. Spontaneous combined gesture use	100/100; Zane, 45/67; Isaiah, 62/67; Graham, 72/67 2. Combined gesture imitation: Noel, 96/100; Gage, 96/67; Zane, 32/0; Isaiah, 69/67; Graham, 36/67 3. Total spontaneous gesture use: Noel, 61/0; Gage, 32/33; Zane, 86/33; Isaiah, 15/0; Graham, 84/100 4. Spontaneous combined gesture use: Noel, 57/0; Gage, 16/0; Zane, 64/0; Isaiah, 23/33; Graham, 79/100	phases are present, but generalization probes infused in acquisition data and not separated. IOA and TI are strong. Social validation is provided.
Tincani (2004)	To compare manual signing with PECS in terms of requesting and speech production	2 children: Carl (5,10; no speech but some imitations) and Jennifer (6,8; imitates words and phrases)	Adapted alternating treatment design	1. Independent requesting 2. Word vocalizations	1. Independent requesting: Carl, 82; Jennifer, 78 2. Word vocalizations: Carl, 100; Jennifer, 100	Preponderant. The natural speech design and the intervention design involved no continuous data collection. IOA and TI were strong.

(Continued)

121

(Continued)

Study	Purpose	Participants (chronological age in years, months; functional speech)	Design	Outcomes	Effect size estimate: Percentage of nonoverlapping data or standard mean difference (Cohen's d and Hedges' g)	Appraisal
Barrera, Lobato-Barrera, & Sulzer-Azaroff (1980)	To compare simultaneous communication, sign-only, and oral communication in terms of expressive sign or spoken labeling	1 child (4,6; history of mutism)	Adapted alternating treatment design	Expressive sign or spoken labeling	Sign alone: 56 Simultaneous: 89 Oral: 67	Suggestive. Both sequence and carryover effects were minimized with the design and procedural safeguards. Sets were equated but only through informal means and without considering all known variables contributing to learning difficulty. IOA is good but TI is lacking. (For a more detailed appraisal see Schlosser, 2003.)
Carr, Binkoff, Kologinsky, & Eddy (1978)	To evaluate if prompting, fading, and stimulus rotation alone improve expressive signs	4 children: Bob (15; no functional speech and few sounds), Dan (15; no functional	Multiple baseline design across object labels taught	Expressive sign labeling	Bob, 100; Dan, 100; Doug, 100; Patrick, 100	Suggestive. Strong design and IOA, but TI is missing.

Study	Purpose	Subjects	Design	Dependent variable	Results	Conclusions
		speech and few sounds), Doug (14; no functional speech and few sounds), Patrick (10; no functional speech and few sounds)				
Carr & Dores (1981)	To evaluate the effects of simultaneous communication training on receptive signing and receptive speech	3 children: Jon (10), Len (11); Mel (11); all with no intelligible speech	Multiple baseline design across object labels taught	Correct responses on receptive language task (receptive speech or receptive signing)	Jon, 100; Mel, 100; Len, 100	Suggestive. A strong design with solid IOA, but TI is not reported.
Carr & Kemp (1989)	To determine whether leading can be replaced with pointing as a means of requesting	4 children: Cal (5), Jim (3), Sue (3), Mike (5); all with no functional speech, but vocalizations	Multiple baseline design across subjects	Generalized (new adults, new settings, new reinforcers) requesting via 1) pointing and 2) leading	1. Pointing: Cal, 100; Jim, 100; Sue, 100; Mike, 100 2. Leading: Cal, 100; Jim, 100; Sue, 100; Mike, 100	Suggestive. Sound design, excellent IOA, but TI is lacking.
Carr & Kologinsky (1983), Experiment 1	To evaluate whether a combination of prompting, fading, differential reinforcement and incidental teaching results in the acquisition of spontaneous requesting and generalization across partners	3 children: John (9; no functional speech and no sounds), Mike (10; no functional speech and no sounds), Bob (14; no functional speech and no sounds)	Multiple baseline design combined with a reversal design	1. Acquisition of spontaneous requests 2. Generalization of requests across partners	1. Acquisition: John, 100; Mike, 100; Bob, 100 2. Generalization: John, 100; Mike, 100; Bob, 100	Suggestive. Acquisition and Generalization: Strong intervention, generalization design, and IOA, but no TI.

(Continued)

Study	Purpose	Participants (chronological age in years, months; functional speech)	Design	Outcomes	Effect size estimate: Percentage of nonoverlapping data or standard mean difference (Cohen's *d* and Hedges' *g*)	Appraisal
Carr & Kologinsky (1983), Experiment 2	To evaluate whether targeted prompting and reinforcement results in greater signed requesting and generalization across adults and settings	3 children: Tom (10; lack of speech), Andy (11; lack of speech), Len (14; lack of speech)	ABCBCD, where B = only sign 1 treated; C = only sign 2 treated; D = both signs treated	1. Acquisition of spontaneous requests 2. Generalization of requests across a) partners and b) settings	1. Acquisition: Tom, 100; Andy, 91; Len, 100 2a. Setting generalization: Tom, 100; Andy, 100; Len, 100 2b. Partner generalization: Andy, 100; Len, 83	Suggestive. Strong design (order effects are not a problem here because it is the same treatment, only a different sign across phases) and IOA, but no TI.
Carr, Kologinsky, & Leff-Simon (1987)	To examine the effects of prompting, fading, stimulus rotation, and differential reinforcement on descriptive signing of action–object phrases	3 children: Ron (15), Dave (16); Rick (11); all no functional speech, only babbling	Multiple baseline design across three actions	Expressively signed novel (i.e., generalized) action–object phrases	Ron, 92; Dave, 100; Rick, 95	Suggestive. Design is strong, IOA is excellent, but TI is lacking.
Keogh, Whitman, Beeman, Halligan, & Starzynski (1987)	To evaluate the effects of verbal prompts, modeling, physical	1 child (14; occasional vocalizations)	Multiple probe design across dialogue situations	1. Acquisition and 2. Generalization to client–client interaction: sign	1. Acquisition: 100 2. Generalization: 40	Suggestive. Strong intervention and generalization

				Dependent variables	Outcomes	Appraisal
	guidance, positive reinforcement, fading, and chaining procedures on sign initiations, signed responses, and nonsigning responses			initiations, responsive signs, and nonsigning responses		designs, IOA excellent, but TI is lacking. In addition, all three dependent variables were added together in the graph, making it difficult to determine specific effects.
Remington & Clarke (1983)	To compare simultaneous communication training with sign-alone training on expressive sign labeling and comprehension	2 children: Diane (10; no functional speech and babbling sounds) and John (15; some nonfunctional verbal speech)	Adapted alternating treatment design	1. Expressive sign labeling 2. Speech comprehension	1. Expressive sign labeling: Diane, 100; John, 100 2. Speech comprehension: Diane, 100; John, 100	Suggestive. Both sequence and carryover effects have been minimized through the design and procedural safeguards. The within-subject replication strengthens the internal validity of findings. Sets were equated using objective methods. IOA is excellent, but TI is lacking. (For a more detailed appraisal see Schlosser, 2003.)

(Continued)

Study	Purpose	Participants (chronological age in years, months; functional speech)	Design	Outcomes	Effect size estimate: Percentage of nonoverlapping data or standard mean difference (Cohen's *d* and Hedges' *g*)	Appraisal
Schepis, Reid, Fitzgerald, Faw, VanDen-Pol, & Welty (1982)	To evaluate the effects of modified incidental teaching strategies on sign acquisition	4 children: Participant 1 (11; occasionally verbalized), Participant 2 (7; no intelligible speech), Participant 3 (9; no intelligible speech), and Participant 4 (11; no intelligible speech)	Multiple baseline design across time of day and subjects	1. Expressive signing (the communicative function is unclear) 2. Vocalizations	1. Expressive signing: Participant 1, 29; Participant 2, 83; Participant 3, 92; Participant 4, 59 2. Vocalizations: Not calculated because there were no time-series data	Expressive signing: suggestive. The design and IOA are strong; TI is lacking. Vocalizations: inconclusive. Data are collapsed into means.
Sommer, Whitman, & Keogh (1988)	To examine the effects of a program that teaches severely developmentally disabled individuals to sign with one another	1 child (14; occasional vocalizations)	Multiple probe design across subjects	1. Acquisition 2. Generalization across situations: sign initiations, responsive signs, and nonsigning responses	1. Acquisition: 67 2. Generalization: 67	Suggestive. Strong design and excellent IOA, but TI is lacking. In addition, all three dependent variables were added together in the graph, making it difficult to determine specific effects.

Study	Purpose	Participants	Design	Outcome measure	Results	Conclusions
Sundberg, Endicott, & Eigenheer (2000)	To compare the efficacy of the standard procedure and the intraverbal procedure in training object naming (tacting) using manual signs	2 children: Participant 1 (5; limited speech) and Participant 2 (4; limited vocal abilities)	Alternating treatments design[l] with baseline and embedded reversal design	Percent of correct tacts using 1) standard procedure and 2) intraverbal procedure	1. Standard procedure. Acquisition: Participant 1, 85; Participant 2, 87. Maintenance: Participant 1, 67; Participant 2, 100 2. Intraverbal procedure. Acquisition: Participant 1, 96; Participant 2, 97 Maintenance: Participant 1 (100) Participant 2 (100)	Suggestive. Appropriate design and IOA is strong, but TI is lacking; no quantitative follow-up data and small sample size are further limitations.
Yoder & Layton (1988)	To examine the effects of pre-treatment verbal imitation abilities and training conditions: 1) speech alone, 2) sign alone, 3) alternating, and 4) simultaneous on the use of verbal communication during treatment	60 children: average age = 5 years; ≤ 25 words based on parent report	Randomized controlled trial	Number of different child-initiated spoken words (echolalia or responses were not counted) under four different treatment conditions	1) versus 2): d = .73; g = .19 1) versus 3): d = .43; g = .11 1) versus 4): d = .33; g = .09 2) versus 4): d = −.33; g = −.09 2) versus 3): d = −.30; g = −.08 No significant difference between conditions	Suggestive. Strong design but lack of TI data.

(Continued)

Study	Purpose	Participants (chronological age in years, months; functional speech)	Design	Outcomes	Effect size estimate: Percentage of nonoverlapping data or standard mean difference (Cohen's *d* and Hedges' *g*)	Appraisal
Brady & Smouse (1978)	To compare the effects of simultaneous communication, sign-alone, and oral training in terms on receptive speech	1 child (6,4; spontaneous unintelligible vocalizations)	Alternating treatments design with most effective treatment in third phase	Receptive speech	Not calculated because the evidence was inconclusive	Inconclusive. The design (using the same words and objects across conditions) does not rule out carryover effects. TI is lacking as well. (See also Schlosser, 2003.)
Hundert (1981)	To compare multiple stimulus training with single stimulus training in terms of expressive sign labeling	1 child (10; no functional speech)	Adapted alternating treatments design	Expressive sign labeling	Not calculated due to inconclusive evidence	Inconclusive. Although random assignment was used, no evidence is provided that the sets were truly equated.
Oxman, Konstantareas, & Liebovitz-Bojm (1979)	To assess the effects of simultaneous communication training on vocal responding	10 children (average age 9,3; minimal or no speech skills)	Pre-post control group design	Presence of first-trial response, articulatory correctness	Not calculated because of inconclusive evidence	Inconclusive. The design is fatally flawed because the control group children were not all children with autism; small sample size; no TI.

| Saraydarian (1994) | To evaluate whether the use of simultaneous communication to model referents enhances referent recognition and production abilities | Experimental group: 10 children (mean age 6,2; nonspeaking or severely delayed in oral/gestural language development). Control group: children with other disabilities | Randomized controlled trial | 1. Receptive speech 2. Expressive labeling (using sign, speech, or both) | Not calculated because of inconclusive evidence | Inconclusive. The design is fatally flawed because the control group children were not all children with autism; no TI. |

Key: IOA, interobserver agreement; TI, treatment integrity.

Overview and Appraisal of Studies Involving Graphic Symbols

Study	Purpose	Participants (chronological age in years, months; functional speech)	Design	Graphic symbols	Outcomes	Effect size estimate: Percentage of nonoverlapping data or MBR	Appraisal
Johnston, Nelson, Evans, & Palazolo (2003)	To determine if creating communicative opportunities, modeling, prompting, and providing natural consequences are effective in terms of requesting	3 children: Brad (4,3; autism + cognitive delay + dysmorphic features + 1- to 2-word utterances), Alex (5,3; pervasive developmental disorder + cognitive delay + 4- to 6-word utterances), Billy (5,1; autism + multiple disabilities + jargon speech)	Multiple-probe design across subjects	PCS on a flash-card	Correct requests to play (graphic symbol or verbal; acquisition, maintenance, generalization)	Requesting, acquisition: Brad, 95; Alex, 53; Billy, 45 Maintenance: Brad, 100; Alex, 100; Billy, 100 Generalization: not calculated, inconclusive	Acquisition: conclusive. Sound design; solid IOA and excellent TI. Generalization: inconclusive. No baseline.
Bryan & Gast (2000)	To evaluate the effectiveness of visual activity schedules in increasing on-task and on-schedule behavior	4 children: Allen (8,11), Tim (8,0), Jack (7,4), Jenny (8,6); with autism, no information about speech skills	A-B-A-B withdrawal design	2-inch by 2-inch line-drawn pictures in a photo album	1. On schedule (completion of each step in a task analysis) 2. On-task with scheduled materials (on schedule	Acquisition/maintenance/generalization: 1. Allen, 100; Tim, 100; Jack, 100; Jenny, 100 2. Allen, 100; Tim, 100;	Preponderant. Sound design but little control on carry-over effects. IOA and TI are good but no blinding of interventionist. Provision

132

				and transitioning between or performing activities) 3. Reduction of on-task with nonscheduled materials (not on schedule and transitioning between or performing activities)	Jack, 100; Jenny, 100 3. Allen, 100; Tim, 100; Jack, 100; Jenny, 100 (all MBR)	of social validity data is a strength.
Hetzroni & Shalem (2005)	To evaluate the effectiveness of mutilevel software in teaching identification of orthographic symbols	6 children: Max (11,0; few 1-word utterances), Bob (11,0; no speech), Gina (13,0; no speech), Lara (10,0; no vocalizations), Sara (10,0; no functional speech and echolalia), Al (10,0; no functional speech and moderate intellectual disability	Multiple-probe design across subjects	Orthographic symbols on computer monitor / Number of correctly matched orthographic symbols to corresponding logos	Max, 67; Bob, 70; Gina, 88; Lara, 60; Sara, 82; Al, 50	Preponderant. The design is sound; it is unclear whether the intervention phase reports probe or training data. IOA is good but was collected only during generalization tasks and is not representative of all probes. TI is excellent.

(Continued)

Study	Purpose	Participants (chronological age in years, months; functional speech)	Design	Graphic symbols	Outcomes	Effect size estimate: Percentage of nonoverlapping data or MBR	Appraisal
Dettmer, Simpson, Myles, & Ganz (2000)	To evaluate the effectiveness of visual supports (schedules, boxes, timers) in facilitating transitions	2 children: Jeff (7,0) and Josh (5,0); with autism, no information about speech skills	A-B-A-B withdrawal design	Visual schedule and album with line drawings	1. Latency to begin new activity 2. Number of physical removals 3. Number of verbal and physical prompts	1. Latency: Jeff, 100; Josh, 100 Not calculated for 2. and 3. because of only 1 data point	Suggestive. Design is appropriate; IOA is good but based on only 15% of sessions; TI is not reported.
Kozleski (1991)	To compare the effectiveness and efficiency of request training using various graphic sets/systems in terms of requesting	4 children: Kevin (7,10), Jessica (12,7), Brian (7,7), Malay (13,6); with autism and no speech	Multiple-baseline design across subjects with multiple interventions introduced in counterbalanced order across subjects	Premack, colored photographs, Blissymbolics, Orthography, Rebus	1. Requesting: Premack 2. Requesting: colored photographs 3. Requesting: Blissymbolics 4. Requesting: Orthography 5. Requesting: Rebus	1. Kevin, 100; Jessica, 100; Brian, 100 2. Kevin, 100; Malay, 100 3. Kevin, 100; Brian, 100; Malay, 100 4. Jessica, 100; Malay, 100 5. Jessica, 100; Brian, 100	Suggestive. The comparative design relies on between-subject control of sequence effects; sets were equated through informal means; TI is not reported; IOA is excellent.

Study	Purpose	Participants	Design	Symbol/Mode	Dependent variables	Results	Comments
Reichle et al. (2005)	To teach requesting assistance and independent task completion	1 adult (40,0); no functional speech, only loud vocalizations, with autism and severe intellectual disability	Multiple-probe design across three components of task completion	Colored PCS on communication card	1. Correct requests by touching "help" symbol 2. Correct completion of task components	1. Requesting: 53 2. Task completion: 100	Suggestive. Appropriate design, but sample size is limited to 1. Strong IOA but no TI.
Sigafoos (1998)	To evaluate the effects of differential reinforcement of reaching and requesting on conditional requesting	1 child (6,0); occasional babbling with autism	A-B-A-C (B = request training; C = conditional request training)	Black-and-white line drawing of symbol for "want"	Aided requesting and conditional requests (reaching versus pointing to symbols)	Requests: pointing to symbol, 83 (PND); reaching, 89 (MBR). Conditional requests: PND and MBR not calculated	Suggestive. Sequence effects are not controlled (minor flaw). The change from "assessment B" to "conditional use" does not demonstrate a functional relation between the independent and dependent variable

(Continued)

Study	Purpose	Participants (chronological age in years, months; functional speech)	Design	Graphic symbols	Outcomes	Effect size estimate: Percentage of nonoverlapping data or MBR	Appraisal
Spillane (1999)	To investigate the effects of discrete trial versus incidental teaching on graphic symbol acquisition	2 children: John (10,0; autism, no speech), Tom (10,0; severe intellectual disability, no speech); Tom was excluded because of no autism diagnosis	Alternating treatment design nested within multiple-baseline design	PCS with Velcro on display board	Correct item labeling demonstrated by selecting corresponding symbol from display and handing to interventionist	Acquisition, discrete trial: John, 18 Acquisition, incidental teaching: John, 30	Suggestive. Appropriate design, but only 1 replication with nonautistic participant. IOA is excellent, but TI is missing.
Stiebel (1999)	To study the effects of teaching parents the problem solving strategy of spontaneous picture card use	3 children: Steven (4,2; autism and hypotonia, lack of spontaneous language), Tommy (6,8; autism, 3- to 5-word vocalizations), Jose (4,6; autism, vocalizations)	Nonconcurrent multiple-baseline design across subjects	Colored photographs	Spontaneous picture card use (pointing to, handing over, or attempting to hand a card to an interactant for unspecified communicative function)	Acquisition: Steven, 100; Tommy, 57; Jose, 78 Follow-up: Steven, 100; Tommy, 80; Jose, 40	Suggestive. Nonconcurrent multiple-baseline design is less convincing than multiple-baseline design. In addition, there are no TI data available. IOA is excellent.

Study	Purpose	Participants	Design	Intervention	Dependent measures	Effect size	Notes
Dexter (1998)	To evaluate the effects of aided language stimulation in terms of imitative and spontaneous communicative behaviors	6 children: Andre (8,1), Tony (9,2), Peter (9,3), Carl (9,0), Sam (7,2), Brad (6,5); with pervasive development disorder-not otherwise specified and limited verbal output	Multiple-baseline design across subjects	PCS in aided language stimulation	1. Number of spontaneous PCS uses during joint book reading 2. Number of spontaneous spoken outputs 3. Mean length of utterances	Not calculated because of inconclusive evidence	Inconclusive. Baseline data are followed by intervention data rather than probe data, making a comparison tedious.
Hamilton & Snell (1993)	To study the effects of milieu teaching on use of a communication book across environments	1 child (15,0; no speech) with autism and severe intellectual disability	Changing criterion design within a multiple-probe design	Communication book: PCS plus photos	Correct responses using communication book	Not calculated because of inconclusive evidence	Inconclusive. Increases in the untreated baselines and training performance could be just a continuation of a trend. No probe data are reported during training phases. IOA and TI are excellent (based on a small percentage of observations).

(Continued)

137

Study	Purpose	Participants (chronological age in years, months; functional speech)	Design	Graphic symbols	Outcomes	Effect size estimate: Percentage of nonoverlapping data or MBR	Appraisal
Reichle & Brown (1986)	To teach the use of a multipaged communication wallet for requesting and providing information	1 adult (23,0; no speech) with autism	A-B phases arranged in multiple-baseline sequence across behaviors	Rebus and Picline drawings in communication wallet	Correct requests; correct item labeling; correctly discriminating between requesting/labeling; correctly locating symbols; explicit requesting (using *want* plus *object name*)	Not calculated because of inconclusive evidence	Inconclusive. No experimental control due to changing dependent variable across replications; both IOA and TI are lacking.
Reichle, Sigafoos, & Remington (1991)	To teach requesting via pointing to symbol	1 adult (AI [27,0], no speech) with autism	A-B-A-C (B = request training; C = seek attention and request training)	Line drawings	Correct requests by pointing to symbol of desired item (either radio or Diet Coke)	Not calculated because of inconclusive evidence	Inconclusive: no return to baseline; both TI and IOA are lacking.
Sigafoos, Laurie, & Pennell (1996)	To demonstrate the use of graphic symbols to teach requesting	Study 1: Two girls with Rett syndrome, Cleo (17,0) and Karen (12,0); both with no speech	A-B phases arranged in multiple-probe/baseline sequence across subjects and behaviors	Study 1: black-and-white line drawing of *want* Study 2: logo of potato chips	Correct requests by touching symbol (Milli was later taught to use a switch to play music when requesting task became too difficult)	Not calculated because of inconclusive evidence	Inconclusive. Lack of experimental control; change of independent variable; TI was vague; IOA was strong.

Source	Purpose	Participants	Design	Conditions	Dependent variable	Effect size	Comments
		Study 2: Two girls with Rett syndrome, Jane (7,0) and Milli (12,0); both with no speech					
Spencer (2002)	To compare the effectiveness and efficiency of static pictures and video modeling on request behavior	4 children: Tom (7,0; verbal + echolalia), Nathan (7,0; verbal + echolalia + perseverations), Donald (7,0; minimally verbal + 1- to 2-word utterances); Chase (9,0; vocalization + 1-word utterances); all with severe autism	Adaptive alternating treatment design combined with a multiple-probe design across subjects	1. Static: digital photographs 2. Dynamic: video modeling	Number of requests (spoken, pointing to, or touching the symbol of an object)	Not calculated because of inconclusive evidence	Inconclusive. Although the design is appropriate, the procedure of providing only the static photos as a response option biased the results in favor of this condition. IOA is excellent, but TI is not reported.

[a] An MBR index for reaching could not be calculated because the conditional use phase does not supply reaching data; a PND for pointing to the symbol when the object was out of reach could not be calculated due to a ceiling effect in the preceding baseline ("assessment B").

Key: IOA, interobserver agreement; MBR, mean baseline reduction; PND, percentage of nonoverlapping data; TI, treatment integrity.

5

Speech Output and Speech-Generating Devices in Autism Spectrum Disorders

RALF W. SCHLOSSER, JEFF SIGAFOOS, AND RAJINDER K. KOUL

Many individuals with autism spectrum disorders (ASDs) have severe communication impairments (i.e., little or no functional speech) to the extent that they may benefit from augmentative and alternative communication (AAC) intervention. Depending on the source consulted, up to 50% of individuals with ASDs fail to develop functional speech skills (Peeters & Gillberg, 1999). These individuals are potential candidates for AAC interventions. AAC refers to an area of educational and clinical practice that aims to supplement or replace an individual's natural speech and/or handwriting through unaided approaches such as manual signing and gestures, as well as aided approaches such as graphic symbols, communication boards, and speech-generating devices (Beukelman & Mirenda, 2005; Lloyd, Fuller, & Arvidson, 1997).

Some scholars have emphasized that AAC might be effective for individuals with ASDs because their characteristics are a good match to the skills needed for AAC use (Mirenda & Schuler, 1988). For example, children with autism are often considered to be visual learners and therefore good candidates for using AAC because it is primarily visual in nature (e.g., manual signs, graphic symbols). In the 1980s, there was a need to justify the use of AAC rather than continuing with traditional speech therapy for some children with severe communication impairments. Hence, these timely and useful arguments mostly juxtaposed AAC with natural speech therapy. Manual signs seemed to be treatment method most heavily researched during these early years (e.g.,

Carr, Binkoff, Kologinsky, & Eddy, 1978). Compared to manual signing, graphic symbols are a relatively newer AAC mode for individuals with ASDs in practice as well as in the development of a research base. However, as early as the 1980s, authors drew attention to the potential benefits of graphic symbols due to their nontransient nature (e.g., Schuler & Baldwin, 1981). Even though manual signs are transmitted in the visual modality as well, they tend to be much more transient.

In the past two decades, AAC intervention research with individuals with ASDs has increased steadily and has broadened in scope to include other AAC modes and intervention strategies. Among these are a variety of selection-based approaches such as nonelectronic communication boards, communication wallets, and communication books. These modes do not rely on technology and require the individual to select symbols on displays to transmit messages to the listener. Among these low-tech options are exchange-based approaches, whereby the individual hands over a graphic symbol (e.g., on a flashcard) and in return gains access to a desired object. The most widely used exchange-based approach is the Picture Exchange Communication System (Frost & Bondy, 2002), a manualized treatment for beginning communicators (see Chapter 10).

Speech-generating devices (SGDs; also known as voice output communication aids) and SGD software (e.g., talking word processors) represent some of the more recent additions to the repertoire of AAC options. Unlike nonelectronic communication methods or typical word processors, SGDs and SGD software provide auditory stimuli via speech output as an added component. SGDs and SGD software have changed the service provision of aided communication. A number of case studies and quasi-experimental reports have described SGD use in one or more individuals with ASDs (Bornman & Alant, 1999; Light, Roberts, Dimarco, & Greiner, 1998; Mirenda, Wilk, & Carson, 2000; Romski & Sevcik, 1996; Thunberg, Ahlsen, & Dahlgren Sandberg, 2007). Because of their nonexperimental nature, they will not be reviewed further in this chapter, which will examine the research on SGD effectiveness for individuals with ASDs.

TYPES OF SPEECH OUTPUT

Most of the currently available SGDs have built-in technology that allows an individual to use either synthesized or digitized speech. *Digitized speech* is based on the conversion of an analog speech waveform into digits and the reconversion of these digits into a speech waveform. In contrast, *synthesized speech* involves converting real-time text into speech using acoustic information and parametric speech coding techniques (Venkatagiri & Ramabadran, 1995).

Digitized Speech

Digitized speech is produced by recording speech in its analog format and then converting it into numbers using a process called *quantization.* Quantization involves sampling the speech waveform at equal intervals and storing it in the computer's memory as a series of numbers. The major limiting factor of digitization used to be that it required a large amount of computer memory. However, more recently, several data compression techniques that reduce memory demands without compromising accuracy of speech output (e.g., delta modulation) have become available.

One of the advantages of using digitized speech is that it is highly intelligible and natural sounding. Nonetheless, Schlosser and Blischak (2001) cautioned that the quality of digitized speech is only as good as its recording, which may be affected by background noise, natural voice quality, and machine noise introduced during recording. Individuals with communicative impairments who are in clinical and educational settings, with objectives limited to meeting basic communication needs, often benefit from digitized speech. For example, SGDs such as the AlphaTalker (Prentke Romich Company, Wooster, OH), DynaMyte (DynaVox, Pittsburgh, PA), and MACAW (ZYGO Industries, Portland, OR) all use digitized speech to record and replay preselected sentences, phrases, or words. Although digitized speech is highly intelligible, one of its drawbacks is that it limits output to a set of prestored messages.

Synthesized Speech

Text-to-speech synthesis involves converting typed words and sentences into speech waveforms. The conversion includes processing the text to identify syntactic and lexical components to generate proper phrase level pronunciation. Additionally, synthesizers maintain a large pronunciation dictionary that includes several thousand words and an "exception dictionary" of words that do not follow normal pronunciation rules based on spellings (Bruckert, 1984). For example, the exception dictionary is used to pronounce English words like *city*, in which the letter *c*, typically pronounced as /k/, is pronounced as /s/. Prosody is assigned to textual input by applying rules that affect duration, pitch, and stress (Allen, Hunnicutt, & Klatt, 1987).

Research has indicated that the intelligibility of the best synthesizers approaches that of natural speech (Duffy & Pisoni, 1992; Koul, 2003; Koul & Allen, 1993; Koul & Hester, 2006; Mirenda & Beukelman, 1987). Although SGDs with synthesized speech offer additional input and feedback that is not possible with nonelectronic communication systems, the inclusion of speech also adds to the cost of these devices.

Table 5.1 offers a summary comparison of digitized and synthetic speech output in terms of acoustic features, programming, messages, cost, and additional device features.

An examination of data on the perception of synthetic speech for single words and sentences reveals that individuals with developmental disabilities such as intellectual impairments seem to identify and respond to synthetic speech stimuli more accurately and quickly as a

Table 5.1. Comparison of digitized and synthesized speech output

Comparison feature	Synthesized speech	Digitized speech
Acoustic	Computer-generated voice	Recorded human voice
	Artificial, "robotic" quality	Natural speech
	Limited number of "voices" to choose from among those provided by the manufacturer	Any voice that is appropriate to age, gender, personality, language, dialect may be recorded
	No need to select natural speaker to record	Potential difficulty in selecting natural speaker to record
	Unnatural prosody and intonation	Natural prosody and intonation
	Permitted changes in rate, loudness, and pitch affect all utterances	Individual utterances may be varied in rate, pitch, loudness, intonation to signal emotion and communicative function (e.g., question, command)
	Speech is consistent	Potential for inconsistency as new messages are added, unless the same voice is used each time; addition of intonation differences contributes to inconsistency
	Not available in all languages	Any language may be produced
Programming	Relatively more difficult to program	Relatively easier to program
	Programmer must be literate	Programmer does not need literacy skills
	May store messages in any environment	Requires a quiet environment for storing messages
Messages	User may produce messages spontaneously	User may produce only those messages that have been stored
	Virtually unlimited number of messages may be stored	Limited message storage
	Only speech may be produced and stored	Nonspeech sounds (e.g., music) may be stored
Additional device features	Print output via built in display or printer	No print output
	Additional features available (e.g., calculator, notepad)	No additional features unless device offers synthesized speech as well

From Schlosser, R.W., Blischak, D.M., & Patel, R. (2007). *Selection and use of speech output for communication and learning: What does the research tell us?* Manuscript in preparation.

result of repeated and systematic exposure to it (Koul & Hester, 2006; Koul & Clapsaddle, 2006). These findings indicate that individuals who use SGDs become more proficient at recognizing synthetic speech over a period of time. In addition, research has shown that there are no significant differences in the perception of repeated and novel repeated synthetic speech by individuals with intellectual disabilities in either the severe range (Koul & Hester, 2006) or the mild to moderate range (Koul & Clapsaddle, 2006). This suggests that, like individuals without disabilities, these individuals are able to generalize their knowledge of the acoustic-phonetic properties of synthetic speech to novel synthetic stimuli.

Additionally, Willis, Koul, and Paschall (2000) observed that individuals with mild to moderate intellectual impairments use the same strategies and make similar errors in answering questions after listening to discourse passages in synthetic and natural speech. These results indicate that individuals with intellectual impairment are able to apply both—world knowledge and information—presented in spoken passages to comprehend text that is presented in synthetic speech. Although none of these studies included individuals with ASDs, it seems plausible that these findings may generalize to those individuals with ASDs who also have intellectual disabilities.

REVIEW OF THE EVIDENCE BASE
AND IMPLICATIONS FOR PRACTICE AND RESEARCH

Speech output in AAC has been studied in at least four ways (Schlosser, 2003):

1. SGDs were part of a larger treatment package being evaluated for its effectiveness, such as SGDs introduced as part of a naturalistic language intervention.

2. A treatment package with an SGD has been compared to a package without an SGD.

3. Speech output has been isolated as an independent variable to study its specific impact when comparing the presence versus absence of speech output.

4. The conditions under which speech output or SGDs are effective have been studied when comparing, for example, digitized versus synthetic speech or speech with high versus low intelligibility.

Several systematic reviews (e.g., Wendt, 2006) as well as narrative reviews (Schlosser, 2003; Schlosser & Sigafoos, 2006) are included in this chapter. Studies discussed herein had to meet the following criteria: 1) investigate the effects of speech output as part of a treatment package or as an independent variable, 2) involve participants with either autism or pervasive developmental disorders-not otherwise specified and little or no functional speech, and 3) use quasi-experimental group designs or single-subject experimental designs.

None of the studies that met these criteria involved group designs. For single-subject experimental designs, the percentage of nonoverlapping data (PND) was applied as an outcome metric (Scruggs, Mastropieri, & Casto, 1987). The PND method requires the calculation of nonoverlap between baseline and successive intervention (or generalization) phases by identifying the highest data point in baseline and determining the percentage of data points during intervention (or generalization or maintenance) exceeding this level. PND scores can range from 0% to 100% and can be interpreted using the conventions set by Scruggs, Mastropieri, Cook, and Escobar (1986). A PND greater than 90% is considered highly effective, a PND between 70% and 90% reflects fair effectiveness, a PND between 50% and 70% is considered of questionable effectiveness, and a PND less than 50% reflects unreliable or ineffective treatments.

For studies that aimed to decrease challenging behaviors, the percentage of zero data (PZD) was calculated. The PZD is computed by finding the first data point in the treatment phase that equals zero and calculating the percentage of data points obtained in the treatment phase, including the first zero, that stay at zero (Scotti, Evans, Meyer, & Walker, 1991). PZD scores can range from 0% to 100% and can be interpreted using the conventions set by Scotti et al. (1991). A PZD greater than 80% is considered highly effective, a PZD between 55% and 80% reflects fair effectiveness, a PZD between 18% and 54% is considered of questionable effectiveness, and a PZD less than 18% reflects ineffectiveness.

Each included study was assessed in terms of the certainty framework suggested and used by several authors (e.g., Granlund & Olsson, 1999; Millar, Light, & Schlosser, 2006; Schlosser & Sigafoos, 2006). This framework classifies the certainty of evidence into four groupings from conclusive to preponderant, and from suggestive to inconclusive, based on three dimensions: 1) design, 2) interobserver agreement (IOA) of the dependent variable, and 3) treatment integrity (TI). *Conclusive evidence* establishes that the outcomes are undoubtedly the results of the intervention based on a sound design and at least adequate IOA and TI. *Preponderant evidence* ascertains that the outcomes are not only plausible but that they are also more likely to have occurred than not due to minor design flaws, with at least adequate IOA and TI. *Suggestive evidence* establishes that the outcomes are plausible and within the realm of possibility, with either a strong design but inadequate IOA and/or TI or with minor design flaws and inadequate IOA and/or TI. *Inconclusive evidence* ascertains that the outcomes are not plausible due to fatal flaws in the research design.

Introducing SGDs as Part of a Treatment Package

Table 5.2 provides a summary of nine studies in which researchers evaluated the effects of SGDs as part of a treatment package in individuals with ASD (Brady, 2000; Durand, 1999; Dyches, 1998; Olive et al., 2007; Schepis, Reid, Behrmann, & Sutton, 1998; Sigafoos, Drasgow et al., 2004; Sigafoos, O'Reilly, Ganz, Lancioni, & Schlosser, 2005; Sigafoos, O'Reilly, Seely-York, & Edrisinha, 2004; Son, Sigafoos, O'Reilly, & Lancioni, 2006). Only studies that yielded suggestive or better results are discussed here.

Durand (1999) provided conclusive evidence that functional communication training using an SGD resulted in successful decreases in challenging behaviors and increases in appropriate communication in two children with autism. The results were obtained in both classroom and community settings. Although the PZD value of 27 for one child in the classroom is not convincing, there was a considerable reduction in challenging behavior over baseline. However, despite this reduction, many of the data points did not reach a zero level.

Schepis et al. (1998) offered suggestive evidence indicating that the use of naturalistic teaching strategies combined with SGDs results in increases in the number of communicative interactions by four young children with autism. The strategy included teaching the classroom teacher and three aides to use child-preferred stimuli available within the natural routine and child-initiated responses as the point of intervention; provide verbal and gestural prompts with minimal use of physical guidance; and use natural cues such as physical approach, expectant delay, questioning looks, and eye contact. The PNDs were consistently 100 across all participants or initiations made by the child participants. The results also showed increases in interactions by classroom staff (i.e., partner outcomes), ranging in PND terms from 83 for one child to 100 for the other three children. The primary reason this study was rated at the suggestive level relates to the lack of treatment integrity data and a relatively minor design flaw. The participants were exposed to the SGD only during intervention and not during baseline; hence, it is difficult to attribute changes in dependent measures to the treatment involving the SGD rather than the mere novelty of the SGD.

Although Schepis et al. (1998) observed that there was no reduction in other communication modalities (e.g., gestures) as a result of introducing the SGD, these data could not be verified through PND

Table 5.2. Studies on the effects of speech-generating devices (SGDs) as part of a treatment package: Summary and appraisal

Study	Purpose	Participants (chronological age in years, months)	Design	SGD (speech type)	Outcomes	Percentage of nonoverlapping data or zero data (%)	Appraisal
Durand (1999), Study 2	To determine the effects of functional communication training on requesting and challenging behaviors in the classroom	2 children: Ron (9,6), David (11,6)	Multiple-baseline design across subjects	IntroTalker; digitized	Unprompted requesting Challenging behavior	Ron (94) David (97) Ron (100) David (27)	Conclusive: strong design, treatment integrity, and interobserver agreement
Durand (1999), Study 3	To determine the effects of functional communication training on requesting and challenging behaviors in community settings	2 children: Ron (9,6), David (11,6)	Multiple-baseline design across subjects	IntroTalker; digitized	Unprompted requesting Challenging behavior	Ron (100) David (100) Ron (100) David (82)	Conclusive: strong design, treatment integrity, and interobserver agreement
Olive et al. (2007)	To study the effects of enhanced milieu teaching to introduce an SGD on elicited vocalizations and independent requesting	3 children: Mickey (4,0), Rocky (4,0), Terrence (5,6)	Multiple-baseline design across subjects	CheapTalk 4 – Inline Direct; digitized speech	Elicited vocalizations Independent requesting with SGD Independent requesting with gestures and SGD	Mickey (0) Rocky (0) Terrence (83) Mickey (88) Rocky (100) Terrence (92) Mickey (100) Rocky (92) Terrence (83)	Suggestive: Minor design flaws as there were only intervention data and no probe data collected. However, the responses

148

Study	Purpose	Participants	Design	SGD	Dependent measure	Outcome data	Certainty of evidence
							were independent and self-initiated; treatment integrity and interobserver agreement strong
Schepis et al. (1998)	To evaluate the effects of naturalistic teaching strategies and SGD use on communicative interactions	4 children: Ben (5,0), Cory (5,0), Lynn (3,0), Ian (3,0)	Multiple probe design	Cheap Talk 4 or 8 (* Ben also used Black Hawk in last several sessions); digitized	Number of communicative interactions; Number of communicative staff interactions	Ben (100), Cory (100), Lynn (100), Ian (100); Ben (83), Cory (100), Lynn (100), Ian (100)	Suggestive: Sound design, good interobserver agreement, but treatment integrity is missing
Sigafoos, Drasgow et al. (2004)	To evaluate the transfer of SGD use from a clinical setting to home and to evaluate a strategy for repairing communication breakdowns	2 children: Jason (16,0), Megan (20,0)	Multiple-baseline design	BIGMack; digitized speech	Requesting; SGD use repair (The use of an SGD was taught for repairing communication breakdowns.)	Jason (28), Megan (45); Jason (100), Megan (100)	Suggestive: Minor design flaw (only 2 replications), interobserver agreement strong, but treatment integrity missing

(Continued)

149

Table 5.2. *(continued)*

Study	Purpose	Participants (chronological age in years, months)	Design	SGD (speech type)	Outcomes	Percentage of nonoverlapping data or zero data (%)	Appraisal
Sigafoos, O'Reilly et al. (2004)	To evaluate the effects of a least-to-most prompting procedure for locating an SGD	3 youths: Megan (20,0), Jason (16,0), Ryan (12,0)	Delayed multiple-baseline design	TechTalk; digitized speech	Requesting with SGD when device is not visible	Megan (100) Jason (100) Ryan (100)	Suggestive: The delayed baselines in two subjects represent a minor design flaw. Interobserver agreement adequate, but treatment integrity not reported
Brady (2000)	To evaluate the effects of SGD instruction during joint activity routines on requesting and object comprehension	1 child: Amy (5,0)	Multiple-baseline design across activities	Speak Easy via Jellybean switch; digitized	Requesting Object comprehension	Amy (percentage of nonoverlapping data could not be calculated due to baseline ceiling effects) Amy (78)	Suggestive: Minor design flaws with only 2 tiers (i.e., 1 replication); good interobserver agreement and treatment integrity

| Dyches (1998) | To evaluate the effects of switch training on communicative interactions and speech production | 2 children: Alan (11, 2), Nathan (10, 4) | A-B-A-B | Big Red/Jelly Bean switch; digitized speech | Number of communicative interactions[a]
Number of spontaneous communicative interactions
Number of verbalizations
Requesting speech off
Vocalizations speech on/off | Not calculated (see appraisal) | Inconclusive: Design does not rule out sequence effects, compares "apples" in baseline with "oranges" in intervention (switch was not present in baseline); number of obligatory contexts not equated across sessions; no treatment integrity. |

(Continued)

Table 5.2. *(continued)*

Study	Purpose	Participants (chronological age in years, months)	Design	SGD (speech type)	Outcomes	Percentage of nonoverlapping data or zero data (%)	Appraisal
Sigafoos et al. (2005), Study 1	To determine the acquisition of requesting with SGDs and preference for specific devices	1 child: Ryan (12,0)	Multiple-baseline design across subjects	BigMac, TechTalk, Mini-Message-mate (all digitized)	Selecting a device and requesting with that device	Not calculated (see appraisal)	Inconclusive: Multiple-baseline design was run across only two subjects (minor flaw). Introducing the devices in a particular order does not rule out sequence effects. Interobserver agreement was adequate, but treatment integrity was not reported.

Study	Objective	Participants	Design	Device	Dependent variable	Percentage of nonoverlapping data	Appraisal
Sigafoos et al. (2005), Study 2	To determine the acquisition of requesting with SGDs and picture exchange and to assess any preference for one over the other	1 child: Ryan, (12,0)	Multiple-baseline design across subjects	Mini-Message-Mate (digitized)	Selecting an AAC option and requesting with that option	Percentage of nonoverlapping data was not calculated because there was no baseline and because of the appraisal	Inconclusive: No baseline prior to communication board instruction; data for instruction were not reported. Prior instruction on the board alone meant increased exposure relative to the SGD.
Son et al. (2006)	To compare acquisition of requesting behavior using a picture-exchange system versus an SGD and to evaluate the effectiveness of allowing an individual to choose his/her AAC device	3 children: Kim (5,5), Lucy (3,8), Bruce (3,0)	Alternating treatments design	TechTalk (digitized)	SGD use for requesting	Not calculated (see appraisal)	Inconclusive: An alternating treatments design does not rule out carryover effects (same symbols and referents were used across conditions)

[a]Communicative interactions in this experiment were defined as "communicating the desire to obtain a drink." Spontaneous communication interactions were described as "indicating the same desire without being questioned or prompted by others."

Key: IOA, interobserver agreement; TI, treatment integrity.

calculations because no graphic time-series data were available. Nonetheless, at first glance, this appears to be a puzzling finding. After all, several research studies have shown that once a new communicative behavior (such as activating an SGD) is introduced, previously used communicative modalities tend to diminish in frequency (Sigafoos, Drasgow, & Schlosser, 2003). In this study, however, the vocabulary introduced on the SGD was novel and thus did not simply replace vocabulary communicated through another mode. The authors also offered another explanation for this finding. They provided data showing that equal quantities of utterances were reinforced by staff regardless of whether the utterance involved SGD use (74%) or no SGD use (75%). Intermittently, the classroom staff and one unfamiliar person were also asked to rate the contextual appropriateness of SGD use. This social validation effort supported the contextual appropriateness of SGD use; however, the authors cautioned that the familiarity of three of the respondents may have led to a biased rating.

The study by Olive et al. (2007) involved three children with autism and rendered suggestive evidence that enhanced milieu teaching used to introduce an SGD resulted in fairly to highly effective results (varying across participants) for requesting with either the SGD alone or in combination with gestures. Enhanced milieu teaching is a hybrid instructional approach that involves strategies from both an interactive model (Girolametto & Weitzman, 2002) and from milieu teaching (Hancock & Kaiser, 2002).

Enhanced milieu teaching shares several common features with the naturalistic teaching strategy implemented by Schepis et al. (1998). In both approaches, preferred objects or play activities are used. Also, adult prompting is contingent on the child's behavior indications (e.g., reaching) and natural reinforcement is provided (i.e., the child gets what he or she asks for) rather than artificial reinforcement. However, there are also some important differences between these two approaches. First, in enhanced milieu teaching, the adult assumes more of a follower role by using responsive interaction strategies, such as expanding child vocalizations and imitating how a child plays with toys. Second, the adult in enhanced milieu teaching takes the lead occasionally by using shorter utterances to match the complexity of the child utterances. Hence, it is important to realize that although both of these teaching strategies were naturalistic in nature, they also differed to some extent. The primary reason that rendered the Olive et al. (2007) study "suggestive" is the absence of testing data and the use of teaching data instead.

A study of two children with autism by Sigafoos, Drasgow et al. (2004) yielded suggestive evidence that SGD use can be taught successfully (PND of 100) as a repair strategy in situations for which prelinguistic requests are not acknowledged by communication partners. Treatment involved planned ignoring of prelinguistic behaviors and least-to-most prompting in SGD use. It was also noted that once the children had acquired the repair strategy, they began using the SGD to initiate requests rather than continuing to rely on prelinguistic behaviors for this purpose. However, the overall effect on the use of SGD for requests, considering all data points including the ones before the repair strategy was acquired, was questionable.

Finally, a study by Sigafoos, O'Reilly, et al. (2004) yielded suggestive evidence that least-to-most prompting was sufficient to teach three adolescents and young adults with ASDs to locate their SGDs, turn them on, and use them to request access to preferred objects. While simple in nature, the first two of these three skills are essential for successful communication. Anyone who has ever searched for misplaced keys will appreciate the importance of being able to locate something as critical as a device that supports communication. Similarly, the operational competence associated with being able to turn on one's own device has ramifications for both independence and self determination. Individuals who master this skill are in a position to communicate with their SGDs whenever they see fit, rather than having to rely on a teacher or caregiver to turn the device on for them.

Based on the suggestive evidence from three of these studies, it seems plausible that treatment packages involving SGDs can be used to improve a variety of communicative functions and behaviors in children with ASDs. Such behaviors include SGD use as a repair strategy, to request objects and activities, and to engage in communicative interactions with caregivers. Because each of the three studies involved different independent variables (i.e., different treatment packages) and different dependent variables, the PND values were not aggregated across studies.

SGD Studies that Isolated the Effects of Speech Output

In several studies, researchers attempted to isolate the specific effect of providing access to speech output during an intervention. The targeted outcome variables included spelling (Schlosser, Blischak, Belfiore, Bartley, & Barnett, 1998; Schlosser & Blischak, 2004), speech production (Parsons & LaSorte, 1993; Schlosser et al., 2007), and requesting (Schlosser et al., 2007; Sigafoos, Didden, & O'Reilly, 2003). Each of these studies is summarized in Table 5.3. Again, only studies that yielded suggestive or better evidence are discussed here.

Table 5.3. Studies on the effects of speech output as an independent variable: Summary and appraisal

Study	Purpose	Participants (chronological age in years, months)	Design	SGD (speech type)	Outcomes	Percentage of nonoverlapping data or zero data (%)	Appraisal
Schlosser & Blischak (2004)	To evaluate the effects of speech output and orthographic feedback on spelling performance (replication)	4 children: Scott (8,0), Fred (12,0), Justin (9,0), Carl (12,0)	Adapted alternating treatments design	Light-WRITER SL35; synthetic speech	Words spelled correctly with speech feedback	Scott (83) Fred (93) Justin (91) Carl (77)	Conclusive: Sound design, IOA and TI are solid.
					Words spelled correctly with speech–print feedback	Scott (83) Fred (93) Justin (86) Carl (68)	
					Words spelled correctly with print feedback	Scott (100) Fred (93) Justin (91) Carl (63)	
Schlosser et al. (1998)	To evaluate the effects of speech output and orthographic feedback on spelling performance	1 child: Martin (10,0)	Adapted alternating treatments design	Light-WRITER SL35; synthetic speech	Words spelled correctly speech	Michael (100)	Conclusive: Sound design; IOA and TI are solid
					Words spelled correctly speech–print	Michael (84)	
					Words spelled correctly print feedback	Michael (84)	

156

Schlosser et al. (2007)	To evaluate the effects of speech output (with and without) on requesting and elicited vocalizations	5 children: Avery (9,0), Greg (8,0), Matthew (10,0), Michael (8,0), Zachary (10,0)	Adapted alternating treatments design	Vantage; synthetic speech	Requesting with speech on	Avery (65) Greg (32) Matthew (31) Michael (33) Zachary (45)	Preponderant: Strong design, strong IOA and TI; however, training was not continued until the learning criterion was reached.
					Requesting with speech off	Avery (2) Greg (30) Matthew (3) Michael (76) Zachary (80)	
					Elicited vocalization with speech on	Avery (0) Greg (0) Matthew (0) Michael (19) Zachary (0)	
					Elicited vocalizations with speech off	Avery (0) Greg (0) Matthew (0) Michael (5) Zachary (0)	

(Continued)

157

Table 5.3. *(continued)*

Study	Purpose	Participants (chronological age in years, months)	Design	SGD (speech type)	Outcomes	Percentage of nonoverlapping data or zero data (%)	Appraisal
Parsons & LaSorte (1993)	To compare spontaneous utterances using computer-assisted instruction with versus without synthesized speech	6 children: S1 (4,8), S2 (5,1), S3 (5,8), 4 (6,2), 5 (6,7), 6 (6,8)	A-B-BCB-BC and ABC-B-BC (additive and reductive)	Apple II GS + software; synthetic speech	Spontaneous utterances with speech on Spontaneous utterances with speech off	S1 (83) S2 (75) S3 (100) S4 (100) S5 (50) S6 (92) S1 (0) S2 (0) S3 (9) S4 (0) S5 (0) S6 (0)	Suggestive: Speech design was mapped onto intervention design; cannot rule out between-group order effects; no TI
Sigafoos, Didden, et al. (2003)	To evaluate the effects of speech output on the maintenance of requesting following the acquisition of requesting with an SGD	2 children: Michael (13,0), Jason (4,0)	Alternating treatments design	BIGmack; digitized speech	Requesting with speech on Requesting with speech off Vocalizations with speech on Vocalizations with speech off	Not calculated (see appraisal) Not calculated (see appraisal) Not calculated (see appraisal, plus baseline ceiling effect) Not calculated (see appraisal, plus baseline ceiling effect)	Inconclusive: Use of the same symbols and object referents across conditions did not control for carry-over.

Key: IOA, interobserver agreement; SGD, speech-generating device; TI, treatment integrity.

158

Spelling   Some SGDs provide not only the opportunity for additional auditory input and feedback through speech output (digitized or synthesized), but also the possibility to add visual input and/or feedback via liquid crystal displays (LCDs). Determining which feedback mode is most effective and efficient for a learner has implications for how to program an SGD for optimal use. Using an adapted alternating treatments design, two studies examined the effects of three feedback conditions (speech, print from the LCD, and speech plus print) on spelling (Schlosser et al., 1998; Schlosser & Blischak, 2004). In the speech condition, participants received auditory feedback from synthesized speech after each letter that was entered and after the whole word was completed, following activation of the Enter button. In the print condition, learners received visual feedback from the LCD display alone, following each letter and word entered. Finally, in the speech plus print condition, learners received both kinds of feedback.

The two studies provide conclusive evidence that the copy–cover–compare instructional method was effective across all three feedback conditions; all participants achieved the criteria (Schlosser et al., 1998; Schlosser & Blischak, 2004). The PND data (see Table 5.3) revealed that one participant seemed to do better with print feedback alone, two other participants did best with speech feedback alone, and another two participants did equally well across all three conditions. Thus, regardless of feedback mode, the learners all demonstrated acquisition of new spelling words. However, based on the differential number of trials to criteria that were used as a measure of learning efficiency, the authors suggested two distinct learning profiles. Learners who exemplified the *visual profile* spelled words most efficiently when the feedback involved print, whereas learners who exemplified the *auditory profile* spelled words most efficiently when feedback involved speech. Based on this evidence, it seems that the most effective feedback mode will vary across individuals and—like AAC in general—one size does not fit all.

Requesting   One study that rendered preponderant evidence examined the effects of teaching five children with autism to request preferred objects with an SGD in two conditions—speech on and speech off (Schlosser et al., 2007). The teaching method for assisting the children to request was kept constant; the only difference was the presence or absence of synthesized speech output. The authors concluded that the children requested more as a result of intervention, but that there was no consistent pattern of effectiveness with regard to speech output. PND calculations suggest that two children were more effective with speech output, two children were more effective without speech output, and one child did equally well in both conditions. Over-all, however, the PND levels of the more successful condition ranged from questionable effectiveness in one participant (50%–70%) to unreliable effectiveness in the other four (<50%).

A number of variables might have contributed to the low acquisition levels in this study. First, the children were taught arbitrary symbols that bore no resemblance to their referents. Second, the location of the symbols was randomized across exposures, to separate true learning from position-based learning. Third, teaching trials were separated temporally from testing trials. These conditions differ from many previous requesting studies and, although highly desirable from a scientific perspective, they may have increased task difficulty beyond a desirable level, especially given the length of implementation and the density of the treatment schedule.

A second study investigated the effects of speech output on the maintenance of requesting in two children with autism (Sigafoos, Didden, et al., 2003). In other words, the authors examined whether speech output was necessary to maintain requesting after requesting had been acquired with an SGD. Maintenance levels of requesting were above baseline in both conditions, with only small differences between the two. For one participant, maintenance was in the range of questionable effectiveness in both conditions, but was 12.5% better with the speech off than with the speech on. For the other participant, maintenance levels were in the fairly effective range across both conditions, with requesting maintained 12% better with the speech on compared to speech off. These findings should be viewed rather cautiously because the use of the same symbols and object referents in both conditions made it impossible to rule out carry-over effects from one condition to the other.

Speech Production   Two studies examined the effects of speech output (on or off) on speech production during SGD instruction. In a study by Parsons and LaSorte (1993) that yielded suggestive evidence, six learners with autism produced more spontaneous vocalizations when working with software that provided speech output (PND of 50%–100%) compared to software that did not provide speech output (PND of 0% for five learners and 9% for one learner). In a study by Schlosser et al. (2007) rendering preponderant evidence, five children were taught to request preferred objects with an SGD in two conditions (speech on and off, as described earlier) and the effects on elicited vocalizations were monitored. Four of the children remained at 0% for vocalizations, even after intervention. The one child made minimal or unreliable gains; he was also the only child with preexisting vocal imitation skills.

Taken together, these two studies present seemingly contradictory findings. A closer look, however, suggests that a number of methodological differences—either individually or collectively—could account for these discrepant results. In the Parsons and LaSorte (1993) study, all speech productions were counted; in the Schlosser et al. (2007) study, only vocalizations that were directly related to the specific objects the participants had been taught to request with the SGD were counted. In the Parsons and LaSorte (1993) study, the vocalizations counted were spontaneous, whereas in the Schlosser et al. (2007) study, they were elicited. In the Parsons and LaSorte (1993) study, the children were not taught a communicative function with the SGD, but in the Schlosser et al. (2007) study, they were taught requesting. Little information was provided about the preexisting vocal imitation skills of the learners in the Parsons and LaSorte (1993) study, whereas preassessment data in this regard were provided in the Schlosser et al. (2007) study. There were numerous other differences as well; therefore, it is clearly premature to draw implications for practice from these two studies combined.

One additional study examined the effects of speech output on vocalizations during the maintenance phase (Sigafoos, Didden, et al., 2003). Specifically, the investigators monitored speech production when the speech was on or off while the child was making requests with an SGD. Unfortunately, the design did not permit the control of carry-over effects between the speech-on and speech-off conditions. In addition, the participant's high baseline performance made it impossible to demonstrate an effect; in fact, a baseline ceiling effect precluded any calculation of the outcome metric as it would have rendered an automatic PND of 0%. Thus, this study should not impact clinical decision making with regard to speech production concurrent with SGD use.

IMPLICATIONS FOR CLINICAL AND EDUCATIONAL PRACTICE

Based on evidence concerning the use of treatment packages involving SGDs and the specific effects of speech output, it seems imperative that SGDs not be discounted as a viable AAC option for children with ASDs. The common practice of automatically excluding speech output as an option for beginning communicators (both with and without ASDs) appears to be grounded in the widely held belief that these individuals tend to process visual stimuli more readily than auditory stimuli, as discussed earlier. However, the evidence suggests that is plausible that the introduction of SGDs using a variety of treatment packages can yield a range of communicative outcomes with these children. In fact, as some of the studies in which speech output was isolated as an independent variable have shown, it may be much more productive to view the processing strengths of children with ASDs relative to specific task demands (such as spelling; see Schlosser & Blischak, 2004) rather than in general. For example, with regard to spelling, the research indicates that some learners do better when feedback is provided primarily in the visual modality, whereas others are more successful when auditory feedback is provided. Based on this evidence, practitioners are advised to view the evidence presented here as a call for individualized assessment to determine which feedback mode seems to work best for a given individual under varying circumstances. Brief implementation of an adapted alternating treatment design might lend itself to such an assessment.

Based on the evidence reviewed here, some practitioners might feel relieved to learn that the introduction of an SGD does not seem to result in extinction of other valued communication modalities. Certainly, the work of Schepis et al. (1998) demonstrated that this was not the case. At the same time, the evidence also indicates that when communication modalities are not viable—as is the case with inconsistently used and/or idiosyncratic prelinguistic modes—SGDs can successfully replace these behaviors as long as the new communicative behaviors serve the same function as the existing ones (Sigafoos, Drasgow, et al., 2004).

Overall, the "bottom-line" recommendation is that SGDs are viable options for individuals with ASDs who require AAC. The available evidence, although limited, is nonetheless sufficient to conclude that SGD use can be taught to individuals with ASDs. Effective procedures for teaching SGD use include a number of empirically validated instructional techniques. Specifically, the evidence suggests that interventions to teach SGD use should 1) create opportunities for communication, 2) use response and stimulus prompts to occasion SGD use, 3) systematically fade these prompts over successive opportunities, and 4) provide differential reinforcement for SGD use.

This systematic instructional package can often promote rapid acquisition of SGD use. For example, Sigafoos, O'Reilly, et al. (2004) reported that 20 minutes of instruction was sufficient to teach three adolescents and young adults to use an SGD to request access to preferred objects. The acquisition teaching procedures used in this study involved creating opportunities for requesting by offering highly preferred objects. Once the item was offered, the researchers waited for the individuals to demonstrate a behavioral indication (i.e., reaching for the item). As an individual reached for an item, the researchers prompted him or her to touch the corresponding panel on the SGD. Prompting consisted of moving the person's hand to the panel using the least amount of physical guidance necessary. Over subsequent opportunities, the prompt was faded by delaying the physical guidance. Each time the individual selected the correct panel on the SGD, he or she received access to the preferred item. Using these procedures, all three participants reached the acquisition criterion (10 independent, correct responses within a 5-minute session) within 20 minutes of training.

Another area of practical concern is selecting an appropriate AAC option for individuals with ASDs. Some preliminary research suggests that these individuals may prefer to use SGDs over alternative low-tech options, such as picture exchange (Sigafoos et al., 2005), although this does not seem to be true of all learners (Son et al., 2006). Because there may be individual differences in preference for various AAC options, it would seem important for clinicians to assess an individual's preference for the use of an SGD over other AAC options, such as manual signs or picture exchange. Doing so will enable individuals to exert some control and self-determination with respect to AAC system selection.

Sigafoos et al. (2005) described a potentially promising methodology for enabling students with disabilities to indicate their preference for communication devices. The approach involves first teaching the individuals to use each communication device to a high and equal level of proficiency. Following this initial exposure and acquisition phase, opportunities to communicate are created, but the individual must first select from among the previously acquired AAC options. To date, this "teach and choose" approach has been used to assess preferences that range from SGDs to low-tech communication boards to picture exchange systems (Sigafoos et al., 2005; Son et al., 2006). This approach is a potentially useful methodology that might enable students with ASDs and other developmental disabilities to participate in communication device selection. However, it is unclear whether this approach could be adapted to assess preferences between, for example, manual signs and SGDs.

DIRECTIONS FOR FUTURE RESEARCH

Great strides have been made in empirically examining the effects of SGDs and speech output for children with ASDs. Nonetheless, there are still many areas that require future research. For example, while the data show that SGD use can be rapidly acquired, most studies to date have focused on teaching behavior regulation functions, such as requesting access to preferred objects or activities. Of course, requesting access to preferred objects and activities is a functional and important skill; however, communication does not end with having ones wants and needs met. It remains to be determined if individuals with ASDs can be taught to use SGDs for accomplishing social communicative functions, such as initiating greetings or commenting on the environment. Future research should focus on developing and evaluating procedures to extend the functional benefits of SGDs.

Similarly, the effects of specific treatment packages involving SGDs and the effects of speech output on speech production are still unclear. Although speech production is not the primary aim of AAC intervention, it remains an important and desirable outcome for many AAC stakeholders. Although there are no studies showing a decline in speech production concurrent with SGD use, little is known about the extent to which SGD and speech output use promotes speech production; the only study to date in this regard provided equivocal outcomes (Olive et al., 2007). Similarly, the only two studies that examined the specific effects of synthesized speech output on speech production presented contradictory findings (Parsons & LaSorte, 1993; Schlosser et al., 2007); a number of important procedural and methodological differences could explain these different outcomes, as discussed earlier.

For future research to advance the existing knowledge base, it is imperative to develop lines of research within which the dependent variable (i.e., speech production) is defined in the same way. In addition, the teaching procedures used in these studies should be either held constant or varied systematically to allow meaningful comparisons and aggregation across studies. For example, even though many of the existing studies focused on requesting as an outcome, they could not be aggregated because the interventions varied considerably (e.g., from functional communication training to enhanced milieu teaching). Similarly, to devise these lines of research, future studies should be theoretically grounded. Toward this end, Blischak, Lombardino, and Dyson (2003) offered several compelling theoretical reasons why speech output might benefit natural speech production.

The evidence to date is based exclusively on single-subject experimental design methodology. The strengths of this methodology include a generally more comprehensive description of individual participants (compared to group studies) and the fact that individual performance differences tend to be revealed more readily. Thus, we know that SGD use and speech output seem to work better for some individuals than for others—an often-observed phenomenon, especially with adapted alternating treatment designs that involve a comparison of two or more interventions (Yoder & Compton, 2004). Future research should be directed to identify participant characteristics that serve as predictors of treatment outcomes using group designs. Specifically, the use of randomized control trials and growth curve analyses based on participant characteristics, as exemplified by Yoder and Stone (2006a, 2006b), could guide future research on SGDs.

Finally, the continued comparison of treatment approaches using SGDs versus other beginning communication strategies such as the Picture Exchange Communication System represents another critical area for future research. Such direct comparisons have the potential to illuminate the benefits (if any) of having early access to speech output for functional communication purposes. Along these same lines, it might be possible to promote greater self-determination in AAC system selection by setting up choice-making opportunities so that the individuals can choose which AAC system (e.g., SGD versus manual sign versus picture exchange) he or she prefers to use.

LIMITATIONS

In this chapter, each study met specific criteria for inclusion and data were extracted systematically—whenever possible, by consistently applying a metric of effectiveness. Nonetheless, there are a number of important limitations to this review (see Schlosser, Wendt, & Sigafoos, 2007) of which the reader should be aware. First, although the studies were drawn from previously conducted systematic reviews, a new systematic search for evidence was not conducted. Hence, a few studies may be missing from this discussion. Second, interrater agreement on inclusion and data extraction was not collected, so the reliability of the process is unknown. Finally, several of the studies were implemented by two of the authors of this chapter; therefore, some bias may be present.

CONCLUSIONS

Based on the appraised evidence concerning the use of treatment packages involving SGDs and the evidence concerning the specific effects of speech output, SGDs are a viable and effective AAC option for individuals with ASDs. However, future research is needed to more fully understand the range of benefits associated with SGD use and speech output.

REFERENCES

Allen, J., Hunnicutt, S., & Klatt, D.H. (1987). *From text to speech: The MITalk system.* Cambridge, England: Cambridge University Press.
Beukelman, D.R., & Mirenda, P. (2005). *Augmentative and alternative communication: Supporting children and adults with complex communication needs* (3rd ed.). Baltimore: Paul H. Brookes Publishing Co.

Blischak, D.M., Lombardino, L., & Dyson, A. (2003). Use of speech-generating devices: In support of natural speech. *Augmentative and Alternative Communication, 19,* 29–35.

Bornman, J., & Alant, E. (1999). Training teachers to facilitate interaction with autistic children using digital voice output devices. *South African Journal of Education, 19,* 364–373.

Brady, N.C. (2000). Improved comprehension of object names following voice output communication aid use: Two case studies. *Augmentative and Alternative Communication, 16,* 197–204.

Bruckert, E. (1984, Jan./Feb.). A new text-to-speech product produces dynamic human quality voice. *Speech Technology, 2,* 114–119.

Carr, E.G., Binkoff, J.A., Kologinsky, E., & Eddy, M. (1978). Acquisition of sign language by autistic children: I. Expressive labeling. *Journal of Applied Behavior Analysis, 11,* 489–501.

Duffy, S.A., & Pisoni, D.B. (1992). Comprehension of synthetic speech produced by rule: A review and theoretical interpretation. *Language and Speech, 35,* 351–389.

Durand, V.M. (1999). Functional communication training using assistive devices: Recruiting natural communities of reinforcement. *Journal of Applied Behavior Analysis, 32,* 247–367.

Dyches, T.T. (1998). Effects of switch training on the communication of children with autism and severe disabilities. *Focus on Autism and Other Developmental Disabilities, 13,* 151–162.

Frost, L.A., & Bondy, A.S. (2002). *The Picture Exchange Communication System training manual* (2nd ed.). Newark, DE: Pyramid Educational Consultants.

Girolametto, L., & Weitzman, E. (2002). Responsiveness of child-care providers in interactions with toddlers and preschoolers. *Language, Speech, and Hearing Services in Schools, 33,* 268–280.

Granlund, M., & Olsson, C. (1999). Efficacy of communication intervention for presymbolic communicators. *Augmentative and Alternative Communication, 15,* 25–37.

Hancock, T.B., & Kaiser, A.P. (2002). The effects of trainer implemented enhanced milieu teaching on the social communication of children with autism. *Topics in Early Childhood Special Education, 22,* 39–54.

Koul, R.K. (2003). Perception of synthetic speech in individuals with and without disabilities. *Augmentative and Alternative Communication, 19,* 49–58.

Koul, R.K., & Allen, G.D. (1993). Segmental intelligibility and speech interference thresholds of high quality synthetic speech in the presence of noise. *Journal of Speech and Hearing Research, 36,* 790–798.

Koul, R.K., & Clapsaddle, K. (2006). Effects of repeated listening experiences on the recognition of synthetic speech by individuals with mild to moderate intellectual disabilities. *Augmentative and Alternative Communication, 22,* 112–122.

Koul, R.K., & Hester, K. (2006). Effects of repeated listening experiences on the recognition of synthetic speech by individuals with severe intellectual disabilities. *Journal of Speech-Language and Hearing Research, 49,* 47–57.

Light, J.C., Roberts, B., Dimarco, R., & Greiner, N. (1998). Augmentative and alternative communication to support receptive and expressive communication for people with autism. *Journal of Communication Disorders, 31,* 153–180.

Lloyd, L.L., Fuller, D.R., & Arvidson, H.H. (Eds.). (1997). *Augmentative and alternative communication: A handbook of principles and practices.* Boston: Allyn & Bacon.

Millar, D., Light, J.C., & Schlosser, R.W. (2006). The impact of augmentative and alternative communication intervention on the speech production of individuals with developmental disabilities: A research review. *Journal of Speech, Language, and Hearing Research, 49,* 248–264.

Mirenda, P., & Beukelman, D.R. (1987). A comparison of speech synthesis intelligibility with listeners from three age groups. *Augmentative and Alternative Communication, 3,* 120–128.

Mirenda, P., & Schuler, A. (1988). Augmenting communication for persons with autism: Issues and strategies. *Topics in Language Disorders, 9,* 24–43.

Mirenda, P., Wilk, D., & Carson, P. (2000). A retrospective analysis of technology use patterns in students with autism over a five-year period. *Journal of Special Education Technology, 15,* 5–16.

Olive, M., de la Cruz, B., Davis, T.N., Chan, J.M., Lang, R.B., O'Reilly, M.F., & Dickson, S.M. (2007). The effects of enhanced milieu teaching and a voice output communication aid on the requesting of three children with autism. *Journal of Autism and Developmental Disorders, 37,* 1505–1513.

Parsons, C.L., & La Sorte, D. (1993). The effect of computers with synthesized speech and no speech on the spontaneous communication of children with autism. *Australian Journal of Human Communication Disorders, 21,* 12–31.

Peeters, T., & Gillberg, C. (1999). *Autism: Medical and educational aspects.* London: Whurr.

Romski, M.A., & Sevcik, R.A. (1996). *Breaking the speech barrier: Language development through augmented means.* Baltimore: Paul H. Brookes Publishing Co.

Schepis, M.M., Reid, D.H., Behrmann, M.M., & Sutton, K.A. (1998). Increasing communicative interactions of young children with autism using a voice output communication aid and naturalistic teaching. *Journal of Applied Behavior Analysis, 31,* 561–578.

Schlosser, R.W. (2003). Roles of speech output in augmentative and alternative communication: Narrative review. *Augmentative and Alternative Communication, 19,* 5–28.

Schlosser, R.W., & Blischak, D.M. (2001). Is there a role for speech output in interventions for persons with autism? A review. *Focus on Autism and Other Developmental Disabilities, 16,* 170–178.

Schlosser, R.W., & Blischak, D.M. (2004). Effects of speech and print feedback on spelling in children with autism. *Journal of Speech, Language and Hearing Research, 47,* 848–862.

Schlosser, R.W., Blischak, D.M., Belfiore, P.J., Bartley, C., & Barnett, N. (1998). The effects of synthetic speech output and orthographic feedback on spelling in a student with autism: A preliminary study. *Journal of Autism and Developmental Disorders, 28,* 319–329.

Schlosser, R.W., & Sigafoos, J. (2006). Augmentative and alternative communication interventions for persons with developmental disabilities: Narrative review of comparative single-subject experimental studies. *Research in Developmental Disabilities, 27,* 1–29.

Schlosser, R.W., Sigafoos, J., Luiselli, J., Angermeier, K., Schooley, K., Harasymowyz, U., & Belfiore, J. (2007). Effects of synthetic speech output on requesting and natural speech production in children with autism. *Research in Autism Spectrum Disorders, 1,* 139–163.

Schlosser, R.W., Wendt, O., & Sigafoos, J. (2007). Not all systematic reviews are created equal: Considerations for appraisal. *Evidence-Based Communication Assessment and Intervention, 1,* 138–150.

Schuler, A.L., & Baldwin, M. (1981). Nonspeech communication and childhood autism. *Language, Speech, and Hearing Services in Schools, 12,* 246–257.

Scotti, J.R., Evans, I.M., Meyer, L.H., & Walker, P. (1991). A meta analysis of intervention research with problem behavior: Treatment validity and standards of practice. *American Journal on Mental Retardation, 96,* 233–256.

Scruggs, T.E., Mastropieri, M.A., & Casto, G. (1987). The quantitative synthesis of single subject research methodology: Methodology and validation. *Remedial and Special Education, 8,* 24–33.

Scruggs, T.E., Mastropieri, M.A., Cook, S.B., & Escobar, C. (1986). Early intervention for children with conduct disorders: A quantitative synthesis of single-subject research. *Behavioral Disorders, 11,* 260–271.

Sigafoos, J., Didden, R., & O'Reilly, M. (2003). Effects of speech output on maintenance of requesting and frequency of vocalizations in three children with developmental disabilities. *Augmentative and Alternative Communication, 19,* 37–47.

Sigafoos, J., Drasgow, E., Halle, J.W., O'Reilly, M.O., Seely-York, S., Edrisinha, C., & Andrews, A. (2004). Teaching VOCA use as a communicative repair strategy. *Journal of Autism and Developmental Disorders, 34,* 411–422.

Sigafoos, J., Drasgow, E., & Schlosser, R.W. (2003). Strategies for beginning communicators. In R.W. Schlosser (Ed.), *The efficacy of augmentative and alternative communication: Towards evidence-based practice* (pp. 324–346). San Diego: Academic Press.

Sigafoos, J., O'Reilly, M., Ganz, J., Lancioni, G., & Schlosser, R.W. (2005). Supporting self-determination in AAC interventions by assessing preference for communication devices. *Technology & Disability, 17,* 143–153.

Sigafoos, J., O'Reilly, M., Seely-York, S., & Edrisinha, C. (2004). Teaching students with developmental disabilities to locate their AAC device. *Research in Developmental Disabilities, 25,* 371–383.

Son, S.H., Sigafoos, J., O'Reilly, M., & Lancioni, G.E. (2006). Comparing two types of augmentative and alternative communication for children with autism. *Pediatric Rehabilitation, 9,* 389–395.

Thunberg, G., Ahlsen, E., & Dahlgren Sandberg, A. (2007). Children with autistic spectrum disorders and speech generating devices: Communication in different activities at home. *Clinical Linguistics and Phonetics, 21,* 457–479.

Wendt, O. (2006). *The effectiveness of augmentative and alternative communication for individuals with autism spectrum disorders: A systematic review and meta-analysis* [doctoral dissertation]. West Lafayette, IN: Purdue University.

Venkatagiri, H.S., & Ramabadran, T. (1995). Digital speech synthesis: A tutorial. *Augmentative and Alternative Communication, 11,* 14–25.

Willis, L.H., Koul, R.K., & Paschall, D.D. (2000). Discourse comprehension of synthetic speech by individuals with mental retardation. *Education and Training in Mental Retardation and Developmental Disabilities, 35,* 106–114.

Yoder, P.J., & Compton, D. (2004). Identifying predictors of treatment response. *Mental Retardation and Developmental Disabilities Research Reviews, 10,* 162–168.

Yoder, P.J., & Stone, W.L. (2006a). A randomized comparison of the effect of two prelinguistic communication interventions on the acquisition of spoken communication in preschoolers with ASD. *Journal of Speech, Language, and Hearing Research, 49,* 698–711.

Yoder, P.J., & Stone, W.L. (2006b). Randomized comparison of two communication interventions for preschoolers with autism spectrum disorders. *Journal of Consulting and Clinical Psychology, 74,* 426–435.

6

Effects of AAC on the Natural Speech Development of Individuals with Autism Spectrum Disorders

DIANE C. MILLAR

Recent reports have suggested that approximately 1 in 150 children are diagnosed with an autism spectrum disorder (ASD; Centers for Disease Control and Prevention, 2007). Some have estimated that as many as one half of individuals with autism never develop speech to the level that they are functionally able to use it as an adequate means of communication (National Research Council, 2001; Wing & Attwood, 1987). Despite current eligibility models that support the practice of providing augmentative and alternative communication (AAC) to individuals with a discrepancy between their communication needs and abilities (e.g., Zangari & Kangas, 1997), many individuals with autism who are unable to use speech as their primary means of communication are denied access to such supports.

A decision to introduce AAC is contentious with regard to young children with ASDs, perhaps more so than for children with other developmental disabilities. Unlike children with significant physical impairments (e.g., cerebral palsy), many children with ASDs present with gross and fine motor abilities that appear to be comparable to their typically developing peers, although research suggests that

subtle but important motor planning and/or coordination impairments may be present (Baranek, Parham, & Bodfish, 2005). In the
absence of obvious physical impairments to account for a lack of
speech, many parents believe their children would be considered typically developing if they would simply "choose" to speak (Lord & Paul,
1997). In addition, many parents and professionals believe that they
have to choose between pursuing either speech or AAC—but not
both—with children with ASDs. As a result, they often adopt a "wait
and see" approach for children who have yet to acquire functional
speech and language, out of concern that AAC may become a "crutch"
or that it might even inhibit development in these areas (e.g.,
Beukelman, 1987; Cress & Marvin, 2003; Dowden & Marriner, 1995;
Zangari & Kangas, 1997). Exacerbating the hesitancy to introduce
AAC, many children with ASDs demonstrate echolalia. Their abilities
to echo adult syntactic forms of language using speech may reinforce
decisions to delay the introduction of AAC because speech is thought
to be emerging. However, although some authors have suggested that
many children with ASDs who eventually develop functional speech
go through a period of echolalia, this is not a proven predictor of functional speech potential (National Research Council, 2001).

The hesitancy to introduce AAC to children with ASDs is understandable; nevertheless, there are serious risks in delaying children's
access to functional communication. If speech is the only mode of
communication made available to young children with ASDs but it
does not satisfy their communication needs, the children are likely to
experience difficulty acquiring language, building social relationships,
and meeting educational goals (Light, Collier, & Parnes, 1985). Moreover, without access to communication, children often develop problem behaviors (e.g., self-injurious behaviors, aggression) in response to
their frustration with the inability to communicate (National Research
Council, 2001).

The benefits of AAC for improving the receptive and expressive
language skills and the communicative competence of individuals with
developmental disabilities have clearly been documented (e.g., Light,
Binger, Agate, & Ramsay, 1999; Light, Roberts, DiMarco, & Greiner,
1998; Romski & Sevcik, 1996). Furthermore, research has demonstrated
that AAC can be highly effective in reducing challenging behaviors. For
example, the use of both functional communication training that incorporates AAC and visual schedules that use graphic symbols have been
well supported in the literature (e.g., Bopp, Brown, & Mirenda, 2004;
Mirenda, 1997, 2001). In addition, some authors have argued that AAC
techniques (especially graphic symbols) are particularly suited to the
unique learning challenges faced by individuals with ASDs because
they enable language to be presented in a visual format that is both

static and predictable, as well as minimize the need for complex motor movements and motor planning (National Research Council, 2001).

Several researchers have also proposed that AAC may enhance speech production in individuals with developmental disabilities and significant speech impairments by reducing the motor and cognitive demands associated with speech production (Lloyd & Kangas, 1994; Romski & Sevcik, 1996). Similarly, others have argued that AAC may reduce the pressure placed on individuals to produce speech; this reduction in the stress related to speech production may indirectly facilitate speech development (Lloyd & Kangas, 1994). Finally, others have proposed that the behavioral theory of automatic reinforcement may explain why the introduction of AAC may result in increased speech (Mirenda, 2003). According to the principle of automatic reinforcement, if AAC and speech are presented together (e.g., a manual sign representing COOKIE along with the spoken label) and then followed by a reinforcer (e.g., a cookie), the frequency of both the AAC mode and the spoken label should increase.

Given the potential advantages of introducing AAC to children with ASDs who are unable to meet their communication needs via speech and the potential negative consequences of withholding access to communication, it is imperative that parents and professionals are familiar with published research documenting the relationship between AAC and natural speech development in individuals with ASDs. This chapter will focus on a discussion of this research, its clinical implications, and directions for future research in this area.

THE EFFECTS OF AAC ON THE SPEECH OF INDIVIDUALS WITH DEVELOPMENTAL DISABILITIES

Although there has been a great deal of speculation about the impact of AAC on the speech development of individuals with developmental disabilities, few research studies have specifically studied this relationship (e.g., Yoder & Layton, 1988). In part, this paucity of research may exist because the purpose of implementing AAC is to enhance communication, not to improve speech production (Beukelman & Mirenda, 2005). Enhanced speech production is usually viewed as a "bonus" side effect of AAC use rather than as a primary goal.

Two reviews of the literature documenting changes in speech production with the introduction of AAC have been completed to date. The first, published by Silverman (1995), reported a review of over 100 published and unpublished reports. His conclusion was that there appeared to be a positive relationship between AAC and natural speech production in many children and adults (i.e., at least 40% of the individuals included in the reviewed literature). However, an examination of the primary sources included in the review reveals a number of limitations that may preclude Silverman's conclusions, including a lack of description of the inclusion criteria and search procedures used, as well as the absence of references for approximately two thirds of the 100 reports that were included in the review. Furthermore, the analysis of data that were extracted from a number of the published studies was inaccurate. Finally, the majority of the studies in the review were published prior to 1982, rendering it outdated in light of the many technological advances in AAC and improvements in research design that have occurred since that time.

The second review was aimed at contributing to evidence-based decision making by parents and professionals who are considering the introduction of AAC to individuals with developmental disabilities (Millar, Light, & Schlosser, 2006). Even though many of the individuals included in the review did not have ASDs, a discussion of the effects of AAC on the natural speech development of individuals with developmental disabilities in general is also relevant and is described in the following sections.

Inclusion Criteria and Search Procedures

Studies that were included in the Millar et al. (2006) review met a number of criteria: 1) published between 1975 and 2003; 2) involved individuals with developmental disabilities and significant speech impairments that prevented them from meeting their daily communication needs; 3) included implementation of AAC; 4) documented progress of the participants' acquisition of the use of AAC; and 5) provided data on speech production for participants before, during, and/or after AAC intervention. Studies that included individuals with a primary hearing impairment were excluded because these individuals are typically not considered candidates for AAC intervention (American Speech-Language-Hearing Association, 1991). In addition, studies that included individuals with acquired disorders were excluded because speech recovery (e.g., after stroke or brain injury) is very different from speech development in individuals who never acquire speech as a primary means of communication.

A combination of search methods was used to locate studies that met the inclusion criteria. These included electronic searches of various research databases (e.g., PsycINFO), hand searches and electronic searches of the tables of contents of 46 journals that typically include articles on AAC, and ancestral searches of references cited in studies that met the inclusion criteria. A coding system based on Schlosser and Lee's (2000) meta-analysis was developed to facilitate comparisons across studies. Coding categories included variables such as the number and characteristics of participants, the goal(s) of the study, the research design, and the type of AAC intervention that was implemented.

Results of Search

The search yielded a total of 23 studies that met the inclusion criteria. Of these, 8 were descriptive case studies, 14 were single-subject experimental designs, and 1 was a group pretest-posttest design. There were 67 participants included in the 23 studies; 40% had intellectual disabilities, 31% had autism, and the remainder had various other developmental disabilities (e.g., cerebral palsy). The goal of the majority of studies was to increase expressive vocabulary; 44% of these studies specifically targeted single words and 26% targeted word combinations. The remainder of the studies aimed to teach communicative functions, such as requesting. A total of 61% of the studies introduced unaided AAC interventions (i.e., manual signs), 31% implemented aided AAC without speech output, one study (4%) used a combination of aided AAC with speech output and aided AAC without speech output, and one study (4%) implemented a combination of unaided and aided AAC without speech output.

Best Evidence Results

The quality of the evidence presented in each of the studies was evaluated based on Slavin's (1986) approach to analyzing studies in the absence of a formal meta-analysis. For each study, the methodological rigor and quality of data were reviewed with regard to the relationship between AAC and speech production. Unfortunately, the majority of studies did not evaluate this relationship as a primary dependent variable; rather, data on speech production were often collected as secondary or collateral measures. Therefore, a decision was made to focus on six studies in which researchers did establish experimental control between the AAC intervention and speech production for at least some of the participants. Although these studies lacked data on treatment integrity, they were considered the to be the best available evidence and were the focus of subsequent analyses of the investigation of the effects of AAC on natural speech development.

Participants   There were 17 participants included in the six "best evidence" studies. Four of the 17 participants had autism and 13 had intellectual disabilities, Down syndrome, or developmental delay; 6 of these 13 also had a hearing impairment. Some of the participants were involved in more than one treatment condition (e.g., manual signing and manual signing with positive reinforcement). Because speech production may have varied depending on the treatment condition, each individual's involvement in each treatment was considered as a separate case, resulting in a total of 27 cases across the six studies.

AAC Interventions   Five of the six studies included manual signs. Only one study included aided AAC without speech output; no studies included AAC with speech output. The interventions varied in length, with a mean length of 42 sessions (range, 4–206 sessions). Of the 27 cases, the majority (78%) used a highly structured, clinician-directed format. Only 22% of the cases included child-centered play activities.

Changes in Speech Production   Of the 27 cases in the best evidence group, 89% (24 cases) demonstrated increases in speech production. In the remaining three cases, there was no change in speech production. None of the 27 cases indicated a decrease in speech production as a result of AAC intervention. Of the 24 cases in which there were increases, 12 measured single-word productions (the mean gain was 13 words, with a range of 1–52 words), six measured two-word combinations (the mean gain was 6 two-word phrases, with a range of 4–7 two-word phrases), and six measured the percentage of opportunities in which the participants produced words or word approximations (the mean gain was 77%, with a range of 40%–100%).

In 17 of the 27 cases, ceiling effects were observed in measuring speech production; this suggests that the observed gains may have been limited by the design of the study. Finally, in 19 of the 24 cases in which there was an increase in speech production, the gains occurred immediately following the initiation of the AAC intervention (i.e., within the first 5 sessions). In the remaining five cases, there was a lag observed prior to gains in speech production (i.e., from 6 to more than 25 sessions).

Limitations

There were several limitations to the review. The first limitation was the very small sample of cases considered to offer the best evidence (i.e., 6 studies, 17 participants, and a total of 27 treatment cases). Thus, generalization to the population of individuals with developmental disabilities who may require AAC is limited. Second, only two of the six studies considered in the best-evidence analysis were published after 1990. Hence, recent advances in AAC systems and intervention approaches were not well represented in the review.

Conclusions

The results of the best-evidence analysis in Millar et al. (2006) indicated that AAC interventions do not appear to have a negative impact on speech production. The participants who demonstrated increased speech production ranged widely in age (i.e., 2–60 years). Various AAC intervention approaches were included in the best-evidence group of studies (i.e., both adult-directed and child-directed instruction). The majority of the studies investigated the effects of unaided AAC; only one study included aided AAC systems without speech output. The gains observed in speech production were variable and quite modest (e.g., an average gain of 13 words). In addition, the ceiling effects noted in several studies may have resulted in underestimations of the potential gains in speech production for many participants.

Although these findings should be considered to be preliminary evidence because of limitations in both the quantity and quality of the studies that were included, the results of the review were generally positive regarding the impact of AAC on speech production While Millar et al. (2006) included individuals with a wide range of developmental disabilities, the remainder of this chapter will focus more specifically on individuals with ASDs and will include studies that did not meet the criteria for methodological rigor employed by Millar et al. (2006). The objective is to summarize the literature to explore more generally the effects of AAC on the speech development of individuals with ASDs. Readers can consult Schlosser and Wendt (2008) for a systematic review of the literature with more stringent criteria.

THE EFFECTS OF AAC ON NATURAL SPEECH IN INDIVIDUALS WITH ASD

Of all the studies included in the review by Millar et al. (2006), 10 involved individuals with ASD and only two of those were considered in the best-evidence group. To update the search, two databases (i.e., PsycINFO, ERIC) were used to identify research published between 1975 and 2007 that 1) included AAC implementation with individuals with ASDs, 2) provided documented of participants' progress with their AAC systems, and 3) included data on speech production before, during, and/or after intervention. Ancestral searches of references cited in studies included in the review were also conducted to identify additional studies that met the inclusion criteria. Researchers with expertise in AAC and ASDs were also contacted for suggestions for locating literature.

Manual Signs

Six studies that met the criteria for this review included the implementation of manual signs with children with autism (see Table 6.1). Of the
six, one study (Kouri, 1988) was considered best evidence in the review
by Millar et al. (2006). A second was not included in the previous
review because it did not meet the criteria used (i.e., Yoder & Layton,
1988). The remaining four studies were identified by Millar et al. (2006)
but were not considered best evidence.

    Using a group design, Yoder and Layton (1988) published one of
the studies in which a primary objective was to study the impact of
AAC (i.e., sign language) on the speech production of children with
ASDs. Sixty children with ASDs under 9 years of age with expressive
vocabularies of less than 25 words participated in the study. The children were randomly assigned to one of four treatment groups: speech
alone, sign alone, simultaneous presentation of sign and speech, and
alternating presentation of sign and speech. The results indicated that,
regardless of the group in which the children participated, those with
higher verbal imitation scores tended to produce more spontaneous
spoken words. When the researchers statistically controlled for verbal
imitation ability, the sign-alone group was found to use significantly

Table 6.1.   Studies using manual signs

Study	Participants	Intervention	Outcomes
Yoder and Layton (1988)	Sixty children under 9 years of age	Speech alone, sign alone, speech and sign, or alternating sign and speech	Children with higher verbal imitation scores produced more spontaneous spoken words
Kouri (1988)	One 3-year-old child	Total communication (sign and speech)	Increase in speech production (10 spontaneous words)
Casey (1978)	Four children between 6 and 7 years of age	Total communication (sign and speech)	Increase in speech production
Fulwiler and Fouts (1976)	One 5-year-old child	Total communication (sign and speech)	Increase in signed words/phrases and speech production
Bonta and Watters (1983)	One 11-year-old child	Total communication (sign and speech)	Increase in speech production
Benaroya, Wesley, Ogilvie, Klein, and Meaney (1977)	Six children between 5 and 12 years of age	Total communication (sign and speech)	Increase in speech production for three children, no change for the other three children

fewer spontaneous words than the other three groups, which were not significantly different from one other. The results suggest that children with ASDs who demonstrate good verbal imitation skills may have greater potential for using speech spontaneously, as compared to children with ASDs who lack such skills. There is a critical need for further research in this area to identify additional predictors of speech development in children with ASDs.

Kouri (1988) used a single-subject withdrawal design to investigate a child-directed treatment approach to teach total communication (i.e., simultaneous manual signing plus speech). One of the five preschool-age children in the study had autism, whereas the other four were diagnosed with other developmental disabilities. The child with autism did not use speech to communicate prior to intervention. Following instruction in total communication using a child-oriented model, this child demonstrated increased speech production (i.e., a gain of 10 spontaneous words). Anecdotal data suggested that the child also demonstrated improvements in communication and reductions in challenging behaviors.

Casey's (1978) study used a multiple baseline design and included four children with autism between 6 and 7 years of age, all of whom lacked spontaneous speech. The study investigated the use of a parent-implemented instructional program in which mothers were taught to use Signed English with the children. The children's teachers were also instructed in the use of total communication. All four children demonstrated increases in the frequency of their verbalizations with both their mothers and their teachers over the course of the study.

The three remaining studies that included the implementation of manual signs with children with autism were case studies. Fulwiler and Fouts (1976) conducted a case study with a 5-year-old child with autism who was taught to use signs via a total communication approach. After 20 hours of instruction, the child demonstrated increased production of signed words and phrases as well as increased speech production. The authors also noted positive changes in the child's behavior over the course of the study. Similarly, an 11-year-old child with autism who had not produced any speech prior to intervention demonstrated the ability to provide spoken labels and signs for pictures with an equal proficiency by the end of a second case study (Bonta & Watters, 1983).

Finally, Benaroya, Wesley, Ogilvie, Klein, and Meaney (1977) implemented an instructional program that included total communication with a larger group of subjects compared to the previous studies. The study included six children with autism between the ages of 5 and 12 years. Instructors simultaneously signed and spoke the labels of pictures. Once the children mastered the signs imitatively, they were asked to respond to questions such as *What is this?* when pictures were

presented. Four of the six children were observed using signs spontaneously. Three of these four children demonstrated gains in speech
production at the single-word level, whereas the remaining three
participants showed no change in speech output.

Although these three case studies offer hopeful information about
the potential benefit of implementing sign language with children
with ASDs who are unable to speak, their methodological limitations
prevent definitive conclusions regarding the relationship between
unaided communication and speech development.

A need for additional experimental studies addressing the implementation of sign language with children with ASDs clearly exists. In
addition, given the fact that the majority of unaided AAC interventions
have incorporated structured, adult-directed models of instruction,
further research in child-directed treatment approaches is also warranted. Presently, a continuum of adult- and child-directed treatment
approaches is used with individuals with ASDs, including discrete
trial, naturalistic teaching techniques, and developmentally oriented
approaches (National Research Council, 2001). These approaches may
facilitate speech development with individuals with ASDs to varying
degrees; some may be more effective than others in promoting speech
production in individuals with specific skill profiles.

Aided AAC without Speech Output

In this section, research related to both the Picture Exchange Communication System (PECS) and other aided AAC approaches will be
summarized.

Picture Exchange Communication System Alone   The major-
ity of studies that have investigated the use of aided AAC systems
without speech output have used the Picture Exchange Communication System (Chapter 10; Frost & Bondy, 2002). PECS has been shown
to be successful in promoting the acquisition of requesting and commenting for children with ASDs. Increased speech production has also
been documented in several studies (see Table 6.2).

A number of hypotheses to explain the relationship between PECS
and increased speech production in children with ASDs have been
proposed. The first is that speech increases because the adult communicative partner is taught to pair speech with icons (i.e., graphic
symbols) on a sentence strip that is offered by the child. The adult is
also taught to pause as he or she reads the sentence strip, to provide an
opportunity for the child to complete the sentence verbally (*I want*...);
this may both elicit and reinforce the child's speech productions

Table 6.2.   Studies using the Picture Exchange Communication System alone

Study	Participants	Outcomes
Bondy & Frost (1994)	One 3-year-old child	Increase in speech production
Bondy and Frost (1994)	Eighty-five children	Twenty-nine percent used speech and graphic symbols/words; 48% used speech alone
Kravits, Kamps, Kemmerer, and Potucek (2002)	One 6-year-old child	Increase in speech production
Charlop-Christy et al. (2002)	Three children between 3 and 12 years of age	Increase in speech production in 40%–100% of opportunities
Ganz and Simpson (2004)	One 5-year-old child	Increase in speech production
Tincani, Crozier, and Alazetta (2006)	Two children between 10 and 12 years of age	Increase in vocal approximations for one child, no change for the other child
Tincani, Crozier, and Alazetta (2006)	One 9-year-old child	Increase in vocal approximations
Magiati and Howlin (2003)	Thirty-four children between 5 and 12 years of age	Increase in speech production

(Charlop-Christy et al., 2002; Yoder & Stone, 2006). In addition, the inclusion of highly reinforcing items for instruction in requesting may contribute to the speech initiation (Charlop-Christy et al., 2002).

Originally, Bondy and Frost (1994) presented the results of a single case study and data following the introduction of PECS with a larger group of children. In the discussion of the single case study, which involved a 36-month-old boy with ASD, the authors noted that, after 11 months of using PECS, the boy was able to use speech alone to communicate. The authors also described the outcomes of 85 children with ASDs who were taught to communicate using PECS, all of whom were described as lacking functional speech at the start of the program. Following instruction, 29% of the children were able to communicate with a combination of speech and graphic symbols or printed words; 48% used speech alone to communicate. Several subsequent studies have investigated the effects of PECS on the acquisition of requesting in children with ASDs more systematically. Eight of these studies documented speech production before, during, and/or following intervention and met the criteria for inclusion in this review.

Within a multiple baseline across settings design, Kravits, Kamps, Kemmerer, and Potucek (2002) taught a 6-year-old child with autism to use PECS at home and at school during center and journal time. Prior to intervention, the child was described as having no spontaneous speech and as producing very little speech even with prompting. In addition to increases in the use of PECS for requesting, the child demonstrated increases in intelligible, spontaneous verbalizations during instruction and in social interactions with peers in two of the three settings (i.e., home and journal time).

Charlop-Christy et al. (2002) also investigated the effects of PECS implementation during free play and academic time in a classroom. The impact of PECS on speech production was the primary objective of the study; however, collateral measures included social-communicative behaviors and problem behaviors. Three children with autism between the ages of 3 and 12 years participated in the multiple-baseline, intra-subject study. All three children lacked spontaneous speech but were described as having speech imitation skills. Measures of speech were calculated as the percentage of structured opportunities in which the children produced speech. All three children demonstrated clear increases in spontaneous speech during and following instruction in 40%–100% of opportunities.

Ganz and Simpson (2004) presented similar results for a 5-year-old child diagnosed with severe autism. Prior to instruction, the child was described as having limited immediate and delayed echolalia that she did not use functionally. The participant mastered the use of the PECS and generalized PECS requesting to novel adults and activities. During PECS training, the participant also demonstrated an increase in the average number of intelligible words spoken per trial. In Phase 1 of training, the participant's average words per trial were 0.36 words; by Phase 4, she used an average of approximately 2.7 three-word phrases in each trial.

In a two-part study, Tincani, Crozier, and Alazetta (2006) investigated the effects of PECS implementation with two children with autism between the ages of 10 and 12 years. Neither child demonstrated functional speech prior to the study. Both children learned to make spontaneous requests following PECS instruction. One of the children did not produce speech during any phase of the study. However, the second child produced vocal approximations in 66% of opportunities during baseline; in approximately 30% of opportunities during PECS Phase I; in 6% of opportunities during PECS Phase II; and in approximately 88% of opportunities during PECS Phase IV. This high level was maintained during the generalization phase of the study. The authors suggested that the use of a time-delay procedure in Phase IV might explain his increase in vocal approximations. As described earlier, in this phase, after the child hands a sentence strip to the adult, the adult reads it (e.g., *I want...*) and then waits 3–5 seconds before handing the requested item to the child. The delay may prompt the child to produce a vocal approximation of the adult model.

To explore this hypothesis, Tincani et al. (2006) implemented PECS with a 9-year-old child with autism in the second part of the study. They used an A-B-A-B design during Phase IV of the PECS instructional program. During the two A phases, no time delay was used before the requested item was provided to the child; in the two B phases, a 3- to 5-second delay was implemented. The child produced vocal approximations in 2%–3% of opportunities during the A phases and in 80.5%–83.3% of opportunities in the B phases. However, there was no change in his frequency of requesting with symbols across the four phases. This study provides important evidence for the need to investigate the effectiveness of specific intervention approaches, such as prompting and prompt-fading techniques that are often used with children with ASD, to determine whether there are key instructional strategies that differentially promote speech production in individuals with ASDs.

Unlike the previous studies investigating the use of PECS with children with ASDs, Magiati and Howlin (2003) conducted a study in which teachers were trained to implement PECS. Thirty-four children with ASDs participated in this group design research. Teachers completed a 2-day workshop and six consultations with PECS instructors to learn how to implement instruction using the PECS protocol. The average number of words produced by the participants at baseline ranged from 6 to 10 words; within 6 months after training, the average number of words increased to 11–20 words. This increase, although modest, was determined to be statistically significant. One of the limitations of the study was that the assessment measures consisted primarily of rating scales and other indirect measures that were completed by teachers and parents. In addition, no reliability procedures were reported to strengthen the methodological rigor of the study. However, this study provides preliminary data supporting the use of a model of PECS instruction that is implemented by teachers.

Comparison of Two Approaches Including PECS   In addition to studying the effects of PECS implementation alone for children with ASDs, researchers have also compared the use of PECS plus other AAC interventions. Two studies of this type met the inclusion criteria for this review (see Table 6.3).

Tincani (2004) compared the effectiveness of sign language with PECS in an alternating treatments design for two children with autism. Neither child was able to produce spontaneous speech prior to PECS implementation, but both were described as having some vocal imitation skills. The child whose motor imitation skills were described as moderately good following a motor imitation assessment was more successful in learning to request using sign language compared to

Table 6.3. Comparison between Picture Exchange Communication System (PECS) and a second intervention

Study	Participants	Interventions	Outcomes
Tincani (2004)	Two children between 5 and 6 years of age	PECS and sign language	Increase in speech production with both
Yoder and Stone (2006)	Thirty-six children between 2 and 3 years of age	PECS and RPMT	Increase in speech production with both

Key: RPMT, responsive education and prelinguistic milieu teaching.

PECS. Additionally, although this child demonstrated increased speech production using both modalities, he produced twice as many vocalizations with sign language than with PECS.

The other participant in the Tincani (2004) study was described as having weak motor imitation skills and was only able to imitate 20% of the hand movements modeled during testing for imitation. She was able to request more accurately using PECS compared to sign language. Similar to the subject in the Tincani et al. (2006) study, this child initially produced more vocalizations with sign language compared to PECS. However, there was a marked decrease in her vocalizations during PECS once she began to use PECS independently. Furthermore, once a time-delay procedure was incorporated during Phase IV, her vocalizations increased to an average of 90% of opportunities. The authors suggested that the different outcomes for the two participants were related to differences in their fine motor (hand) skills. The participant with better fine motor imitation skills was more successful with sign language than was the participant with poor fine motor skills. This is congruent with previous suggestions that children who have fine motor deficits may benefit from AAC interventions that require less physical effort and less motor planning (Mirenda & Erickson, 2000). PECS may be one option for minimizing physical effort and fine motor demands for children with ASDs who have deficits in this area.

A second study that compared intervention approaches investigated the effects of PECS and responsive education and prelinguistic milieu teaching (RPMT; Yoder & Stone, 2006). This was a randomized group experiment that included 36 children with autism who had fewer than 20 different words collected from three cumulative communication samples. Children participated in either RPMT or PECS for three 20-minute sessions per week for a total of 6 months. One of the unique aspects of this study was the inclusion of semistructured free play to examine generalization, rather than the highly structured contexts used to assess speech production in most other studies. Overall, children who participated in the PECS group were more successful than those in the RPMT group with regard to the frequency of spontaneous spoken communication acts and the number of spontaneous words produced in semistructured free play following intervention, although both groups demonstrated improvements on both measures. When the authors considered the children's object exploration skills, they found that by 6 months after instruction, children with strong object exploration skills in the PECS group used more spontaneous words than those in the RPMT group. The opposite was true for children with weak object exploration skills; these children used more spontaneous words with RPMT compared to PECS. The authors argued that children who are unable to play with objects may do better with intervention programs that specifically include instruction in object play skills, such as RPMT.

Aided AAC Other Than PECS   PECS is the most common form of aided AAC without speech output that has been studied to date. Only one study of unaided AAC without speech output other than PECS was included in the Millar et al. (2006) review, although it was not considered a best evidence study according to the evaluation criteria used. Garrison-Harrell, Kamps, and Kravits (1997) investigated the use of a peer-mediated intervention with three children with autism between 6 and 7 years of age. The peers were taught to use communication displays during social interactions, using a multiple-probe and multiple-baseline design across settings and subjects to document changes in the frequency and duration of interactions and how the AAC displays were used. Data were also collected on the rate of communicative verbalizations at baseline and during instruction.

All three children in the Garrison-Harrell et al. (1997) study were observed to increase their verbalizations during instruction. Although this is the only study that used a form of aided AAC without voice output that was not PECS, the positive results are encouraging. Given the variety of aided AAC techniques without speech output that are currently available (e.g., topic boards, communication books), research is sorely needed to determine the effects of these techniques on speech development. Additionally, research should investigate the potential advantages of including peers and other facilitators in instruction to aid in generalization.

Aided AAC with Speech Output

Despite technological advances and the variety of electronic AAC devices that are currently available, surprisingly few researchers have documented the effects of aided AAC with speech output on the speech development of individuals with ASDs (see Table 6.4). Two

Table 6.4.   Aided AAC with speech output

Study	Participants	Interventions	Outcomes
Parsons and LaSorte (1993)	Six children between 4 and 7 years of age	Apple IIGS computer with Echo IIb speech synthesizer	Increase in speech production
Olive et al. (2007)	Three children between 3 and 5 years of age	Four-button speech-generating device	Increase in speech production

studies that used speech output met the criteria for this review (Olive et al., 2007; Parsons & LaSorte, 1993).

Parsons and LaSorte (1993) compared the effect of a computer system with and without synthesized speech output on the spontaneous speech production of six children with autism between the ages of 4 and 7 years. The children were described as demonstrating the ability to produce speech but lacking the ability to use speech functionally. Students with no speech at all were not included in the study. The computer system consisted of an Apple IIGS computer with a color monitor and an Echo IIb speech synthesizer [see Parsons and LaSorte (1993) for more details on the equipment]. The software allowed the children to type combinations of letters that were displayed on the monitor and to hear the written text spoken through the speech synthesizer.

An interactional single-subject experimental design was used in the Parsons and LaSorte (1993) study. To reduce order effects, both A-B-BC-B-BC and A-BC-B-BC-B designs were implemented: A represented baseline, B represented use of the computer, and C represented synthesized speech. For the B condition, in which the computer was used without synthesized speech, the computer's speaker volume was turned to the off position. The frequency of spontaneous utterances was calculated for each session. The results showed that when synthesized speech was turned off (i.e., condition B), the children's spontaneous speech productions were at or below baseline (i.e., condition A). When synthesized speech was used on the computer (condition BC), there was an increase in spontaneous speech productions for all six subjects. The authors also made some interesting observations related to the children's behavior during the study, noting that most of them appeared highly motivated to use the computer; that many spontaneously repeated the synthesized speech; and that, in general, the children appeared to benefit from the combination of visual, auditory, and tactile information that was provided. Unfortunately, many of the procedures used in this study were not well-defined and the nature of the task in which the children participated was not well described. Further, descriptions of the children's speech prior to intervention were lacking sufficient detail. Nonetheless, the study provides some preliminary information about the potential positive effects of using computerized speech output with children with ASDs.

Olive et al. (2007) conducted a study investigating the effects of enhanced milieu teaching combined with a speech-generating device with three children with autism between the ages of 3 and 5 years. The children received 5 minutes of instruction per day for a maximum of 19 sessions. The researchers specifically measured the children's use of the speech-generating device, gestures, and vocalizations and verbalizations during play. Using a multiple-probe, intrasubject design, the authors provided data supporting an increase in vocalizations for one of the three children during implementation of the instructional program. In addition, requesting increased for all three children within a very short time period. This study provides preliminary data supporting the use of a speech-generating device in combination with enhanced milieu teaching for children with ASDs, although additional research in this area is needed.

SUMMARY AND CLINICAL IMPLICATIONS

It is essential that professionals and parents who are considering the introduction of AAC to children with ASDs remember that the primary goal of AAC is to improve functional communication. Research clearly supports the use of AAC to enhance the communicative competence and language skills of individuals who are unable to meet their communication needs via speech alone (e.g., Light et al., 1998, 1999). Hesitation about introducing AAC out of fear that AAC will impede speech development is understandable; however, there are serious clinical implications in adopting such a "wait and see" approach, especially with regard to problem behavior and language development.

Although this was not a systematic review that critically evaluated the methodological rigor and quality of research designs, some important preliminary findings are evident. First, as in the Millar et al. (2006) review, no data were found to support the suggestion that AAC implementation negatively affected the speech production of individuals with ASD. In fact, most of the existing research suggests that AAC may enhance speech development in these individuals. Second, this review suggests a number of possible correlations between specific skills and speech development with the implementation of AAC. With regard to manual signing, vocal imitation skills appear to be correlated with speech development (Yoder & Layton, 1988); with regard to PECS, object exploration skills seem to be similarly related (Yoder & Stone, 2006). In addition, some researchers have noted that children who have at least some verbal imitation skills tend to acquire spontaneous speech at a faster rate than those who lack such skills (e.g., Charlop-Christy et al., 2002; Schwartz, Garfinkel, & Bauer, 1998).

Finally, another important finding was that a variety of specific instructional strategies may facilitate speech production in children with ASDs. For example, the results of the study by Tincani et al. (2006) suggest that the time delay that is typically used in Phase IV of PECS may have a positive effect on vocalizations; a similar observation was noted in other studies as well (e.g., Charlop-Christy et al., 2002). Kouri (1988) effectively used a child-directed approach to teach total communication to several children with developmental disabilities, including ASDs. Garrison-Harrell et al. (1997) used peer-mediated instruction in their study and demonstrated positive effects on speech production. Given the breadth of instructional approaches available, specific analyses to determine individual effects on speech development appears to be warranted.

Limitations and Directions for Future Research

The research regarding the effects of AAC on the speech development of individuals with ASDs is quite encouraging, but also has a number of limitations. First, there are very few published studies that include documentation of changes in speech production before, during, and/or after AAC intervention. This restricts the extent to which generalizations of the results to the population of individuals with ASDs can be made. Also, in the majority of the studies, the primary research objectives were to investigate the effects of AAC on the acquisition of language (e.g., single words) and/or specific communicative functions (e.g., requesting). Documentation of changes in speech production was often a secondary or collateral measure. In addition, most of the research studies reviewed in this chapter would not have met the criteria for best evidence that were employed in the Millar et al. (2006) review. Finally, given the variety of AAC systems available today, the research does not reflect many recent technological advances in the field.

Future research is needed to identify specific skills that may serve as predictors of speech development (e.g., speech imitation, echolalia). The effect of various intervention approaches, including specific types of prompting and fading strategies, should be addressed in future studies. Also, it is important that the long-term effects of various intervention approaches on speech development be investigated. Much of the research documented the changes in speech production during or immediately following intervention. Additional research is also needed to document the effects of a wider range of AAC systems—in particular, the inclusion of various forms of AAC with speech output.

Despite the limitations of the studies published to date, the results are nonetheless promising and suggest that AAC may have positive effects on the speech development of individuals with ASDs. As high-quality research on this topic continues to accumulate, the current reluctance among some families and clinicians to introduce AAC to individuals with ASDs is likely to be reduced, so that these individuals can access communication in a timely manner that promotes the development of language, literacy, and other related skills.

REFERENCES

American Speech-Language-Hearing Association. (1991). Report: Augmentative and alternative communication. Committee on Augmentative Communication. *ASHA, 5,* 9–12.

Baranek, G.T., Parham, L.D., & Bodfish, J.W. (2005). Sensory and motor features in autism: Assessment and intervention. In F. Volkmar, A. Klin, & R. Paul (Eds.), *Handbook of autism and pervasive developmental disorders* (3rd ed., pp. 831–857). New York: John Wiley & Sons.

Benaroya, S., Wesley, S., Ogilvie, H., Klein, L.S., & Meaney, M. (1977). Sign language and multisensory input training in children with communication and related developmental disorders. *Journal of Autism and Childhood Schizophrenia, 7,* 23–31.

Beukelman, D.R. (1987). When you have a hammer, everything looks like a nail. *Augmentative and Alternative Communication, 3,* 94–95.

Beukelman, D.R., & Mirenda, P. (2005). *Augmentative and alternative communication: Supporting children and adults with complex communication needs* (3rd ed.). Baltimore: Paul H. Brookes Publishing Co.

Bondy, A.S., & Frost, L.A. (1994). The Picture Exchange Communication System. *Focus on Autistic Behavior, 9,* 1–19.

Bonta, J.L., & Watters, R.G. (1983). Use of manual signs by developmentally disordered speech deficient children in delayed auditory-to-picture matching-to-sample. *Analysis and Intervention in Developmental Disabilities, 3,* 295–309.

Bopp, K.D., Brown, K.E., & Mirenda, P. (2004). Speech-language pathologists' roles in the delivery of positive behavior support for individuals with developmental disabilities. *American Journal of Speech-Language Pathology, 13,* 5–19.

Casey, L.O. (1978). Development of communicative behavior in autistic children: A parent program using manual signs. *Journal of Autism and Childhood Schizophrenia, 8,* 45–59.

Centers for Disease Control and Prevention. (2007). Prevalence of autism spectrum disorders: Autism and developmental disabilities monitoring network—Fourteen sites, United States, 2002. Surveillance Summaries, February 9, 2007. *Morbidity and Mortality Weekly Report, 56,* SS-1.

Charlop-Christy, M.H., Carpenter, M., Loc, L., LeBlanc, L.A., & Kellet, K. (2002). Using the Picture Exchange Communication System (PECS) with children with autism: Assessment of PECS acquisition, speech, social-communicative behavior, and problem behavior. *Journal of Applied Behavior Analysis, 35,* 213–231.

Cress, C., & Marvin, C. (2003). Common questions about AAC services in early intervention. *Augmentative and Alternative Communication, 19,* 254–272.

Dowden, P., & Marriner, N. (1995). Augmentative and alternative communication: Treatment principles and strategies. *Seminars in Speech and Language, 16,* 140–156.

Frost, L.A., & Bondy, A.S. (2002). *The Picture Exchange Communication System training manual* (2nd ed.). Newark, DE: Pyramid Educational Consultants.

Fulwiler, R.L., & Fouts, R.S. (1976). Acquisition of American Sign Language by a noncommunicating autistic child. *Journal of Autism and Childhood Schizophrenia, 6,* 43–51.

Ganz, J., & Simpson, R. (2004). Effects on communicative requesting and speech development of the Picture Exchange Communication System in children with characteristics of autism. *Journal of Autism and Developmental Disorders, 34,* 395–409.

Garrison-Harrel, L., Kamps, D., & Kravits, T. (1997). The effects of peer networks on social-communicative behaviors for students with autism. *Focus on Autism and Other Developmental Disabilities, 12,* 241–254.

Kouri, T.A. (1988). Effects of simultaneous communication in a child-directed treatment approach with preschoolers with severe disabilities. *Augmentative and Alternative Communication, 4,* 222–232.

Kravits, T.R., Kamps, D.M., Kemmerer, K., & Potucek, J. (2002). Increasing communication skills for an elementary-aged student with autism using the Picture Exchange Communication System. *Journal of Autism and Developmental Disorders, 32,* 225–230.

Light, J., Binger, C., Agate, T., & Ramsay, K. (1999). Teaching partner-focused questions to individuals who use augmentative and alternative communication to enhance their communicative competence. *Journal of Speech and Hearing Research, 42,* 241–255.

Light, J., Collier, B., & Parnes, P. (1985). Communication interaction between young nonspeaking physically disabled children and their caretakers: Part 1: Discourse patterns. *Augmentative and Alternative Communication, 1,* 63–74.

Light, J.C., Roberts, B., DiMarco, R., & Greiner, N. (1998). Augmentative and alternative communication to support receptive and expressive communication for people with autism. *Journal of Communication Disorders, 31,* 153–180.

Lloyd, L.L., & Kangas, K. (1994). Augmentative and alternative communication. In G.H. Shames, E.H. Wiig, & W.A. Secord (Eds.), *Human communication disorders* (4th ed.) (pp. 606–657). New York: Merrill/Macmillan.

Lord, C., & Paul, R. (1997). Language and communication in autism. In D.J. Cohen & F.R. Volkmar (Eds.), *Handbook of autism and pervasive developmental disorders* (2nd ed., pp. 195–225). New York: John Wiley & Sons.

Magiati, I., & Howlin, P. (2003). A pilot evaluation study of the Picture Exchange Communication System (PECS) for children with autistic spectrum disorders. *Autism: The International Journal of Research and Practice, 7*(3), 297–320.

Millar, D.C., Light, J.C., & Schlosser, R.W. (2006). The impact of augmentative and alternative communication intervention on the speech production of individuals with developmental disabilities: A research review. *Journal of Speech, Language, and Hearing Research, 49,* 248–264.

Mirenda, P. (1997). Functional communication training and augmentative communication: A research review. *Augmentative and Alternative Communication, 13,* 207–225.

Mirenda, P. (2001). Autism, augmentative communication, and assistive technology: What do we really know? *Focus on Autism and Other Developmental Disabilities, 16,* 141–151.

Mirenda, P. (2003). Toward functional augmentative and alternative communication from students with autism: Manual signs, graphic symbols, and voice output communication aids. *Language, Speech, and Hearing Services in Schools, 34,* 203–216.

Mirenda, P., & Erickson, K. (2000). Augmentative communication and literacy. In S.F. Warren & J. Reichle (Series Eds.) & A.M. Wetherby & B.M. Prizant (Vol. Eds.), *Communication and language intervention series: Vol. 9. Autism spectrum disorders: A transactional developmental perspective* (pp. 333–367). Baltimore: Paul H. Brookes Publishing Co.

National Research Council. (2001). *Educating children with autism.* Washington, DC: National Academies Press.

Olive, M., de la Cruz, B., Davis, T., Chan, J., Lang, R., O'Reilly, M., & Dickinson, S. (2007). The effects of enhanced milieu teaching and a voice output communication aid on the requesting of three children with autism. *Journal of Autism and Developmental Disorders, 37,* 1505–1513.

Parsons, C.L., & La Sorte, D. (1993). The effect of computers with synthesized speech and no speech on the spontaneous communication of children with autism. *Australian Journal of Human Communication Disorders, 21,* 12–31.

Romski, M.A., & Sevcik, R.A. (1996). *Breaking the speech barrier: Language development through augmented means.* Baltimore: Paul H. Brookes Publishing Co.

Schlosser, R.W., & Lee, D.L. (2000). Promoting generalization and maintenance in augmentative and alternative communication: A meta-analysis of 20 years of effectiveness research. *Augmentative and Alternative Communication, 16,* 208–226.

Schlosser, R.W., & Wendt, O. (2008). Effects of augmentative and alternative communication intervention on speech production in children with autism: A systematic review. *American Journal of Speech-Language Pathology, 17*(3), 212–230.

Schwartz, I.S., Garfinkle, A.N., & Bauer, J. (1998). The Picture Exchange Communication System: Communicative outcomes for young children with disabilities. *Topics in Early Childhood Special Education, 18,* 144–159.

Silverman, F. (1995). *Communication for the speechless* (3rd ed.). Boston: Allyn & Bacon.

Slavin, R.E. (1986). Best-evidence synthesis: An alternative to meta-analytic and traditional reviews. *Educational Researcher, 15,* 5–11.

Tincani, M. (2004). Comparing the Picture Exchange Communication System (PECS) and sign language training for children with autism. *Focus on Autism and Other Developmental Disabilities, 19,* 152–163.

Tincani, M., Crozier, S., & Alazetta, L. (2006). The Picture Exchange Communication System: Effects on manding and speech development for school-aged child with autism. *Education and Training in Developmental Disabilities, 41,* 177–184.

Wing, L., & Attwood, A. (1987). Syndromes of autism and atypical development. In D.J. Cohen, & A.M. Donnellan (Eds.), *Handbook of autism and pervasive developmental disorders* (pp. 3–17). New York: John Wiley & Sons.

Yoder, P.J., & Layton, T.L. (1988). Speech following sign language training in autistic children with minimal verbal language. *Journal of Autism and Developmental Disorders, 18,* 217–229.

Yoder, P.J., & Stone, W.L. (2006). A randomized comparison of the effect of two prelinguistic communication interventions on the acquisition of spoken communication in preschoolers with ASD. *Journal of Speech, Language, and Hearing Research, 49,* 698–711.

Zangari, C., & Kangas, K. (1997). Intervention principles and procedures. In L.L. Lloyd, D.R. Fuller, & H.H. Arvidson (Eds.), *Augmentative and alternative communication: A handbook of principles and practices* (pp. 235–253). Boston: Allyn & Bacon.

III

AAC Interventions

7

AAC and the
SCERTS® Model

Incorporating AAC within a Comprehensive,
Multidisciplinary Educational Program

EMILY RUBIN, AMY C. LAURENT,
BARRY M. PRIZANT, AND AMY M. WETHERBY

Positive long-term outcomes for individuals with autism spectrum disorders (ASDs) are strongly correlated with social communicative competence (National Research Council, 2001). Thus, when developing a comprehensive educational program, progress should be measured across everyday social contexts and a range of social partners, not just the initial teaching situation. Although a range of methodologies call for the implementation of supports at specific times of an individual's day, vulnerabilities in social communicative competence are evident across every activity, every social partner, and every social context. Additionally, available curricula may fall short by solely focusing on educational objectives for the individual with ASD.

Setting appropriate targets for the individual with a social disability does not always ensure that social partners will modify their communicative style; consistently provide augmentative and alternative communication (AAC); and modify the environment based upon the individual's unique learning style, family priorities, and the demands of specific social settings across the day (Simpson, de Boer-Ott, & Myles, 2003). The National Research Council (2001) identified these needs for individuals with ASDs and recommended the development of more meaningful outcome measures that specifically document progress in social communicative competence across partners, contexts, and activities.

The SCERTS® Model is a multidisciplinary team approach that provides a comprehensive, curriculum-based assessment to ensure that targeted goals and objectives for the individual with ASD directly affect the core challenges that compromise social communicative competence, while measuring progress in natural contexts across multiple partners and settings (Prizant, Wetherby, Rubin, Laurent, & Rydell, 2005a, 2005b). To do so, progress is documented not only in the individual, but also in how social partners interact with that individual and how the environment is adapted with learning supports and AAC. In other words, objectives are selected not only for the individual with ASD, but also for that individual's social partners. In this approach, the critical role of a partner in fostering more sophisticated language, appropriate social behavior, perspective taking, and the ability to maintain a state of active engagement is recognized.

The assessment process also includes a mechanism to support an educational team and family in connecting assessment with educational planning by embedding target objectives for the individual in natural routines at school, at home, and in community settings. This mechanism holds the social partners accountable for a range of interpersonal and learning supports including, but not limited to, consistent communicative style accommodations and the provision of AAC supports across natural routines and social contexts.

This chapter provides an overview of the SCERTS Assessment Process (SAP) as a tool to facilitate the implementation of the SCERTS Model. Using observational data from everyday social contexts and information gathered directly from everyday social partners, the SAP has been designed to provide a meaningful outcome measure to document 1) progress related to the core challenges of individuals with ASDs in functional activities and 2) generalization of gains and fidelity of programming across communicative partners, activities, and social environments (Prizant et al., 2005a, 2005b). Specifically, this chapter focuses on how AAC is incorporated into the SCERTS Model with regard to assessment and implementation across developmental and curricular stages.

DOCUMENTING PROGRESS
RELATED TO THE CORE CHALLENGES OF ASD

The most critical domains for prioritizing educational goals and documenting progress should relate to the core challenges in ASD, particularly those challenges that compromise an individual's social-adaptive functioning across a range of social partners and within natural routines (American Speech-Language-Hearing Association, 2006; National Research Council, 2001). In fact, longitudinal research has shown that when progress is made in relation to these core challenges of ASD, this progress is predictive of gains in language acquisition, social-adaptive functioning, and academic achievement (National Research Council,

2001). Although heterogeneity is notable across individuals with ASDs, challenges with establishing shared attention and predicting the actions of social partners are considered "hallmark" features of the disorder, regardless of an individual's cognitive abilities or learning style (Volkmar, Lord, Bailey, Schultz, & Klin, 2004). These challenges affect two critical areas of development, namely Social Communication and Emotional Regulation, which are two of the primary domains of the SCERTS curriculum-based assessment.

Social Communication

With respect to social communication, difficulties in the ability to establish shared attention and predict the actions of one's social partners can compromise the ability to initiate bids for communication and appreciate another's intentions and emotional states, affecting developmental achievements in the capacity for joint attention. A limited ability to establish shared attention will also affect an individual's understanding and use of nonverbal communication, understanding and use of language, and ability to follow social conventions or conversational "rules." These latter challenges have an impact on developmental achievements in the capacity for symbol use (Prizant, Wetherby, Rubin & Laurent, 2003).

As an individual matures and benefits from educational programming, these core challenges in social communication will likely take different forms and may be addressed through multimodal communication (e.g., gestures, sign language, object/picture communication supports, spoken language, speech generating devices [SGDs], and/or written language). Thus, decisions regarding appropriate modes of communication should be sensitive to the developmental capabilities of the individual, such as whether that individual is presymbolic, is at an emerging language stage, or is able to use more advanced semantic and syntactic discourse strategies.

In the SCERTS Model, these developmental shifts are addressed through distinct stages of curricula (Prizant et al., 2005a, 2005b). The Social Partner stage curriculum is appropriate for an individual who is predominantly presymbolic, relies on gestures as a primary means of establishing shared attention, and uses concrete objects to comprehend another's intentions (e.g., a juice box to foster recognition of a transition to snack time). The Language Partner stage curriculum is appropriate for an individual who is using symbolic language (e.g., spoken words, sign language, and/or pictures or graphic symbols) as a primary means of communication and is developing a repertoire of single words, multiword combinations, and creative simple sentence structures. Individuals at this stage may also be using echolalia, or phrases that are "borrowed" from previous social contexts, as a means to communicate intentions. The Conversational Partner stage curriculum is appropriate for an individual who is using conversational-level discourse to communicate, while developing an awareness of social perspectives and an understanding of social conventions.

By applying a developmental framework, appropriate goals and objectives can be determined in a manner that is sensitive to an individual's current strengths and functional needs, family priorities, and the demands of everyday social contexts and social partners. Sample educational objectives based on the SCERTS curriculum-based assessment in the domain of Social Communication are outlined in Table 7.1 for the social partner, the language partner, and the conversational partner with respect to the curricular components of joint attention and symbol use.

Table 7.1.   SCERTS® Social Communication curriculum: Sample educational objectives

Social Partner stage

Joint Attention
- Initiating bids for interaction
- Looking toward people
- Sharing positive emotion
- Requesting and protesting desired food or objects
- Requesting comfort
- Requesting social games
- Commenting on objects
- Repeating communication to repair a breakdown

Symbol Use
- Taking turns by repeating own actions or sounds
- Anticipating another's actions in familiar routines
- Using familiar objects in constructive play
- Using conventional gestures to share intentions
- Using words bound to routines
- Responding to a few frequently used phrases

Language Partner stage

Joint Attention
- Engaging in extended reciprocal interaction
- Securing attention prior to communicating
- Requesting help or other actions
- Greeting
- Commenting on actions or events
- Showing off
- Modifying communicative bids to repair breakdowns

Symbol Use
- Imitating familiar actions or words
- Following contact and distal points

- Combining a variety of actions with objects in play
- Using a variety of gestures in coordination with gaze
- Understanding and using a variety of relational meanings in word combinations (e.g., agent + action + object, modifier + object, negation + object)

Conversational Partner stage

Joint Attention

- Modifying language based on what partners have seen or heard
- Describing plausible causal factors for the emotions of self and others
- Sharing intentions for social interaction with peers (e.g., greeting, regulating turns, praising partners, expressing empathy)
- Initiating a variety of conversational topics
- Gauging the length and content of conversational turn based on partners
- Recognizing and repairing communication breakdowns

Symbol Use

- Using behaviors modeled by partners to guide social behavior
- Understanding nonverbal cues of turn taking and topic change
- Taking on a role and cooperating with peers in dramatic play
- Using appropriate body posture and proximity
- Understanding and using a variety of sentence constructions
- Following conventions for initiating and taking turns in conversation

---

From Prizant, B.M., Wetherby, A.M., Rubin, E., Laurent, A.C., & Rydell, P.J. (2005). *The SCERTS® Model: A comprehensive educational approach for children with autism spectrum disorders. Vol. 1: Assessment.* Baltimore: Paul H. Brookes Publishing Co.; adapted by permission.

Emotional Regulation

Difficulties in establishing shared attention and predicting the actions of one's social partners also contribute to challenges in Emotional Regulation, a domain in the SAP. Because the ability to effectively regulate emotional state and behavior supports competent social and communicative exchanges, prioritizing educational goals in this domain is essential (National Research Council, 2000). Active engagement in social situations is dependent, however, on the ability to accurately perceive a social event by predicting social behavior in others. Thus, individuals with ASDs frequently misinterpret social events and may fail to recognize assistance that is offered by social partners due to these core challenges. These patterns affect developmental achievements in the capacity for mutual regulation, leading to increased social anxiety and/or withdrawal.

Limitations in establishing shared attention further compromise the development of emotional regulation by affecting achievements in the capacity for self-regulation. Learning through imitation requires the ability to share an attentional focus. When this is disrupted, behaviors modeled by social partners are often missed. Thus, individuals with ASDs often continue to use early developing and/or idiosyncratic strategies to regulate their emotions and arousal far beyond early childhood. Immature patterns of behavior (e.g., chewing on one's shirt, hoarding preferred items, averting gaze) may be observed, as well as more extreme strategies such as "lashing out" and/or bolting from the social setting. A compromised ability to benefit from models provided by others may also result in the development of language for self-regulation that follows more idiosyncratic patterns. For example, an individual with ASD may initiate a topic of special interest to cope with social anxiety and/or may recite the lines of a favorite movie when faced with distressful social circumstances (Rydell & Prizant, 1995). As these self-regulatory strategies may appear atypical or inappropriate, social partners may impose punitive measures, leading to increased emotional dysregulation or diminished self-esteem.

In a similar manner to social communication, applying a developmental framework is necessary to ensure that appropriate goals and objectives in emotional regulation are determined in a manner that is sensitive to an individual's current strengths and functional needs, family priorities, and the demands of everyday social contexts and social partners. Sample educational objectives based on the SCERTS curriculum-based assessment in the domain of Emotional Regulation are outlined in Table 7.2 for the Social Partner, the Language Partner, and the Conversational Partner with respect to the curricular components of mutual regulation and self-regulation.

DEVELOPING INTERPERSONAL AND LEARNING SUPPORTS

There is a strong relationship between the social communicative competence of an individual with ASD and how communicative partners adapt their communicative styles and modify the environment with learning supports (American Speech-Language-Hearing Association, 2006; National Research Council, 2001). Achievements in social communication and emotional regulation are, in fact, dependent on successful social interactions with partners across a range of social contexts. However, social partners face constant challenges in responding to often subtle and unconventional bids for communication, fostering initiation, and providing AAC supports to foster expressive language and emotional regulation for individuals with ASD.

While a range of methodologies focus on the individual's acquisition of target skills in isolated teaching sessions, the SCERTS Model has been designed to ensure that social partners make adjustments across a variety of activities and social contexts (Prizant et al., 2005a, 2005b). As a result, the SCERTS curriculum-based assessment includes the domain of Transactional Support, which provides ongoing assessment of the

Table 7.2. SCERTS® Emotional Regulation curriculum: Sample educational objectives

---

Social Partner stage

Mutual Regulation

- Expressing happiness and anger
- Soothing when comforted by partners
- Protesting when distressed
- Responding to partner's attempts to reengage in activity or interaction

Self-Regulation

- Noticing people and things in the environment
- Using behavioral strategies to regulate arousal during social interactions
- Using behavioral strategies to regulate arousal during transitions
- Removing self from overstimulating or undesired activity

Language Partner stage

Mutual Regulation

- Understanding and using symbols to express emotions
- Making choices when offered by partners
- Using language strategy to request a break
- Using language strategies to request a regulating activity or input
- Responding to partner's use of language to recover from extreme dysregulation

Self-Regulation

- Persisting during tasks with reasonable demands
- Using behavioral strategies modeled by partners to regulate arousal level
- Using language strategies to engage productively in an extended activity
- Using language strategies to regulate arousal during transitions
- Using language strategies to recover from extreme dysregulation

---

Conversational Partner stage

Mutual Regulation

- Understanding and using graded emotion words to express emotion
- Responding to information or strategies offered by partners to regulate arousal
- Collaborating and negotiating with peers in problem solving
- Requesting assistance to resolve conflict and problem solve situations

Self-Regulation

- Demonstrating ability to inhibit actions and behaviors
- Using behavioral strategies to engage productively in an extended activity
- Using self-monitoring and self-talk to guide behavior
- Identifying and reflecting on strategies to support regulation
- Using planning and rehearsing (i.e., metacognitive strategies) to regulate arousal during new and changing situations

---

From Prizant, B.M., Wetherby, A.M., Rubin, E., Laurent, A.C., & Rydell, P.J. (2005). *The SCERTS® Model: A comprehensive educational approach for children with autism spectrum disorders. Vol. 1: Assessment.* Baltimore: Paul H. Brookes Publishing Co.; adapted by permission.

consistency with which an individual with ASD is provided with inter-personal and learning supports across partners and contexts (i.e., school, home, and community). The interpersonal support component refers to the interactive style modifications that social partners make to foster greater initiation, independence, and competence in the individual with ASD. The learning support component refers to modifications that are made to the environment (e.g., visual and organizational structures) and the provision of AAC supports that foster the ability to establish shared attention, language expression and comprehension, attend to relevant stimuli in the environment, and predict the actions of social partners. Table 7.3 provides a summary of the critical goals in interpersonal and learning supports that are essential for social partners in a comprehensive educational program for individuals with ASDs.

As is evident from Table 7.3, AAC support is embedded within the component of learning support in the transactional support curriculum. Here, AAC refers broadly to the use of unaided approaches such as gestures and sign language, as well as aided approaches such as objects, pictures, graphic symbols, written language, SGDs, and computer-based tools and software. These partner behaviors are included in assessment based on the quality of evidence that is vailable supporting the efficacy of AAC (American Speech-Language-Hearing Association, 2005; Mirenda, 2003)—particularly evidence that highlights how these supports foster communicative competence in individuals with ASDs, not only in isolated teaching sessions but across social partners and social contexts. For example, Schlosser and Lee (2000) conducted a meta-analysis of research studies that were specifically conducted to document the efficacy of AAC. Their research found that the majority of AAC supports were effective at producing changes in social communicative behavior *and* generalization across contexts when partners provided support in natural settings.

There are four primary partner objectives included within the learning support component of the Transactional Support domain. These objectives ensure that progress is tracked with respect to how consistently AAC supports are provided across social partners and whether these supports are available across social contexts and natural activities. Specifically, partner use of AAC is examined according to the extent to which it enhances 1) understanding of communication and expressive language, 2) understanding of language and behavior, 3) expression and understanding of emotion, and 4) emotional regulation. In the sections that follow, these partner objectives are discussed in detail with respect to how they may incorporate AAC for the Social Partner, Language Partner, and Conversational Partner developmental stages in the SAP.

Table 7.3. SCERTS® Transactional Support curriculum: Partner goals and sample objectives

Interpersonal support	Learning support
1. The partner is responsive to the individual (e.g., responding to signals to foster a sense of communicative competence and recognizing signs of dysregulation and offering support).	1. The partner structures activity for active participation (e.g., defining clear beginning and ending to activities, providing predictable sequence of activities).
2. The partner fosters initiation (e.g., offering choices and waiting and encouraging initiations).	2. The partner uses augmentative communication support to foster development (e.g., communication and expressive language, understanding of language, emotional regulation).
3. The partner respects individual's independence (e.g., providing time for individual to solve problems at own pace).	3. The partner uses visual and organizational supports (e.g., using supports to define steps and time for completion of activities).
4. The partner sets stage for engagement (e.g., using appropriate nonverbal behavior to encourage interaction).	4. The partner modifies goals, activities, and learning environment (e.g., arranging the learning environment to promote initiation, adjusting task difficulty for child success).
5. The partner provides developmental support (e.g., providing guidance for success in activities).	
6. The partner adjusts language input (e.g., adjusting complexity of language input to individual's developmental level).	
7. The partner models appropriate behaviors (e.g., modeling appropriate behavior when individual uses inappropriate behavior).	

From Prizant, B.M., Wetherby, A.M., Rubin, E., Laurent, A.C., & Rydell, P.J. (2005). *The SCERTS® Model: A comprehensive educational approach for children with autism spectrum disorders. Vol. 1: Assessment.* Baltimore: Paul H. Brookes Publishing Co.; adapted by permission.

Partner Use of AAC to Enhance Communication and Expressive Language

Social Partner Stage For individuals at the Social Partner stage, the provision of augmentative communication supports to enhance communication and expressive language may involve the use of objects to support the capacity for joint attention (e.g., initiating bids for interaction) and the capacity for symbol use (e.g., using conventional gestures to share intentions). For example, objects can be paired with preferred social routines to support an individual's ability to represent and request a game across contexts. A specific blanket might be used for Peekaboo or a toy rocket might be paired with a *3, 2, 1... blast* *off* routine. Eventually, a basket of these objects can be presented to allow the individual with ASD to make a choice by touching or giving one of these objects to his or her social partner and securing attention with proximity or communicative gaze. Within feeding or snack routines, a communication board might be created with several of the individual's preferred snack items sealed in transparent containers and attached with Velcro to an accessible "menu board." This support can be used to facilitate the use of a conventional gesture, such as a touch paired with communicative gaze or a giving gesture. Both of these are presymbolic communicative bids that provide the early developmental foundation for acquiring symbolic language to serve these same functions (e.g., *Mommy open; Daddy cookie; Help, please*).

The use of AAC supports at these early stages of communicative development can also be an effective means to prevent what has been referred to as "communication failure" by ensuring that an individual has an efficient means of communicating both instrumental and social functions (Romski & Sevcik, 2005, p. 179). By providing an efficient means of communication, AAC has also been shown to be an effective support for preventing or replacing challenging behaviors such as aggression and self-injury (Frea, Arnold, & Vittimberga, 2001; Mirenda, 1997).

Language Partner Stage   Although concerns are often raised as to whether AAC inhibits the development of spoken language as individuals with ASDs enter emerging language stages, empirical evidence to support this notion is not available (see Chapter 6, this volume; Mirenda, 2001, 2003; National Research Council, 2001). In fact, AAC approaches have been shown to provide effective support for promoting social communication and language development with individuals who have limited functional speech, as well as those who are in both early and later stages of acquiring speech as a primary mode of communication (American Speech-Language-Hearing Association, 2006; National Research Council, 2001). However, the National Research Council (2001) recognized that there is limited research available to indicate which forms of AAC will be the most effective for a specific individual. Thus, at the Language Partner stage, the provision of AAC may involve a range of tools, depending upon the unique learning style of the individual with ASD and the unique requirements of specific social contexts. Various forms of AAC may include the use of sign language; photographs or graphic symbols; or SGDs to foster a range of word types, early word combinations, and creative simple sentence structures.

In the SAP, sample objectives at the Language Partner stage related to expressive communication and language might include those supporting the capacity for joint attention (e.g., requesting help or other

actions and commenting on actions or events), as well as those supporting the capacity for symbol use (e.g., using a variety of relational
meanings in word combinations). The use of color coding paired with
photographs and graphics can be incorporated across social partners
and natural routines to foster agent–action–object word combinations.
For example, during lunch at school, a graphic placemat menu might
be available with photographic representations of a student's teachers
(e.g., *Emily, Amy*) enhanced with a thick red border; graphic representations of different actions (e.g., *open, drink, cut, eat*) enhanced with a
thick green border; and graphic representations of different objects in
that activity (e.g., *yogurt, milk, pizza, crackers*) enhanced with a thick
yellow border (see Figure 7.1). The student might then be provided
with a sentence template that includes a blank white box with a red
border, a blank white box with a green border, and blank white box
with a yellow border to elicit an agent–action–object word combination. The student is then supported to match the appropriate symbols
to their appropriate location on the template to make a request for help
and use a developmentally appropriate word combination (e.g., *Emily
open yogurt*). Across social partners and different social contexts, these

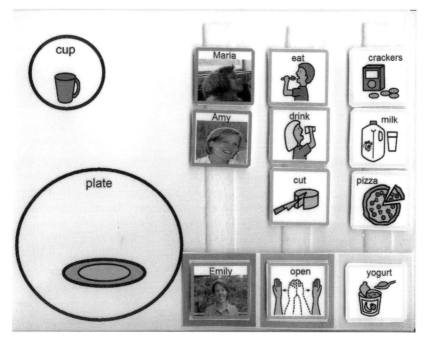

Figure 7.1. Graphic placemat menu for a student at the Language Partner stage. (The Picture Communication Symbols ©1981–2008 by Mayer-Johnson LLC. All Rights Reserved Worldwide. Used with permission.)

AAC supports can be modified to meet the unique demands of the individuals and activities.

Conversational Partner Stage   At the Conversational Partner stage, the provision of AAC to foster expressive communication and language might include the continued use of sign language, pictures, graphic symbols, and written language. In fact, the SAP ensures that social partners continue to provide AAC to foster communication and expressive language regardless of whether an individual has acquired spoken language as a primary mode of communication. Evidence is available that supports the use of both unaided and aided AAC approaches for supporting the capacity for joint attention (e.g., sharing intentions for social interaction with peers) and the capacity for symbol use (e.g., understanding and using a variety of sentence constructions and following conventions for initiating and taking turns in conversation; American Speech-Language-Hearing Association, 2006; Johnston, Nelson, Evans, & Palazolo, 2003; Krantz & McClannahan, 1993).

An individual at the Conversational Partner stage who is learning to initiate conversations during nature walks with his class might be provided with a keychain bracelet with the names or photographs of each of his or her classmates included on separate cards. On the reverse of each of the cards, written conversation starters related to the classmate's preferred topics can be provided. During snack time, this educational objective might be addressed using a placemat containing similar photographic and/or written supports.

Partner Use of AAC to Enhance Understanding of Language and Behavior

Social Partner Stage   For individuals with ASDs who are at the Social Partner stage, AAC supports enhance understanding of language and behavior and contribute to capacity for symbol use. Supports may include gestures, signs, objects, photographic images, or SGDs. The use of AAC for this purpose has been demonstrated in a number of studies that have illustrated the effectiveness of augmenting verbal language with such visual supports and SGDs (Brady, 2000). In the SAP, sample educational objectives for this developmental stage might include anticipating another's actions in familiar routines and responding to a few frequently used phrases. For example, to increase the salience of a greeting routine (e.g., a family member's arrival home from work), the individual with ASD might be shown a photograph of this family member just prior to his or her arrival at the front door. This support may enhance that individual's ability to anticipate social actions, as well as to comprehend a familiar phrase, such as *Mommy's* *home.* Similarly, the use of gestures or concrete manual signs might be used to enhance an individual's ability to respond to familiar phrases across natural routines. Comprehension can be supported by augmenting the verbal instruction (e.g., *open the door*) with the sign for OPEN (i.e., motioning one's hands from midline to an open stance).

Language Partner Stage   For individuals with ASDs who are at the Language Partner stage, the provision of AAC supports to enhance understanding of language and behavior might involve, for example, the use of use of aided language stimulation, in which spoken and visually depicted language are presented simultaneously (see Chapter 8, this volume; National Research Council, 2001). Additional AAC support such as pictures, graphic symbols, or written words to augment verbal language might also be used to enhance the capacity for symbol use.

In the SAP, sample educational objectives for this developmental stage include combining a variety of actions with objects in play and understanding a variety of relational meanings in word combinations. For an individual with ASD at the Language Partner stage engaged in an inclusive classroom environment, the use of written supports might be used to indicate the steps involved within a play sequence and the language that can be used to engage with a peer. Figure 7.2 provides an example of a play script for a "pizza party." Each step is listed on the "to do" or green side of the board. As each step is complete, the written support is moved to the "all done" or red side of the board. Such learning supports have been found to be effective for increasing understanding of sequential play and enhancing responsiveness to the communicative bids of others (Goldstein & Cisar, 1992; Thiemann & Goldstein, 2004).

Conversational Partner Stage   For individuals with ASDs who are at the Conversational Partner stage, the provision of AAC support to enhance understanding of language and behavior provides an effective means for targeting goals related to the capacity for symbol use. Sample educational objectives include—but are not be limited to— understanding nonverbal cues of turn taking and topic change, using appropriate body posture and proximity, and understanding a variety of sentence constructions.

An example of an AAC support for enhancing understanding of nonverbal cues for turn taking in conversation might include the use of a hand signal provided to a class during an academic lesson, which ensures that each student is aware of when it is an appropriate time to initiate a comment or question. An upright palm presented by the teacher can be used to represent *I can talk about this later,* an index finger presented by the teacher can represent *I can talk about this in a minute,* and an open palm presented by the teacher can represent

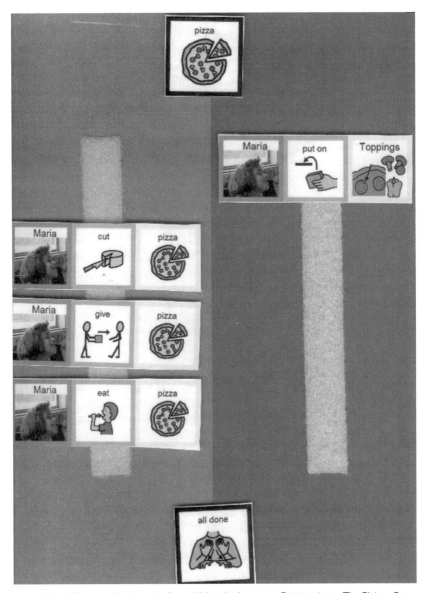

Figure 7.2. "Pizza party" play script for a child at the Language Partner stage. (The Picture Communication Symbols ©1981–2008 by Mayer-Johnson LLC. All Rights Reserved Worldwide. Used with permission.)

This is a good time to talk. Each of these signals could be supported with a written reminder to ensure comprehension (see Figure 7.3). Individuals with ASDs who are at the Conversational Partner stage often have difficulty gauging appropriate timing for these initiations because

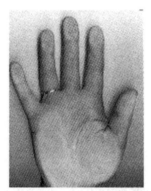

I can talk about this later.

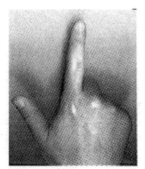

I can talk about this in a minute.

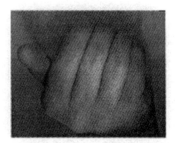

This is a good time to talk.

Figure 7.3. Pictorial reminder of a hand signal used by a teacher, which provides information about appropriate times to initiate a comment or question, for a student at the Conversational Partner stage.

this relies on the ability to establish shared attention and predict the actions of the teacher (i.e., nonverbal social cues). When a clear gesture is provided by the teacher, the social problem-solving demands are reduced and competence in the communicative exchange can be fostered. Importantly, this strategy may accomplish the objective without discouraging a student with ASD through the provision of negative feedback.

Partner Use of AAC to Enhance Expression and Understanding of Emotion

Social Partner Stage   Individuals with ASDs who are at the Social Partner stage tend to share less positive affect (Dawson, Hill, Spencer, Galpert, & Watson, 1990; Wetherby, Prizant, & Hutchinson, 1998) and demonstrate less attention to emotional displays of distress or discomfort than their typically developing peers (Sigman, Kasari, Kwon, & Yirmiya, 1992). Likewise, less emotional reciprocity is often noted following praise (Kasari, Sigman, Baumgartner, & Stipek, 1993). These variables compromise areas of development that are typically associated with social reciprocity and language acquisition (Dawson et al., 2004). In part, this may be due to difficulty in predicting how one's actions affect the emotional responses of others and providing one's social partners with information that allows them to provide mutual regulation.

AAC supports can provide an effective means to enhance expression and understanding of emotion related to the capacity for joint attention and the capacity for mutual regulation. For example, challenging behaviors can be prevented through the provision of communicative tools that serve equivalent functions for the individual (Bopp, Brown, & Mirenda, 2004). Sample educational objectives might include sharing positive emotion, sharing negative emotion, protesting when distressed, requesting comfort, and soothing when comforted by partners. An example of an AAC support to enhance emotional expression at this stage might include the provision of a model for the manual sign ANGRY paired with the sign for ALL DONE. By targeting this objective, the social partner may become more responsive to early signals of distress, will be more likely to honor protests when appropriate, and will be empowered with a behavior to model as a replacement strategy for challenging behaviors, such as pushing away undesired food or more aggressive actions.

Language Partner Stage   For individuals with ASDs who are at the Language Partner stage, the provision of AAC supports to enhance expression and understanding of emotion provides an effective means for targeting goals related to the capacities for joint attention and mutual regulation. A sample educational objective might include understanding and using symbols to express emotions. The use of graphic symbols has been found to enhance the efficiency of word recall and an individual's spontaneous communication (Ganz & Simpson, 2004). Therefore, when these supports are available for emotional expression, individuals with ASDs have access to an efficient tool for communicating through socially appropriate means, a strategy that often prevents unconventional challenging behavior that might be serving the same function (Mirenda, 1997).

During classroom activities, an individual with ASD might be provided with an emotion keyring bracelet that consists of a set of laminated cards representing various emotional states. Graphic symbols with related written labels are on the front of each card (e.g., happy, sad, and angry; Figure 7.4a) and symbols representing words that can be used to request assistance are on the reverse side of each card (e.g., *high five* for happy; *hug* for sad; and *all done* for angry; Figure 7.4b). This support can be modified to suit the unique needs of social partners and activities across natural social contexts (e.g., school, home, and community).

Conversational Partner Stage   For individuals with ASDs who are at the Conversational Partner stage, AAC supports to enhance expression and understanding of emotion provide an effective means for targeting goals related to the capacities for joint attention and mutual regulation. Sample educational objectives might include describing plausible causal factors for the emotions of self and others, understanding and using graded emotion words to express emotion, or responding to information or strategies offered by partners to regulate arousal.

An example of an AAC support for enhancing expression and understanding of emotion might include the use of a pictorially supported Social Story (Gray, 1995). This form of AAC provides the individual with ASD with a written support to both enhance appropriate emotional expression and encourage awareness of the impact of social behaviors on the thoughts and emotional states of others (Barry & Burlew, 2004).

Partner Use of AAC to Enhance Emotional Regulation

Social Partner Stage   For individuals with ASDs who are at the Social Partner stage, the provision of AAC supports to enhance emotional regulation provides an effective means for targeting goals

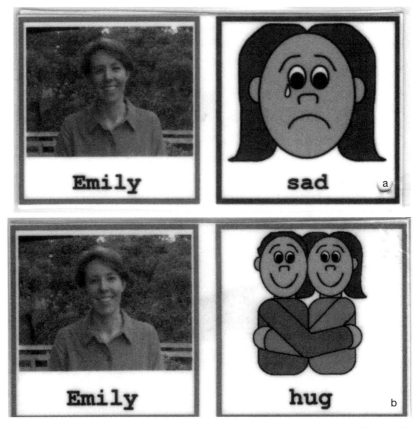

Figure 7.4. *a,* Card with graphic symbol representing "sad." *b,* Reverse side of "sad" card with symbol representing an appropriate request for assistance ("hug"). (From Emotion Ring ©2006–2008 by Communication Crossroads; reprinted with permission.)

related to the capacities for mutual regulation and self-regulation. Sample educational objectives might include protesting when distressed, responding to a partner's attempts to reengage in an activity or interaction, and using behavioral strategies to regulate arousal during transitions. Because individuals with ASDs at this stage are not yet symbolic communicators, the use of simple photographs and/or objects may be useful tools for compensating for the difficulties they experience in predicting social sequences and making transitions (Pierce & Schreibman, 1994).

When preparing for a transition to a community outing such as the swimming pool, giving the individual his or her swimsuit or goggles can provide a concrete indication of the upcoming activity. Similarly, in the classroom, an object-based schedule board to indicate the sequence of activities can be constructed using a transparent shoe rack. Within each "slot," an object can be included to remind the individual of where to go next (e.g., a preferred toy for free choice, a rubber duck for circle time to represent the initial song, a juice box for snack time, and small ball to represent recess). Eventually, these objects can be paired with photographs to introduce graphic symbols that represent the activities in the schedule.

Language Partner Stage   For individuals with ASDs who are at the Language Partner stage, the provision of AAC supports to enhance emotional regulation provides an effective means for targeting goals related to the capacities for mutual regulation and self-regulation. Sample educational objectives might include using specific language strategies to request a break, to request a regulating activity or input, to engage productively in an extended activity, and/or to regulate arousal during transitions.

An AAC support to enhance this aspect of development for a language partner might include the use of both between- and within-activity schedules (Bopp et al., 2004; Bryan & Gast, 2000). For example, an individual with ASD who is participating in a flag-making art project in the classroom can be supported to understand the steps toward task completion through the provison of pictures or graphic symbols that represent the steps within this task (e.g., I find the blue stars, I find the red stripes, I find the glue, I glue the stars on the flag, I glue the stripes on the flag, and I glue the flag on the stick).

Conversational Partner Stage   For individuals with ASDs who are at the Conversational Partner stage, the provision of AAC supports to enhance emotional regulation provides an effective means for targeting goals related to the capacities for mutual regulation and self-regulation. Sample educational objectives might include collaborating and negotiating with peers in problem solving, requesting assistance to resolve conflicts and problem-solve situations, using self-monitoring and self-talk to guide behavior, and identifying and reflecting on strategies to support regulation.

A range of AAC supports has been shown to be effective with respect to these aspects of development. For example, the use of visual and written supports within a comic strip conversation (Gray, 1995) is an effective tool for supporting an individual's recognition of the perspectives of social partners, including their thoughts, feelings, and intentions. This enables an individual with ASD to take in social information that can be used to negotiate with peers and to reflect on whether a specific regulatory strategy is appropriate, given the social contexts and partners involved (Kerr & Durkin, 2004; Parsons & Mitchell, 1999; Wellman et al., 2002).

FUTURE RESEARCH

Longitudinal research documenting outcomes for individuals with ASDs has highlighted the importance of fostering social communicative competence (National Research Council, 2001). Thus, both the SCERTS Model and the related curriculum-based assessment have been derived from descriptive group research studies indicating that developmental achievements in the domains of Social Communication and Emotional Regulation are predictive of gains in language acquisition, social adaptive functioning, and academic achievement—areas that foster social competence (Prizant et al., 2005a, 2005b).

Additionally, there is a strong recognition within this approach that skill acquisition in isolated teaching contexts is not the ultimate goal. Rather, gains related to social communicative competence should be observable across social partners and social contexts. Thus, the Transactional Support domain has been developed to provide a measure of partner behavior and to ensure treatment fidelity and progress across partners and contexts. This domain incorporates evidence-based practices and strategies that have been associated with progress in the domains of Social Communication and Emotional Regulation.

Of the practices and strategies incorporated in the Transactional Support domain of the SCERTS Model, AAC plays a prominent role due to its efficacy for fostering expressive communication and language, understanding of language and behavior, expression of emotion, and emotional regulation (Prizant et al., 2005a, 2005b). The SAP provides a tool to ensure that these supports are infused across social partners and social contexts in a manner that is sensitive to the functional needs of specific situations and the unique learning style of the individual with ASD. Future research is needed to ensure that the SAP is a reliable outcome measurement of progress for the individual with ASD and a reliable indicator of fidelity across social partners and settings. Once the reliability of the SAP has been demonstrated, a next step might include conducting experimental group treatment designs with randomized clinical trials to document group treatment effects under controlled conditions; this could examine the efficacy of the SCERTS Model in comparison with other comprehensive educational programs.

Additionally, the Transactional Support domain of the SAP provides a means to examine the relationship between specific educational/treatment strategies and positive social-communicative outcomes for children with ASDs. Within the assessment process, information can be gathered as to the relative consistency with which social partners modify their communicative styles, consistently provide AAC supports, and modify the environment based on an individual's unique learning style across activities, interactive partners, and social contexts. Thus, the relative impact of the presence or absence of specific interpersonal supports or learning supports can be documented, allowing researchers to examine which variables appear to be the most effective for individual children and then predict specific outcomes. Relationships investigated might include—but would not be limited to—the relationships between 1) AAC provision to enhance expression of emotions and emotional regulation and reductions in challenging behavior, 2) AAC provision to enhance understanding of language and an individual's development of conventional means for initiating and taking turns in conversation, and 3) AAC provision to enhance expressive language and an individual's overall social communicative competence.

REFERENCES

American Speech-Language-Hearing Association. (2005). *Roles and responsibilities of speech-language pathologists with respect to augmentative and alternative communication: Position statement.* Retrieved on December 23, 2007 from http://www.asha.org/members/deskref-journal/deskref/default

American Speech-Language-Hearing Association. (2006). *Guidelines for speech-language pathologists in diagnosis, assessment, and treatment of autism spectrum disorders across the life span.* Retrieved on December 23, 2007, from http://www.asha.org/NR/rdonlyres/8D2CE221-E7E6-4B60-AAF4-76C13BD8B6A6/0/v3GL_autismLSpan.pdf

Barry, L.M., & Burlew, S.B. (2004). Using social stories to teach choice and play skills to children with autism. *Focus on Autism and Other Developmental Disabilities, 19,* 45–51.

Bopp, K., Brown, K., & Mirenda, P. (2004). Speech-language pathologists' roles in the delivery of positive behavior support for individuals with developmental disabilities. *American Journal of Speech-Language Pathology, 13,* 5–19.

Brady, N. (2000). Improved comprehension of object names following voice output communication aid use: Two case studies. *Augmentative and Alternative Communication, 16,* 197–204.

Bryan, L.C., & Gast, D.L. (2000). Teaching on-task and on-schedule behaviors to higher functioning children with autism via picture activity schedules. *Journal of Autism and Developmental Disorders, 30,* 553–567.

Dawson, G., Hill, D., Spencer, A., Galpert, L., & Watson, L. (1990). Affective exchanges between young autistic children and their mothers. *Journal of Abnormal Child Psychology, 18,* 335–345.

Dawson, G., Toth, K., Abbott, R., Osterling, J., Munson, J., Estes, A., & Liaw, J. (2004). Early social attention impairments in autism: Social orienting, joint attention, and attention to distress. *Developmental Psychology, 40,* 271–283.

Frea, W.D., Arnold, C., & Vittimberga, G.L. (2001). A demonstration of the effects of augmentative communication on the extreme aggressive behavior of a child with autism within an integrated preschool setting. *Journal of Positive Behavior Interventions, 3,* 194–198.

Ganz, J.B., & Simpson, R.L. (2004). Effects on communicative requesting and speech development of the Picture Exchange Communication System in children with characteristics of autism. *Journal of Autism and Developmental Disorders, 34,* 395–409.

Goldstein, H., & Cisar, C.L. (1992). Promoting interaction during sociodramatic play. Teaching scripts to typical preschoolers and classmates with disabilities. *Journal of Applied Behavior Analysis, 25,* 265–280.

Gray, C.A. (1995). Teaching children with autism to "read" social situations. In K. Quill (Ed.), *Teaching children with autism: Strategies to enhance communication and socialization* (pp. 219–241). Albany, NY: Delmar.

Johnston, S., Nelson, C., Evans, J., & Palazolo, K. (2003). The use of visual supports in teaching young children with autism spectrum disorder to initiate interactions. *Augmentative and Alternative Communication, 19,* 86–103.

Kasari, C., Sigman, M.D., Baumgartner, P., & Stipek, D.J. (1993). Pride and mastery in children with autism. *Journal of Child Psychology and Psychiatry, 34,* 353–362.

Kerr, S., & Durkin, K. (2004). Understanding of thought bubbles as mental representations in children with autism: Implications for theory of mind. *Journal of Autism and Developmental Disorders, 34,* 637–648.

Krantz, P.J., & McClannahan, L.E. (1993). Teaching children with autism to initiate to peers. *Journal of Applied Behavior Analysis, 26,* 121–132.

Mirenda, P. (1997). Functional communication training and augmentative communication: A research review. *Augmentative and Alternative Communication, 13,* 207–225.

Mirenda, P. (2001). Autism, augmentative communicative and assistive technology: What do we really know? *Focus on Autism and Other Developmental Disabilities, 16,* 141–151.

Mirenda, P. (2003). Toward functional augmentative and alternative communication for students with autism: Manual signs, graphic symbols, and voice output communication aids. *Language, Speech, and Hearing Services in Schools, 34,* 202–215.

National Research Council. (2000). *From neurons to neighborhoods.* Washington, DC: National Academies Press.

National Research Council. (2001). *Educating children with autism.* Washington, DC: National Academies Press, Committee on Educational Interventions for Children with Autism, Division of Behavioral and Social Sciences and Education.

Parsons, S., & Mitchell, P. (1999). What children with autism understand about thoughts and thought bubbles. *Autism, 3,* 17–38.

Pierce, K., & Schreibman, L. (1994). Teaching daily living skills to children with autism in unsupervised settings through pictorial self-management. *Journal of Applied Behavior Analysis, 27,* 471–482.

Prizant, B.M., Wetherby, A.M., Rubin, E., & Laurent, A.C. (2003). The SCERTS® Model: A transactional, family-centered approach to enhancing communication and socioemotional abilities of children with autism spectrum disorder. *Infants and Young Children, 16,* 296–316.

Prizant, B.M., Wetherby, A.M., Rubin, E., Laurent, A.C., & Rydell, P.J. (2005a). *The SCERTS® Model: A comprehensive educational approach for children with autism spectrum disorders. Vol. I: Assessment.* Baltimore: Paul H. Brookes Publishing Co.

Prizant, B.M., Wetherby, A.M., Rubin, E., Laurent, A.C., & Rydell, P.J. (2005b). *The SCERTS® Model: A comprehensive educational approach for children with autism spectrum disorders. Vol. II: Intervention.* Baltimore: Paul H. Brookes Publishing Co.

Romski, M., & Sevcik, R.A. (2005). Augmentative communication and early intervention: Myths and realities. *Infants and Young Children, 18,* 174–185.

Rydell, P., & Prizant, B. (1995). Assessment and intervention strategies for children who use echolalia. In K. Quill (Ed.), *Teaching children with autism: strategies to enhance communication and socialization* (pp. 105–129). Albany, NY: Delmar.

Schlosser, R.W., & Lee, D. (2000). Promoting generalization and maintenance in augmentative and alternative communication: A meta-analysis of 20 years of effectiveness research. *Augmentative and Alternative Communication, 16,* 208–227.

Sigman, M., Kasari, C., Kwon, J.H., & Yirmiya, N. (1992). Responses to negative emotions of others by autistic, mentally retarded, and normal children. *Child Development, 63,* 796–807.

Simpson, R.L., de Boer-Ott, S.R., & Myles, B.S. (2003). Inclusion of learners with autism spectrum disorders in general education settings. *Topics in Language Disorders, 23,* 116–133.

Thiemann, K., & Goldstein, H. (2004). Effects of peer training and written-text cueing on social communication of school-age children with pervasive developmental disorder. *Journal of Speech, Language, and Hearing Research, 47,* 126–144.

Volkmar, F.R., Lord, C., Bailey, A., Schultz, R.T., & Klin, A. (2004). Autism and pervasive developmental disorders. *Journal of Child Psychology and Psychiatry, 45,* 145–170.

Wellman, H., Baron-Cohen, S., Caswell, R., Gomez, J.C., Swettenham, J., Toye, E., & Lagatutta, K. (2002). Thought bubbles help children with autism acquire an alternative to theory of mind. *Autism, 6,* 343–363.

Wetherby, A.M., Prizant, B.M., & Hutchinson, T. (1998). Communicative, social/affective, and symbolic profiles of young children with autism and pervasive developmental disorders. *American Journal of Speech-Language Pathology, 7,* 79–91.

8

The System for Augmenting Language

Implications for Young Children with Autism Spectrum Disorders

MARYANN ROMSKI, ROSE A. SEVCIK, ASHLYN SMITH, R. MICHEAL BARKER, STEPHANIE FOLAN, AND ANDREA BARTON-HULSEY

One striking hallmark of autism spectrum disorders (ASDs) is specific difficulty in the social-communicative aspects of language development (Lord, 2000; Wetherby, Prizant, & Hutchinson, 1998). In concert with these difficulties, some children with ASDs exhibit such severe language delays that they do not speak at all or are at the very beginning stages of speech and language development. In fact, recent estimates assert that between one third (Bryson, 1996) and one half (Lord & Paul, 1997) of children and adults with ASDs do not use speech functionally (i.e., their speech is echolalic or they speak only a few words; National Research Council, 2001). Unfortunately, these estimates do not specify the ages of these children and do not indicate whether or not they participated in interventions aimed at developing their speech and language skills.

Lord, Risi, and Pickles (2004) argued that the patterns of language change over time in children with ASDs and must be examined. It is unclear whether young children who are described as nonspeaking will remain so throughout their lives, whether interventions directed toward the development of speech and language skills are likely to be successful, and which children are most likely to have good outcomes

The authors thank the parents, teachers, and children who participated in these studies for their cooperation and support; and Lisa Wiggins for her input on how to determine the retrospective inclusion of children who may be appropriate for the analyses. Research reported in this manuscript was funded by grants from the National Institutes of Health (HD-06016 and DC-03799).

in this regard. Thus, "nonspeaking" should not be seen as a static state; rather, it should be viewed as a characteristic that can change over time as a result of maturity, intervention, or both.

When a child is not speaking, there are a range of language intervention strategies that may help facilitate the child's language development (e.g., Mirenda, 2003; Mirenda & Erickson, 2000; Sevcik & Romski, 1999). This chapter explores the implications of a specific type of augmentative and alternative communication (AAC) intervention known as the System for Augmenting Language (SAL) for beginning communicators, including exploratory data from SAL studies with school-age children with autism and toddlers at risk for ASDs. In relation to the SAL, it also provides a brief review of the literature on AAC interventions for beginning communicators with ASDs.

PROFILES OF BEGINNING COMMUNICATORS

Beginning communicators are children who come to the task of learning language with a spoken and/or symbol vocabulary of less than 50 words (Romski, Sevcik, & Fonseca, 2003). The upper limit of 50 words marks an important shift that occurs in typical language development—the vocabulary growth spurt. For beginning communicators to develop functional language and communication skills, they must be able to comprehend *and* produce language so that they can take on the roles of both listener and speaker in conversational exchanges (Sevcik & Romski, 2002).

Young, typically developing children learn to speak before the age of 2 years. They do so after spending more than a year being exposed to spoken language input from their caregivers. Prior to actually uttering their first words, these children comprehend about 50 words and develop an intentional communicative repertoire of vocalizations and gestures that they use to request and refer to objects and events in their environments (Chapter 3; Adamson, 1996). During this period from birth to approximately 18–21 months of age, typically developing children advance through the prelocutionary and illuctionary stages of communication development. Around 9 months of age, they begin to comprehend the speech of others in context; by 12 months of age, they understand approximately 50 words.

Somewhere between 12 and 15 months of age, young children begin to produce first word approximations and then slowly start to develop a vocabulary. At about the same time that they attain a 50-word vocabulary (18–21 months of age), they also begin to combine words. Prior to the time that most children have a 50-word vocabulary, the focus of their communication development is on the pragmatic (i.e., intentional communication and communication functions such as requesting and commenting) and the semantic (i.e., vocabulary and later semantic relations) aspects of language, rather than on the grammatical aspect.

The early word learning of typically developing children appears to be couched in their ability to extract relevant information from their linguistic environment and to associate it with their own developing vocal forms to express wants and needs (Baldwin & Markman, 1989; Golinkoff, Mervis, & Hirsh-Pasek, 1994; Mervis & Bertrand, 1993). Most children begin talking by gradually building individual vocabularies composed of a range of words (e.g., objects, actions, emotions; Nelson, 1973) until they evidence the important vocabulary growth spurt at about 18–21 months of age (Golinkoff et al., 1994). With this spurt, their rate of vocabulary acquisition increases dramatically and they also begin to combine words to express semantic relations.

This initial period of communication and language development is rich with opportunities for young children to develop a firm communication and language foundation, even though they are not yet talking. This foundation includes opportunities to communicate via vocalizations, gestures, and other means—even before the child uses a conventional output mode such as speech, manual signing, or graphic symbols and develops language comprehension skills. The literature on typically developing children's communication language development strongly suggests that these early types of experiences are important for later receptive and expressive language development. It also illustrates the integrated development of communication, language, and speech—three separate but related processes.

Beginning communicators with disabilities or delays encompass a broad range of communicative profiles during this developmental period that vary widely, depending on a combination of their biological status, the environments in which they function, and their experiences. Depending on the child's chronological age and disability severity, communication profiles may range from unintelligible speech and/or echolalic speech to a very limited number of words (e.g., fewer than 10) or no speech at all. Individual child profiles will interact differentially with various language intervention strategies to influence intervention outcomes. Among the individual factors that contribute to an individual's beginning communicative profile are his or her intellectual development, related disabilities, and communicative experiences (which includes factors such as chronological age, vocal and gestural production skills, and speech comprehension skills; Romski, Sevcik, Cheslock, & Hyatt, 2002; Sevcik & Romski, 2002). Children with ASDs exhibit profiles that are influenced by the specific characteristics of ASDs, such as marked difficulties with social communication and the development of joint attention (Adamson, Bakeman, Deckner, &

Romski, in press; Paparella & Kasari, 2004; Mundy & Stella, 2000, Wetherby et al., 1998). Difficulties with the development of joint attention in particular may have a number of influences on the speech and language profiles of children with ASDs, including their abilities to use language for communication.

To address the needs of beginning communicators, AAC interventions must integrate communication experiences with receptive and expressive language activities. This integration requires approaches that incorporate technology and are developmental in nature, such as the SAL (Romski, Sevcik, Cheslock, & Barton, 2006).

THE SYSTEM FOR AUGMENTING LANGUAGE

The SAL (Romski & Sevcik, 1996; Romski, et al., 2006) is an AAC intervention approach originally developed as part of a longitudinal research study of the language development of school-age beginning communicators with moderate to severe intellectual disabilities. It was designed to supplement beginning communicators' natural— albeit severely limited—receptive and expressive language abilities and to facilitate their ability to communicate in a conventional manner in everyday environments, primarily home and school. The children in the original SAL project had at least primitive intentional communication skills, spoken language vocabularies of less than 10 intelligible words or word approximations, and gross pointing skills, along with histories that included a number of years of unsuccessful communication experiences and/or interventions prior to their participation in the study.

Components of the SAL

The SAL consists of five integrated components: 1) a speech-generating device (SGD); 2) individually chosen vocabulary words and the visual-graphic symbols to represent them; 3) natural everyday environments that encourage, but do not require, the child to produce symbols; 4) models of symbol use by communicative partners; and 5) an ongoing resource and feedback mechanism. The SAL is implemented in natural environments that include home, school, and community settings, as well as a variety of communication partners such as parents, siblings, peers, classroom teachers, speech-language pathologists, and others with whom the child interacts. This intervention approach was termed a *system* because the five organized components must work in concert. One component alone, such as a speech-generating device, is not sufficient. We believe that it is the integration of the five components that facilitates the language learning process (Romski et al., 2006).

Component 1: Speech-Generating Devices   The first component of the SAL is an SGD, also known as a computer-based speech-
output communication device or a voice output communication aid
(VOCA). Over the past decade, there has been a substantial increase in
the quantity and quality of reasonably priced SGDs on the commercial
market (McBride & Rush, 2007). The specific SGD can vary, depending
on the individual needs of the child and the range of available technology. From our perspective, the critical feature of this SAL component
is the speech output and the child's ability to access it. The device is
simply the tool.

Speech output is a critical component of the SAL because the
SGD serves as the medium for language experiences. The computer-
generated voice permits the child to compensate for the use of a visual
communication system. Use of a synthetic or digitized auditory signal
permits partners to both hear the speech output that is produced when
the child activates a symbol and to comprehend the message immediately. This feature is particularly important when children are integrated in general community settings and interact with a broad range
of both familiar and unfamiliar communicative partners. The SGD
automatically links the child's visual symbol communication with a
familiar auditory modality in social interaction contexts. It permits the
child to use a multimodal form of communication, including a voice
(albeit not his or her own), while retaining access to the visual modality (Romski & Sevcik, 1996; Romski et al., 2006).

Component 2: Lexicon and Symbols   The second component
of the SAL has two prongs: a relevant lexicon or vocabulary and the
visual-graphic symbols used to represent the lexicon. The lexicon that
is available for understanding and expression plays a very important
role in language learning by providing a foundation on which communicative interactions are built. Although individuals with little or no
functional speech are often exposed to a spoken input vocabulary that
is comparable to that of a speaking child, their output vocabulary is
likely to be externally constrained by the visual-graphic symbol items
that are available on an AAC display. One of the same features that
has been proposed to facilitate their learning via augmented means—
namely, that fact that graphic symbol use relies on their relatively
strong recognition memory rather than their relatively weak recall
memory (Fristoe & Lloyd, 1979)—may also serve to limit their symbol
use because it places restrictions on the number and range of vocabulary items that can be made available to them at any one time.

The second prong of this component is the visual-graphic symbol
set that is used to represent the lexicon. The issues regarding which

symbol set to employ with an individual are complex (for detailed discussions, see Mineo-Mollica, 2003; Sevcik, Romski, & Wilkinson, 1991). Symbols that are arbitrary do not visually resemble the vocabulary items they represent, whereas nonarbitrary symbols resemble the meanings they represent to varying degrees. For example, the printed English word *cap*—an arbitrary symbol—does not resemble the piece of clothing that is worn on the head, whereas the Picture Communication Symbol (PCS) for *cap* is a line drawing of the object it represents.

Over the course of the SAL's history, there has been a shift in use from arbitrary symbols (i.e., lexigrams) to pictographic symbols such as PCSs to represent the lexicon. When the authors began studying the communication development of toddlers, a conscious decision was made, based on input from the children's parents, to employ visual-graphic symbols, which are perceived as more age appropriate for young children than arbitrary symbols (Sevcik, Romski, & Adamson, 2004). Mineo-Mollica (2003) suggested that the skills a child brings to the task, the type of symbol representation, the number of representations that are presented simultaneously, and the arrangement of representations must all be considered when determining which symbol set(s) to use.

Component 3: Teaching Through Natural Communicative Exchanges
Components 3 and 4 focus on the teaching dimensions of the SAL. Component 3 specifies both where and how children will experience communication opportunities with their SGDs. Loosely structured, naturalistic communicative experiences are provided to encourage, but not require, children's use of the symbols during daily activities. These natural communicative experiences are embedded in routines in which the children engage during the course of their daily activities. Such an approach is consistent with contemporary research and theories that recommend the implementation of AAC interventions in natural environments to emphasize the functional nature of language, facilitate the generalization of communicative routines to diverse contexts, and increase the spontaneity of communicative exchanges (for a review, see Romski, Sevcik, & Fonseca, 2003).

Although traditional, structured interventions have often occurred in isolated settings in which practitioners and children interact, natural settings such as homes, schools, and community venues provide familiar locations for the occurrence of shared communicative experiences. Natural settings also provided numerous daily routines for the child's engagement (e.g., meals, bath time, bed time) that can be used to provide communicative opportunities.

Component 4: Partner's Use of the Device   The partner's active role in communicative interactions is the fourth component of the SAL. Partners play two rather obvious roles in the communication exchange: they are speakers who provide communicative input to the children and listeners who respond to the children's communications. Because their child partners use visual-graphic symbols, the way the partners communicate must be modified. Thus, an instructional focus that encompasses partners must include considerations of both their roles, as a speaker and listener. Additionally, partners must be comfortable with the SGD used by the child. Romski, Sevcik, Adamson, Cheslock, and Smith (2007) reported that parents who were given structured experiences were able to learn to use SGDs to communicate with their children.

In the SAL, communicative partners are encouraged to integrate use of the SGD into their own spoken language communications by employing augmented language input. *Augmented language input* refers to the communication/language input provided by a child's communicative partner, which includes speech supplemented by AAC symbols, the speech output produced by the SGD, and the environmental context (Romski & Sevcik, 2003). In the example *Tommy, let's go* outside *and ride your* bike, *outside* and *bike* are symbols spoken by the SGD after the partner activates them; the remaining words are produced as verbal speech by the adult. This permits each family member or teacher to incorporate SGD use into ongoing communicative interactions, while at the same time providing spoken language models.

Partner augmented input, in turn, serves several functions for the participant. First, it provides a model for how the SAL can be used, in what contexts, and for what purposes. When the child's communicative partners employ SAL as augmented input, the simultaneous pairing of visual symbols and synthetic speech output may permit the child to extract spoken words from the language-learning environment. The specific way in which the symbols are both produced and paired with synthetic speech can serve to segment the critical word/symbol from the natural stream of speech (e.g., *Let's see your* dress) and may facilitate the child's ability to match the symbol/word with its physical referent. Second, this technique has the potential to reinforce the effectiveness of using the SGD; when a partner incorporates the SAL in successful communicative exchanges, the child is provided with real-world experiences that illustrate both symbol meanings and the varied functions each symbol can serve. This allows the child to experience the potential utility and power of the SAL. Finally, and perhaps most importantly, partner augmented input makes an implicit statement to the child that the SGD provides an acceptable vehicle for communicating—a vehicle that the partner is also willing to use (Romski & Sevcik, 2003; Sevcik & Romski, 2002; Sevcik, Romski, Watkins, & Deffebach, 1995).

Component 5: Monitoring Ongoing Use   The fifth and final component of the SAL is a resource and feedback mechanism that is used to monitor the child's and partner's ongoing use. This mechanism consists of gaining regular information from the child and his or her primary communicative partners. This information, coupled with various assessment tools, can help the clinician gain insights into the child's patterns of communicative use, accomplishments and/or difficulties that might be experienced, and operational challenges that might be present in the settings of use. Regular meetings can also be held with the child's communicative partners to provide opportunities for face-to-face interactions to discuss progress and problems.

THE AAC LITERATURE AND CHILDREN WITH ASD

As this book highlights, the AAC literature includes numerous intervention strategies aimed at teaching various aspects of language and communication to children with ASDs. Some of these studies have examined the responsivity of children with ASD to individual components of the SAL (e.g., SGDs, augmented communication input). In this section, we provide a brief overview of findings from these reports to illustrate how existing research has incorporated individual components of the SAL, as well as the degree to which they have been successful for children with ASDs.

Speech-Generating Devices

In their review, Schlosser and Bischak (2001) argued that speech output can play an important role in interventions for children with ASD. They concluded, however, that there is little clear and consistent evidence about the exact nature of that role. Lancioni et al. (2007) provided an updated review of the literature on the use of SGDs (which they referred to as voice output communication aids or VOCAs). Three of the studies they reviewed included at least some children with ASDs. The outcomes they reported suggested that SGDs resulted in gains in either receptive or expressive language skills, most often in the area of requesting.

Light, Roberts, Dimarco, and Greimer (1998) also presented a case report of a 6-year-old boy with autism who had severe receptive and expressive language difficulties. After the child had 2 years of experience with a Macintosh Powerbook computer with Write:OutLoud software, he was able to respond appropriately to questions (who, what, when, where) about stories read in class and at home. The child was also able to follow orally presented one-step instructions involving prepositions, as well as two- and three-step instructions presented either orally or in writing. Although this boy used speech as his primary mode of communication, the Powerbook augmented his speech when he needed to communicate more complex information.

Overall, the literature indicates that both simple and more complex SGDs may be appropriate tools for language and communication interventions for children with ASDs. Additional research is required to determine the specific roles that such SGDs can play (see Chapter 5 for a complete review and discussion of these issues).

The Lexicon and Symbols

There is little comparative literature on the development of a functional lexicon for children with ASDs. Most of the lexicons that have been used to date in research studies are limited to objects (e.g., car, book) or other nouns (e.g., foods, drinks) that serve the function of requesting (e.g., *I want [object]*). In addition, Mirenda (2003) suggested that there is a dearth of evidence about the type(s) of symbols (i.e., arbitrary, pictographic) that best facilitate symbol learning by children with ASDs.

Augmented Input

The enhanced input to which children who use AAC are typically exposed to has been termed augmented input (Romski & Sevcik, 2003), aided language stimulation (Goossens' & Crain, 1986) and aided language modeling (Drager et al., 2006). These three approaches differ slightly.

Augmented input, described earlier in this chapter, is characterized as the incoming communication/language from a child's communicative partner that includes speech; it is supplemented by AAC symbols, the speech output produced by an SGD when symbols are activated, and the environmental context (Romski & Sevcik, 2003). *Aided language stimulation* is a broader term that is somewhat analogous to total communication and simultaneous communication (e,g., manual signing plus speech). *Aided language modeling* incorporates components of both of these strategies and involves engaging the child in interactive play activities while providing models of AAC symbol use on a language display without speech output.

All three of these interventions highlight the role of partners in communication interactions with children with ASDs and target the importance of comprehension in the language development process (Romski & Sevcik, 2003). A few studies have examined the effectiveness of augmented input communication for beginning communicators with ASDs.

Peterson, Bondy, Vincent, and Finnegan (1995) assessed the effects of interventions in three communicative input modalities on the task performance and frequency of target behaviors in two boys with autism and challenging behaviors (ages 7 and 9 years). The three different communicative inputs were spoken language alone, pictorial or gestural input alone, and a combination of pictorial or gestural input plus spoken input. The authors reported that spoken input alone did not enhance the boys' performances, especially compared to the combination input strategy. In fact, they suggested that spoken input alone resulted in increased challenging behaviors.

Over a 22-month period, Cafiero (2001) examined the effect of a natural aided language intervention on the communication, behavior, and academic program of a 13-year-old nonverbal adolescent with autism. During a 3-month period initially following the introduction of graphic symbol displays, the adolescent showed increases in his functional lexicon. He was able to use this lexicon to initiate requests, make comments, and combine 2 or 3 words to form multiword utterances. His lexicon decreased over the summer months when natural aided language strategies were not used, but increased again when the school year resumed. This finding suggests that continuous use of natural aided language techniques may be required to maintain the communicative lexicon and stimulate language growth.

Drager et al. (2006) examined the effectiveness of aided language modeling on both symbol comprehension and production in two preschool-age children with ASDs who used fewer than 30 functional words. Aided language modeling included components of both aided language stimulation and augmented input and incorporated graphic symbol displays for communication. Both children showed substantial increases in symbol comprehension and elicited symbol production, although comprehension skills increased more than production skills.

As a whole, evidence from this modest set of studies suggests that augmenting communication input for children with ASDs can be effective in increasing both symbol comprehension and production. Clearly, further examination of this intervention approach is needed.

Parent Instruction for Children with ASDs

Another component of the SAL is the role of the parent as communication partner. Partner instruction is not a new concept in either AAC

(Light & Binger, 1998) or in interventions with children with ASDs. Parent instruction can take many different forms. We use four representative studies to illustrate how parents can learn to be successful at learning and using early language and communication intervention strategies with their children with ASDs.

Laski, Charlop, and Schreibman (1988) taught parents to support the communication of their children with autism (ages 5.0 to 9.6 years) using the Natural Language Paradigm (NLP). Parent instruction consisted of three components: a discussion of NLP procedures, observations of trained interventionists conducting NLP with a child, and continuous observation and feedback during the parent's administration of NLP. Following the second parent training session, parents conducted four NLP interventions per week at home in addition to those conducted in a clinic. Following completion of parent training instruction, parents conducted NLP interventions in the home only. Results indicated that after their parents were taught to implement NLP, all of the children demonstrated increases in at least one of the following domains: imitating, answering, spontaneous speech, or vocalizing.

Kaiser, Hancock, and Nietfeld (2000) examined the effects of teaching six parents how to use enhanced milieu teaching with their preschool children with ASDs. The parents learned to use the intervention techniques and maintained them at low levels at home 6 months later. The children achieved a variety of communication targets; four of the six children maintained these communication skills at the 6-month follow-up assessment.

Kashintath, Woods, and Goldstein (2006) taught the parents of five toddlers with ASDs to use specific strategies within daily routines to support communication. The strategies included arranging the environment, using natural reinforcement, using time delay when providing labels for objects, and using contingent imitation. Results indicated that all five parents increased their use of the strategies in daily routines and that all children demonstrated increases in expressive communication.

Finally, Grela and McLaughlin (2006) investigated parent instruction as part of a focused stimulation intervention for a 3-year-old boy with ASDs. The intervention focused on supporting the child's comprehension of *What is X doing?* questions and simple one-step commands. Researchers met with the parents for 1 hour each week for 4 weeks. Parents were taught techniques such as following the child's lead, commenting on the child's activities, and using focused stimulation to support communication intervention goals. Three weeks into the intervention, the child's responses to target questions and target commands increased by 75% and 20%, respectively. By completion of the intervention, the child responded to 80% of target questions and 30% of target commands.

Summary

These selected examples support the suggestion that children with ASDs can benefit from SGDs, augmented input techniques, and parent-implemented instruction directed toward language development. These findings, albeit with a small set of children, suggest that children with ASDs can benefit from the individuals components that make up the SAL.

PHASES OF SAL RESEARCH

The SAL intervention has been developed as one component in a program of research designed to examine the factors that impact communication development for children with significant developmental delays. The first set of studies was a longitudinal investigation of SAL use by 13 school-age children (Romski & Sevcik, 1996), followed by a number of exploratory studies that examined extensions of the SAL intervention to preschoolers and toddlers (Sevcik, Romski, & Adamson, 2004).

The authors' exploration of SAL use with preschoolers and toddlers led to the examination of the receptive and expressive components of SAL separately; then the components were contrasted with a spoken communication intervention in a randomized control study of 60 toddlers with developmental delays who were at significant risk for developing difficulties with spoken language skills (Romski et al., 2008). This section briefly describes the outcomes of this series of studies, as well as reports of SAL use with school-age children with ASDs and a retrospective examination of toddlers who received diagnoses of ASDs as preschoolers.

School-Age Children: Communication Gains with SAL

Thirteen school-age children (mean chronological age of 12 years 8 months) who received SAL intervention integrated the use of SGDs into their extant vocal and gestural repertoires (Romski, Sevcik, Robinson, & Bakeman, 1994). The result was a rich, multimodal means of communication that they employed to successfully and effectively communicate with both adults (Romski, Sevcik, Robinson, et al., 1994) and peers (Romski, Sevcik, & Wilkinson, 1994). Individual participant achievements ranged from use of a modest set of 20–35 symbols to the use of more than 100 symbols to convey referential and social-regulative symbolic messages in varied daily contexts with adults (Adamson, Romski, Deffenbach, & Sevcik, 1992). Some of the youth also developed combinatorial symbol skills (Wilkinson, Romski, & Sevcik, 1994), as well as the ability to produce intelligible spoken words and rudimentary reading skills (Romski & Sevcik, 1996).

Two categories of communication achievement were identified in these youngsters. One group was described as having an advanced achievement pattern, whereas the second group was described as having a beginning achievement pattern. The nine advanced achievers comprehended and produced most of their symbol vocabularies and rapidly acquired other symbolic skills. The four beginning achievers initially comprehended their symbols better than they used them in production. Their overall vocabulary was smaller (i.e., 35 symbols or less) and their overall progress was slower than that of the advanced group.

After 5 years of SAL experience, Romski, Sevcik, and Adamson (1999) employed a repeated measures design and systematically controlled the 13 SAL users' access to their SGDs in a conversational study with an unfamiliar adult partner. The participants were able to convey more conversationally appropriate, less ambiguous, and more specific information to the unfamiliar adult partner with their SGDs than without them.

Similarly, Romski, Sevcik, Adamson, and Bakeman (2005) used a group design to compare the skills of the 13 SAL users to 13 youth with intellectual disabilities who spoke and 13 others who did not speak and had no SAL experience. The SAL-experienced individuals were able to convey more appropriate, less ambiguous, and more specific information than comparable individuals who were symbol-naïve and unable to speak. In addition, their communication patterns were similar in several ways to those of the individuals who spoke, although they still lacked the ability to convey information about past and future events. The comparison group design allowed a confirmation of the initial hypothesis that the SAL intervention produced outcomes that were better than those that would have occurred in the absence of intervention. It was found that the SAL experience enhanced the communication skills of the 13 participants in interactions with unfamiliar partners; they functioned more like individuals with intellectual disabilities who spoke than like individuals who were unable to speak.

SAL Intervention for Toddlers and Preschoolers with Developmental Delays

SAL intervention was also explored with preschoolers (Sevcik, Romski, & Adamson, 2004). This section will briefly summarize the outcomes of a parent-implemented language intervention study (Romski et al., 2008) on the use of various SAL components with 60 toddlers (mean chronological age of 29.5 months) with developmental delays who had less than 10 spoken words or word approximations. The vocabulary development of these toddlers was compared across three interventions: augmented communicative input, augmented communicative output, and speech communication intervention. The ability of the children to transfer their vocabulary to home settings was also examined.

Given the young age of the children in this study, we separated the comprehension (i.e., augmented language input) and production components of the SAL into two separate interventions: augmented communicative input and augmented communicative output. Augmented communicative input included the receptive components of the SAL and augmented communicative output included the expressive components; both included SGDs with digitized speech. Parent–child pairs were randomly assigned to one of the three interventions.

For augmented communicative input, each child's interventionist and parent used an SGD and individualized target vocabulary of visual-graphic symbols and spoken words to provide communication input via vocabulary models (Romski & Sevcik, 2003). Symbols were also positioned in the environment to mark referents. For augmented communicative output intervention, the interventionist and parent used an SGD and individualized target vocabulary of visual-graphic symbols and spoken words to encourage the child to produce communications using the device. For the spoken communication intervention, which served as a contrast condition to augmented communicative input and augmented communicative output, children's interventionists and parents employed individualized target vocabularies and both encouraged and prompted the children to produce spoken words.

All three interventions were parent-implemented in home settings. In addition, prior to beginning the interventions, the three groups were well-matched and there were no significant differences between the groups. Female interventionists with a bachelor's degree in psychology or communication disorders were taught to implement all three intervention protocols and were supervised by a certified and licensed speech-language pathologist.

Although the three interventions differed in terms of the specific mode of delivery, they shared a number of common features. Each intervention was designed to be 24 sessions (or 12 weeks) in length with 18 sessions (or 9 weeks) occurring in a laboratory setting and 6 sessions (or 3 weeks) taking place in each child's home. Each session was 30 minutes in length and consisted of three 10-minute blocks of play, book reading, and snack, in that order. A set of targeted vocabulary words was individually chosen for each child by his or her parent, in collaboration with the project's speech-language pathologist.

The goal of all three interventions was parent implementation. Parents first received an intervention protocol manual with weekly materials that included goals for the parent, interventionist, and child (Romski & Cheslock, 2000). During the first 8 sessions (4 weeks), the parent and the speech-language pathologist observed the interventionist implement the intervention with the child. While they observed, the speech-language pathologist highlighted strategies that the interventionist was using and answered the parent's questions about the interaction. Beginning in the ninth session, the parent joined the session for the last 10 minutes (snack) and received ongoing coaching by the interventionist to implement the intervention protocol. By the 16th session, the parent led the entire 30-minute session. The last 3 weeks were led by the parents and conducted at home. All intervention sessions were videotaped.

All children showed evidence of significant intervention gains as a result of the parent-implemented language interventions. Parents readily and reliably learned to use the three intervention protocols, including those that involved SGDs, with their children (Romski et al., 2008). Both of the augmented language interventions (augmented communicative input and augmented communicative output) provided a way for the children to communicate via visual-graphic symbols plus digitized speech after only 18 sessions (or 9 weeks) of intervention; the children continued to use their SGDs at home after 24 sessions.

Compared to the speech communication intervention, augmented communicative output and, to a lesser extent, augmented communicative input substantially increased the likelihood that children would produce a modest number of spoken words for the target vocabulary after just 18 sessions of parent-implemented intervention. These gains were maintained with the parent in the home at 24 sessions. Both the augmented communicative input and augmented communicative output interventions permitted a specific focus on the target vocabulary and provided additional supports to both the child and parent. In addition, children in the augmented communicative input and augmented communicative output groups also showed a larger type-token ratio and produced significantly more intelligible communicative utterances than the children in the speech communication intervention group. This finding suggests that the use of an SGD plus speech may contribute to the intelligibility of child communications (for a detailed report of this study, see Romski et al., 2008).

SAL Use for Children with ASDs

Two studies investigated SAL use with children with ASDs. In the first (Romski and Sevcik, 1996), two of the children had dual diagnoses of severe intellectual disabilities and autism. In the early intervention study with toddlers (Romski et al., 2008), 12 of the 60 toddlers received diagnoses of ASDs once they entered preschool.

School-Age Children   Two school-age children with dual diagnoses of severe intellectual disabilities and autism (chronological ages of 16 years 7 months and 7 years 3 months) learned to communicate via the SAL and were characterized as advanced achievers (Romski & Sevcik, 1996). These two participants showed evidence of a fairly swift rate of acquisition of symbols, followed by the emergence of symbol combinations and other symbol skills (e.g., printed word recognition). Although their performance and learning appeared comparable to the other 11 participants, Romski and Sevcik (1996) reported that "...the 2 participants with autism, gave us the impression that they were more interested in the mechanical operation of the speech-output device itself than in using it to communicate (p. 106)."

Exploring Receptive and Expressive SAL Use with Young Children At Risk for ASDs   Children with diagnoses of ASDs were not included in the Romski et al. (2008) study because we believed that their families might have expectations that could complicate the children's responsivity to intervention. However, by the 12-month follow-up assessment, parents of 14 of the 60 children who had completed the study as toddlers reported that their children had received diagnoses of autism after they completed the intervention. Given our positive intervention outcomes, we retrospectively explored how these children in particular benefited from the interventions.

While 2 of these 14 children had formal diagnoses of ASDs using an appropriate testing protocol, the remaining 12 children did not. Their parents reported that a professional had assigned a diagnosis of autism, but no standard assessment protocol was reported. Thus, two of our staff with experience in ASDs (a speech language pathologist and a special educator) reviewed the assessment reports of these 12 children and also viewed a 30-minute videotape of each child and his or her parent interacting during a follow-up assessment. They then independently rated each child against the criteria from the *Diagnostic and Statistical Manual of Mental Disorders, Fourth Edition, Text Revision* for autistic disorder or pervasive developmental disorder-not otherwise specified (PDD-NOS) (American Psychiatric Association, 2000).

Using both of these categories provided a broad net for including children in this exploratory analysis. Of the 12 children, 10 independently received the same ratings from both staff members: 9 of the 12 met the criteria for Autistic Disorder or PDD-NOS and 1 child did not. The reviewers also disagreed on the ratings for two remaining children, so we did not include them in the subsequent analyses. Thus, the data from a total of 11 children were examined.

Of the 11 children, 6 children had been randomly assigned to one of the augmented language interventions (3 to augmented communicative input and 3 to augmented communicative output); however, for the purpose of this review, we grouped them together. The remaining 5 children had been randomly assigned to the speech communication intervention. Table 8.1 provides a description of the 11 children at the onset of the intervention study.

Each child's individualized target vocabulary consisted of both routine-specific and core vocabulary items that were available for use during the intervention sessions. Core vocabulary items were available across routines and routine-specific vocabulary items were available only during specific routines. The majority of the vocabulary items consisted of social-regulative words (e.g., mine, my turn, what's this, more), action words (e.g., jump, eat, play, open, clean up) and objects (e.g., toothbrush, fish, book, cookie, puzzle, bubbles). As shown in Table 8.2, after 18 sessions, the children in the augmented communicative input or output interventions and the speech communication intervention had a mean of 15.7 (range, 12–21) and 15 target vocabulary items (range, 13–16) available for use, respectively. They maintained these target vocabulary items through session 24.

Table 8.2 also shows the percentage of target vocabulary items that were used after 18 sessions (i.e., those conducted in the laboratory) and 24 sessions (including sessions 19–24, which were conducted at home) for all 11 children by their assigned intervention. At 18 sessions, the six children in the augmented language interventions were using a mean of 71% of their symbols on an SGD; five of the six children used a majority of their symbols. After transfer to the home environment during sessions 19–24, five of the six children continued to use their symbols (mean, 68.5%). With regard to spoken word target vocabulary, one child in the speech communication intervention and two children in augmented communicative input or output intervention used words for a very small percentage of their target vocabulary at 18 sessions. Two of these three children maintained word usage at 24 sessions, whereas an additional child in speech communication intervention had started use a small percentage of words by this time.

Table 8.1. Participants' demographic information at the start of intervention

Participant number	Group	Age (months)	Sex	Ethnicity	Mullen standard score	SICD receptive language age (months)	SICD expressive language age (months)	MCDI item C.1[a]	Vineland standard score
1	ACI	24	M	Caucasian	64	8	10	0	64
2	ACI	26	M	Caucasian	58	16	16	0	65
3	ACI	26	M	Caucasian	48	16	8	1	66
4	ACO	38	M	Hispanic	48	16	12	0	62
5	ACO	34	M	Asian	48	12	8	0	62
6	ACO	24	M	Caucasian	54	12	8	1	66
Mean		28.7			53.33	13.33	10.33	0.33	64.17
7	SCI	21	F	Asian	51	10	10	0	69
8	SCI	32	M	Hispanic	54	12	12	0	69
9	SCI	30	M	African American	67	20	16	0	66
10	SCI	37	M	Caucasian	57	20	16	0	63
11	SCI	38	M	Asian	48	16	8	0	57
Mean		31.6			55.40	15.60	12.40	0.00	64.40

Key: Mullen, Mullen Scales of Early Learning (Mullen, 1995); SICD, Sequenced Inventory of Communication Development (Hendrick, Prather, & Tobin, 1984); MCDI, MacArthur-Bates Communication Development Inventory (Fenson et al., 1985); Vineland, Vineland Scales of Adaptive Behavior (Sparrow, Balla, & Cicchetti, 1993); ACI, augmented language input; ACO, augmented language output; SCI, spoken communication intervention.

[a]For item C.1, 0 = never; 1 = sometimes.

Table 8.2.   Percentage of target vocabulary usage (total vocabulary)

		Symbols		Words	
Child	Group	Session 18	Session 24	Session 18	Session 24
1	ACI	95% (21)	76% (21)	0% (21)	0% (21)
2	ACI	29% (14)	0% (14)	0% (14)	0% (14)
3	ACI	83% (12)	92% (12)	17% (12)	0% (12)
4	ACO	81% (15)	94% (15)	13% (15)	6% (15)
5	ACO	53% (16)	93% (16)	0% (16)	0% (16)
6	ACO	88% (16)	56% (16)	0% (16)	0% (16)
	Mean	72% (15.7)	69% (15.7)	5% (15.7)	1% (15.7)
7	SCI	N/A	N/A	0% (16)	0% (16)
8	SCI	N/A	N/A	0% (13)	15% (13)
9	SCI	N/A	N/A	0% (16)	0% (16)
10	SCI	N/A	N/A	7% (15)	7% (15)
11	SCI	N/A	N/A	0% (15)	0% (15)
	Mean	N/A	N/A	1% (15)	4% (15)

Note: All values represent percentage of the total available vocabulary words that are presented in parentheses.

Key: ACI, augmented language input; ACO, augmented language output; SCI, spoken communication intervention.

As part of the larger study, all sessions were videotaped. We transcribed the 30-minute sessions at baseline, 18, and 24 sessions using Systematic Analysis of Language Transcripts (SALT) software (Miller & Chapman, 1985). Table 8.3 presents the children's mean length of utterance in morphemes (MLU), type-token ratio, percent of intelligible utterances, utterance rate, mean length of turns, and total turns at each of these time points. Consistent with the general study findings, the children who received augmented communicative input or output interventions showed greater increases in their type-token ratio and proportion of intelligible utterances at 18 and 24 sessions than the children who participated in the speech communication intervention. Unlike the overall findings, the children in the speech communication intervention took more total turns than the children in the augmented communicative input or output interventions.

Table 8.4 presents the parents' MLU, mean turn length, and total turns. The parents' data are again consistent with the larger study. The parents in the augmented communicative input/output interventions reduced the mean length of their turns from baseline to 18 and 24 sessions, whereas the speech communication parents did not do so consistently.

At the completion of intervention, on the receptive and expressive scales of the Sequenced Inventory of Communication Development (SICD; Hendrick, Prather, & Tobin, 1984), the children in the

Table 8.3. Child transcript measures

Child	Group	Mean length of utterance (morphemes)			Type-token ratio			Percentage of intelligible utterances			Utterance rate			Mean length of turn in utterances			Total turns		
		S-00	S-18	S-24	S-00	S-18	S-24	S-00	S-18	S-24	S-00	S-18	S-24	S-00	S-18	S-24	S-00	S-18	S-24
1	ACI	0.94	0.96	0.96	0.13	0.30	0.24	0.00	0.68	0.54	0.54	2.57	2.43	1.14	1.10	1.07	14	70	68
2	ACI	1.00	1.00	1.00	0.04	0.17	0.13	0.00	0.26	0.29	0.83	1.93	1.03	1.09	1.26	1.15	23	46	27
3	ACI	0.86	1.00	1.00	0.17	0.10	0.10	0.00	0.86	0.81	0.23	3.67	4.03	1.00	1.93	1.75	7	57	69
4	ACO	1.00	0.99	0.95	0.05	0.10	0.12	0.00	0.34	0.53	0.74	9.37	7.90	1.00	1.60	1.44	22	176	165
5	ACO	0.98	0.99	0.99	0.02	0.12	0.12	0.00	0.43	0.79	2.00	3.90	4.30	1.09	1.14	1.05	55	103	123
6	ACO	1.00	0.99	1.01	0.01	0.20	0.26	0.00	0.80	0.84	2.63	2.83	2.27	1.03	1.18	1.10	77	72	62
	Mean	0.96	0.99	0.99	0.07	0.17	0.16	0.00	0.56	0.63	10.16	4.05	3.66	1.06	1.37	1.26	33.0	87.3	85.7
7	SCI	1.00	0.99	1.00	0.07	0.07	0.04	0.05	0.07	0.00	1.47	2.40	1.77	1.10	1.13	1.04	40	64	51
8	SCI	1.00	1.00	1.09	0.08	0.05	0.06	0.03	0.08	0.24	2.07	4.30	13.0	1.22	1.28	1.54	51	101	254
9	SCI	0.97	1.02	1.05	0.11	0.09	0.07	0.08	0.30	0.30	1.30	5.27	3.83	1.08	1.24	1.19	36	127	97
10	SCI	1.00	1.06	1.12	0.11	0.18	0.11	0.21	0.33	0.43	5.55	6.83	6.37	1.44	1.38	1.58	112	149	121
11	SCI	1.00	1.00	1.00	0.04	0.02	0.04	0.00	0.00	0.00	0.77	1.43	0.77	1.00	1.02	1.00	23	42	23
	Mean	0.99	1.01	1.05	0.08	0.08	0.06	0.07	0.16	0.19	2.23	4.05	5.15	1.17	1.21	1.27	52.4	96.6	109.2

Key: ACI, augmented language input; ACO, augmented language output; SCI, spoken communication intervention; S-00, baseline observation session; S-18, intervention session 18; S-24, intervention session 24.

Table 8.4. Parent transcript measures

Child	Group	Mean length of utterance (morphemes)			Mean length of turn in utterances			Total turns		
		S-00	S-18	S-24	S-00	S-18	S-24	S-00	S-18	S-24
1	ACI	3.04	2.69	2.73	20.12	6.65	5.46	17	69	90
2	ACI	2.34	3.21	2.88	14.91	10.81	11.35	35	53	54
3	ACI	2.7	3.11	3.46	15.09	6.02	7.03	34	91	73
4	ACO	2.97	3.43	3.25	29.05	2.48	3.29	21	179	166
5	ACO	3.07	3.53	3.48	18.40	6.09	7.10	42	101	115
6	ACO	3.12	3.25	3.02	10.32	10.43	9.97	69	69	75
	Mean	2.87	3.20	3.14	17.98	7.08	7.37	36.33	93.67	95.50
7	SCI	2.96	2.69	2.59	16.95	10.84	12.03	38	61	60
8	SCI	3.54	3.33	3.52	13.34	6.44	2.36	50	87	236
9	SCI	3.31	3.23	3.53	16.38	5.27	6.02	37	117	99
10	SCI	2.53	2.23	2.19	3.43	3.15	2.48	120	152	131
11	SCI	4.02	2.39	2.96	40.05	18.05	38.72	22	40	25
	Mean	3.27	2.77	2.96	18.03	8.75	12.32	53.40	91.40	110.20

Key: ACI, augmented language input; ACO, augmented language output; SCI, spoken communication intervention; S-00, baseline observation session; S-18, intervention session 18; S-24, intervention session 24.

239

augmented communicative input or output interventions had scores of 17.33 and 13.33—an average gain of 4 and 3 months, respectively, although only four of the six children accounted for these gains. Children in the speech communication intervention had scores of 16.4 and 16 on the receptive and expressive scales of the SICD, respectively—an average gain of 0.5 (accounted for by one child) and 3.6 months, with all five children contributing to the gains. It is difficult to know if these gains were a result of the intervention or maturation.

These exploratory data about the use of the SAL with young children later diagnosed with ASDs suggest that the children who received either augmented communicative input or output interventions were able to communicate using symbols after 18 sessions and maintained this level of symbol use when the intervention was taken home. By 18 sessions, only some of the children who received the speech communication intervention produced spoken words or word approximations for a very small percentage of their target vocabularies. They had no other conventional way to communicate while they were learning to speak. Of course, these exploratory findings are to be interpreted cautiously; there were only a small number of children in each intervention group and the data are meant only to illustrate the potential of SAL intervention outcomes.

In general, these descriptive findings suggest that the response of the children with ASDs to the intervention was comparable to the other children in the study. Furthermore, they suggest that SGDs may play an important role in early communication intervention for children with ASDs. This type of intervention provides the children with an immediate way to communicate with their parents and other communication partners.

Being able to communicate at a very young age may help children with ASDs to gain control over their environments and thus decrease the likelihood that challenging behaviors will emerge early in life. Our results also suggest that SGDs did not hinder speech development in these young children with ASDs, although speech development was slow to emerge.

These comparative data are preliminary and are based on retrospective analyses. They support the need for further exploration of the use of parent-implemented augmented language interventions to specify their role in language and communication development. There is also a need for a larger-scale prospective study of children with ASDs to determine if the positive trend in this analysis is supported. We are now following these children into elementary school and will assess their speech, language, AAC, and literacy skills between 6 and 9 years of age. Given their early experience with the parent-implemented

SAL intervention, it will be important to examine how their communication skills continue to develop and to identify their communication strengths and weaknesses during elementary school.

Yoder and Stone (2006) reported successful outcomes using PECS in children with ASDs in a randomized control study comparing PECS to a prelinguistic milieu teaching approach. Similarly, a comparison of SAL and PECS outcomes in a randomized control study would be useful to determine which components of the two interventions may contribute to improved language and communication skills in children with ASDs.

CONCLUSIONS

The SAL has been shown to be a successful language intervention approach for toddlers, preschoolers, and school-age children with development disabilities and their families. Although it has not been examined specifically for use with children with ASDs, the preliminary data presented in this chapter suggest that it shows promise. The SAL may be a viable language intervention strategy for young children at risk for ASDs because it serves to compensate for their lack of speech and language skills and because it provides supports to parents and other communicative partners.

REFERENCES

Adamson, L.B. (1996). *Communication development during infancy.* Boulder, CO: Westview.

Adamson, L.B., Bakeman, R., Deckner, D., & Romski, M.A. (in press). Joint engagement and the emergence of language in children with autism and Down syndrome. *Journal of Autism and Developmental Disorders.*

Adamson, L.B., Romski, M.A., Deffenbach, K., & Sevcik, R.A. (1992). Symbol vocabulary and the focus of conversations: Augmenting language development for youth with mental retardation. *Journal of Speech and Hearing Research, 35,* 1333–1334.

American Psychiatric Association. (2000). *Diagnostic and statistical manual of mental disorders* (4th ed., Text rev.). Washington, DC: American Psychiatric Association.

Baldwin, D.A., & Markman, E.M. (1989). Establishing word-object relations: A first step. *Child Development, 60,* 381–398.

Bryson, S.E. (1996). Brief report: Epidemiology of autism. *Journal of Autism and Developmental Disorders, 26,* 165–167.

Cafiero, J.M. (2001). The effect of an augmentative communication intervention on the communication, behavior, and academic program of an adolescent with autism. *Focus on Autism and Other Developmental Disabilities, 16,* 179–189.

Drager, K.D.R., Postal, V.J., Carrolus, L., Catellano, M., Gagliano, C., & Glynn, J. (2006). The effect of aided language modeling on symbol comprehension and production in 2 preschool children with autism. *American Journal of Speech-Language Pathology, 15,* 112–125.

Fenson, L., Dale, P., Reznick, S., Thal, D., Bates, E., Hartung, J., Pethick, S., & Reilly, J. (1993). *MacArthur Communicative Development Inventories: User's guide and technical manual.* San Diego: Singular.

Fristoe, M., & Lloyd, L. (1979). Nonspeech communication. In N.R. Ellis (Ed.), *Handbook of mental deficiency: Psychological theory and research* (2nd ed., pp. 401–430). Mahwah, NJ: Laurence Erlbaum Associates.

Golinkoff, R.M., Mervis, C.B., & Hirsh-Pasek, K. (1994). Early object labels: the case for a developmental lexical principles framework. *Journal of Child Language, 1,* 125–155.

Goossens', C., & Crain, S. (1986). *Augmentative communication intervention resource.* Lake Zurich, IL: Don Johnston.

Grela, B.G., & McLaughlin, K.S. (2006). Focused stimulation for a child with autism spectrum disorders: A treatment study. *Journal of Autism and Developmental Disorders, 36,* 753–756.

Hendrick, D., Prather, E., & Tobin, A. (1984). *Sequenced Inventory of Communication Development.* Los Angeles: Western Psychological Services.

Kaiser, T., Hancock, T., & Nietfeld, J. (2000). The effects of parent-implemented enhanced milieu teaching on social communication of children who have autism. *Early Education and Development, 11,* 423–446.

Kashinath, S., Woods, J., & Goldstein, H. (2006). Enhancing generalized teaching strategy use in daily routines by parents of children with autism. *Journal of Speech, Language, and Hearing Research, 49,* 466–485.

Lancioni, G., O'Reilly, M., Cuvo, A., Singh, N., Sigafoos, J., & Didden, R. (2007). PECS and VOCAs to enable students with developmental disabilities to make requests: An overview of the literature. *Research in Developmental Disabilities, 28,* 468–488.

Laski, K.E., Charlop, M., & Schreibman, L. (1988). Training parents to use the natural language paradigm to increase their autistic children's speech. *Journal of Applied Behavior Analysis, 21,* 391–400.

Light, J.C., & Binger, C. (1998). *Building communicative competence with individuals who use augmentative and alternative communication.* Baltimore: Paul H. Brookes Publishing Co.

Light, J.C., Roberts, B., Dimarco, R., & Greiner, N. (1998). Augmentative and alternative communication to support receptive and expressive communication for people with autism. *Journal of Communication Disorders, 31,* 153–180.

Lord, C. (2000). Communication intervention research in communication and autism spectrum disorders. *Journal of Autism and Developmental Disorders, 30,* 393–398.

Lord, C., & Paul, R. (1997). Language and communication in autism. In F.R. Volkmar & D.J. Cohen (Eds.), *Handbook of autism and pervasive developmental disorders* (2nd ed., pp. 195–225). New York: John Wiley & Sons.

Lord, C., Risi, S., & Pickles, A. (2004). Trajectory of language development in autistic spectrum disorders. In M.L. Rice & S.F. Warren (Eds.), *Developmental language disorders: From phenotypes to etiologies* (pp. 7–29). Mahwah, NJ: Lawrence Erlbaum Associates.

McBride, D., & Rush, L. (2007). Types of digitized SGDs. *Augmentative Communication News, 19,* 5–7.

Mervis, C.B., & Bertrand, J. (1993). Acquisition of early object labels: The roles of operating principles and input. In A. Kaiser & D.B. Gray (Eds.), *Enhancing children's communication: Research foundations for intervention* (pp. 287–316). Baltimore: Paul H. Brookes Publishing Co.

Miller, J., & Chapman, R. (1985). *Systematic analysis of language transcripts.* Madison, WI: University of Wisconsin.

Mineo-Mollica, B. (2003). Representational competence. In & D.R. Beukelman & J. Reichle (Series Eds.) & J.C. Light, D.R. Beukelman & J. Reichle (Vol. Eds.), *Augmentative and alternative communication series. Communicative competence for individuals who use AAC: From research to effective practice* (pp. 107–145). Baltimore: Paul H. Brookes Publishing Co.

Mirenda, P. (2003). Toward functional augmentative and alternative communication for students with autism: Manual signs, graphic symbols, and voice output communication aids. *Language, Speech and Hearing Services in Schools, 34,* 203–216.

Mirenda, P., & Erickson, K.A. (2000). Augmentative communication and literacy. In S.F. Warren & J. Reichle (Series Eds.) & A.M. Wetherby & B.M. Prizant (Vol. Eds.), *Communication and language intervention series: Vol. 9. Autism spectrum disorders: A transactional developmental perspective* (pp. 333–367). Baltimore: Paul H. Brookes Publishing Co.

Mullen, E., (1995). *Mullen Scales of Early Learning.* Circle Pines, MN: American Guidance Service.

Mundy, P., & Stella, J. (2000). Joint attention, social orienting, and nonverbal communication in autism. In S.F. Warren & J. Reichle (Series Eds.) & A.M. Wetherby & B.M. Prizant (Vol. Eds.), *Communication and language intervention series: Vol. 9. Autism spectrum disorders: A transactional developmental perspective* (pp. 55–77). Baltimore: Paul H. Brookes Publishing Co.

National Research Council. (2001). *Educating children with autism.* Committee on Educational Interventions for Children with Autism, Division of Behavioral and Social Sciences and Education. Washington, DC: National Academies Press.

Nelson, K. (1973). Structure and strategy in learning to talk. *Monographs of the Society for Research in Child Development, 38*(1–2, Serial No. 149).

Paparella, T., & Kasari, C. (2004). Joint attention skills and language development in special needs populations: Translating research to practice. *Infants & Young Children, 17,* 269–280.

Peterson, S., Bondy, A., Vincent, Y., & Finnegan, C. (1995). Effects of altering communicative input for students with autism and no speech: Two case studies. *Augmentative and Alternative Communication, 11,* 93–100.

Romski, M.A., & Cheslock, M. (2000). *Technical report #1: Intervention manual.* Georgia State University, Atlanta.

Romski, M.A., & Sevcik, R.A. (1996). *Breaking the speech barrier: Language development through augmented means.* Baltimore: Paul H. Brookes Publishing Co.

Romski, M.A., & Sevcik, R.A. (2003). Augmented input: Enhancing communication development. In D.R. Beukelman & J. Reichle (Series Eds.) & J.C. Light, D.R. Beukelman & J. Reichle (Vol. Eds.), *Augmentative and alternative communication series. Communicative competence for individuals who use AAC: From research to effective practice* (pp. 147–162). Baltimore: Paul H. Brookes Publishing Co.

Romski, M.A., Sevcik, R.A., & Adamson, L.B. (1999). Communication patterns of youth with mental retardation with and without their speech-output communication devices. *American Journal on Mental Retardation, 104,* 249–259.

Romski, M.A., Sevcik, R.A., Adamson, L.B., & Bakeman, R. (2005). Communication patterns of individuals with moderate or severe cognitive disabilities: Interactions with unfamiliar partners. *American Journal on Mental Retardation, 110,* 226–238.

Romski, M.A., Sevcik, R.A., Adamson, L.B., Cheslock, M., & Smith, A. (2007). Parents can implement AAC interventions: Ratings of treatment implementation across early language interventions. *Early Childhood Services, 1,* 249–261.

Romski, M.A., Sevcik, R.A., Adamson, L.B., Cheslock, M., Smith, A., Barker, R., & Bakeman, R. (2008). *Comparison of parent-implemented augmented and non-augmented language interventions for toddlers with developmental delays.* Manuscript submitted for publication.

Romski, M.A., Sevcik, R.A., Cheslock, M., & Barton, A. (2006). The System for Augmenting Language: AAC and emerging language intervention. In R.J. McCauley & M. Fey (Eds.), *Treatment of language disorders in children* (pp. 123–147). Baltimore: Paul H. Brookes Publishing Co.

Romski, M.A., Sevcik, R.A., Cheslock, M.B., & Hyatt, A. (2002). Enhancing communication competence in beginning communicators: Identifying a continuum of AAC language intervention strategies. In D.R. Beukelman & J. Reichle (Series Eds.) & J. Reichle, D.R. Beukelman, & J.C. Light (Vol. Eds.), *Augmentative and alternative communication series. Exemplary practices for beginning communicators* (pp. 1–23). Baltimore: Paul H. Brookes Publishing Co.

Romski, M.A., Sevcik, R.A., & Fonseca, A.H. (2003). Augmentative and alternative communication for persons with mental retardation. In L. Abbeduto (Ed.), *International review of research in mental retardation: Language and communication* (pp. 255–280). New York: Academic Press.

Romski, M.A., Sevcik, R.A., Robinson, B.F., & Bakeman, R. (1994). Adult-directed communications of youth with mental retardation using the system for augmenting language. *Journal of Speech and Hearing Research, 37,* 617–628.

Romski, M.A., Sevcik, R.A., & Wilkinson, K.M. (1994). Peer-directed communicative interactions of augmented language learners with mental retardation. *American Journal on Mental Retardation, 98,* 527–538.

Schlosser, R.A., & Bischak, D.M. (2001). Is there a role for speech output in interventions for persons with autism? *Focus on Autism and Other Developmental Disabilities, 15,* 170–178.

Sevcik, R.A., & Romski, M.A. (1999). Issues in augmentative and alternative communication in child psychiatry. In R. Paul (Ed.), *Child and adolescent psychiatric clinics of North America* (pp. 77–87). Philadelphia: W.B. Saunders.

Sevcik, R.A., & Romski, M.A. (2002). The role of language comprehension in establishing early augmented conversations. In D.R. Beukelman & J. Reichle (Series Eds.) & J. Reichle, D.R. Beukelman, & J.C. Light (Vol. Eds.), *Augmentative and alternative communication series. Exemplary practices for beginning communicators* (pp. 453–474). Baltimore: Paul H. Brookes Publishing Co.

Sevcik, R.A., Romski, M.A., & Adamson, L.B. (2004). Augmentative communication and preschool children: Case example and research directions. *Disability and Rehabilitation, 26,* 1323–1329.

Sevcik, R.A., Romski, M.A., Watkins, R., & Deffebach, K. (1995). Adult partner-augmented communication input to youth with mental retardation using the system for augmenting language (SAL). *Journal of Speech and Hearing Research, 38,* 902–912.

Sevcik, R.A., Romski, M.A., & Wilkinson, K. (1991). Roles of graphic symbols in the language acquisition process for persons with severe cognitive disabilities. *Augmentative and Alternative Communication, 7,* 161–170.

Sparrow, S., Balla, D., & Cicchetti, D. (1985). *Vineland Adaptive Behavior Scales.* Circle Pines, MN: American Guidance Service.

Wetherby, A.M., Prizant, B.M., & Hutchinson, T.A. (1998). Communicative, social/affective and symbolic profiles of young children with autism and pervasive developmental disorders. *American Journal of Speech-Language Pathology, 7,* 79–92.

Wilkinson, K.M., Romski, M.A., & Sevcik, R.A. (1994). Emergence of visual-graphic symbol combinations by youth with moderate or severe mental retardation. *Journal of Speech and Hearing Research, 37,* 883–895.

Yoder, P., & Stone, W.L. (2006). A randomized comparison of the effect of two prelinguistic communication interventions on the acquisition of spoken communication in preschoolers with ASD. *Journal of Speech, Language, and Hearing Research, 49,* 698–711.

9

Using AAC Technologies to Build Social Interaction with Young Children with Autism Spectrum Disorders

KATHRYN D.R. DRAGER, JANICE C. LIGHT, AND ERINN H. FINKE

Autism affects nearly all aspects of development. In particular, children with autism spectrum disorders (ASDs) are at risk for delays or disorders in social, cognitive, language, and literacy development. The introduction of augmentative and alternative communication (AAC) and appropriate intervention at an early age can provide children with ASDs both the means and the opportunities to engage in communication for a variety of purposes, including social interaction, which may significantly impact language opportunities and development.

This chapter focuses on using AAC technologies as a means to build social engagement with young children with ASDs. In this chapter, the term *AAC system* is used to refer to both unaided AAC systems (e.g., gestures, signs) and aided AAC systems, and as well as to both low-tech (e.g., nonelectronic communication boards and books) and high-tech electronic systems (e.g., speech-generating devices or

This chapter was supported in part by the Communication Enhancement Rehabilitation Engineering Research Center (AAC-RERC). The AAC-RERC is a virtual research center that is funded by the National Institute on Disability and Rehabilitation Research (NIDRR) of the U.S. Department of Education under Grant H133E030018. The opinions contained in this publication are those of the grantees and do not necessarily reflect those of the Department of Education.

SGDs). AAC technologies refer specifically to electronically aided AAC systems (e.g., SGDs).

ASDs are characterized in part by deficits in social interaction. Social competence has a significant impact on language learning and development of communicative competence. There are several hypotheses as to why children with ASDs have difficulty with social interaction. Communication for social interaction requires a fundamental desire to interact with others and obtain new information and perspectives. This desire may be impacted in children with ASDs as a result of a deficit in theory of mind (Astington & Baird, 2005), which relates to the ability to understand that others have differing perspectives. Tager-Flusberg (1996) and Mundy and Stella (2000) have suggested that deficits in the acquisition of a theory of mind prevent children with ASDs from being internally motivated to initiate communicative acts for social interaction, which require a desire to understand the thoughts and ideas of others.

Alternatively, Stone, Ousley, Yoder, Hogan, and Hepburn (1997) hypothesized that social interaction is less common in children with ASDs than in typically developing children because children with ASDs find the experience of sharing attention with adults to be less rewarding. As a result, children with ASDs participate less in commenting because the outcome of commenting behavior tends to be social in nature. In contrast, according to results obtained by Stone et al. (1997), children with ASDs as young as 2–3 years of age show relative strengths in using communication for needs and wants as compared to communication to attract or maintain the attention of others. Children with ASDs in the Stone et al. (1997) study communicated less often than language- and age-matched children in a structured activity designed to elicit either requesting or commenting. When the children with ASDs did communicate, they more frequently requested objects or actions; they were less likely to comment on an object or an activity.

Quill (1997) presented another hypothesis about the social impairments of children with ASDs. She noted that both requesting and rejecting (i.e., communication of needs and wants) are linked to tangible contextual cues. She argued that the presence of visual retrieval cues, such as preferred objects, serves as a prompt for requesting behavior. Social contexts, in contrast, do not typically provide such concrete visual cues. As a result, impairments in social behavior may be, in part, a function of the inability of individuals with ASDs to extract relevant information in the absence of visual cues.

Regardless of the mechanism, children with ASDs have great difficulty with initiating communication for social interaction. Many children with ASDs are also at risk for speech development. It has been estimated that approximately 14%–20% of children with ASDs will not develop speech and language skills that will be functional for meeting their everyday communication needs (Lord, Risi, & Pickles, 2004). Without access to communication, children with ASDs are at continued risk for impairments in language, cognitive, and social development. In an effort to increase the communication skills of children with ASDs who do not develop functional speech for daily communication, AAC systems and technologies have been implemented through a variety of means.

AAC AND INDIVIDUALS WITH ASD

AAC approaches for individuals with ASDs have consisted of both unaided and aided approaches. Unaided approaches include gestural communication, such as signing, which is fast, portable, and cost-efficient. Some children with ASDs maintain relative strengths in motor skills. Chapter 4 in this volume addresses the research and clinical practice related to the use of unaided modes of communication. Numerous studies also demonstrate the effectiveness of aided AAC systems (often nonelectronic) in increasing functional communication. Among the more popular aided approaches is the Picture Exchange Communication System (PECS) for children with ASDs (Chapter 10; Bondy & Frost, 1994).

Limited empirical evidence exists on the comparative effectiveness of various types of AAC systems for children with ASDs. Both aided and unaided approaches have been shown to be effective for many individuals in this population, particularly for the function of requesting (Mirenda, 2003). Individuals with ASDs can learn to use unaided and aided AAC systems when they are provided with appropriate opportunities and instruction to do so. Much less evidence is available to support the use of assistive technologies, especially SGDs, for individuals with ASD. In addition, little research has addressed implementing any form of AAC (i.e., unaided, nonelectronic aided, or SGDs) for children with ASDs in terms of effectiveness in teaching functions other than requests (Mirenda, 2003). Communication interventions for children with ASDs need to be expanded from this limited focus to a broader focus on the core deficits of the communication disorder, specifically social interaction (National Research Council, 2001).

AAC TECHNOLOGIES TO ENHANCE
SOCIAL INTERACTION OF CHILDREN WITH ASD

The overarching goal of this chapter is to consider the use of AAC technologies as a means of enhancing the social interaction of children with ASDs. Specifically, this chapter will 1) review the research related to the design and customization of appropriate AAC technologies for children with ASDs, 2) review the research on intervention to promote social interaction, 3) present a case study to illustrate the clinical implications of implementing AAC technologies to enhance social interaction, and 4) discuss priorities for future research to advance understanding and improve practice for children with ASDs who require AAC.

As with other groups, there are two essential components in intervention to enhance social interaction for children with ASDs who require AAC: AAC systems and AAC intervention/instructional techniques. AAC systems are the tools to ensure effective communication. These tools must be designed to meet the needs and accommodate the skills of young children with ASDs given their deficits in communication, particularly social communication. However, the tools for communication alone will not be sufficient to meet the communication needs of children with ASDs. It is also important to consider interventions to build social interaction skills and the impact of these intervention strategies on the development of social communication for children with ASDs. Each of these components—appropriate AAC technologies and appropriate intervention strategies—will be discussed in turn.

SELECTING AND CUSTOMIZING
APPROPRIATE AAC TECHNOLOGIES

Communication for all persons is multimodal, with both unaided and aided techniques. Different modes are chosen depending on the context, environment, and communication partner. Although there is limited evidence supporting the use of high-tech AAC technologies, these systems have the potential to facilitate social communication for individuals with ASDs.

High-tech AAC technologies may be a good match for the skills and needs of children with ASDs for several reasons. First, SGDs provide a means to augment not only expression but also comprehension of messages produced by other partners (Light, Roberts, DiMarco, & Griener, 1998). Supporting the comprehension of language may be necessary when children with ASDs present with a need for increased time in processing language input and when cognitive deficits are concomitant with the ASD diagnosis. Additionally, high-tech AAC systems present language through the visual channel using static visual pictures or symbols. This use of the visual channel has potential benefits for children with ASDs who have been reported to evidence relative strength in visual processing skills (Wetherby, Prizant, & Schuler, 2000), although there is little research evidence available to support this proposition. Mirenda (2001) has further suggested that SGDs carry an advantage for children with ASDs in that they provide speech output and thus have the potential to be integrated easily into environments with unfamiliar people. Because of the speech output, SGDs may facilitate natural social communication. Speech output offers individuals increased power over their environment and allows them to be able to obtain someone's attention and communicate across a distance. There may be other advantages as well; many children with ASDs demonstrate an interest in technology and find computer activities to be reinforcing (Stromer, Kimball, Kinney, & Taylor, 2006).

A few studies have addressed the use of SGDs to teach a variety of specific skills to children with ASDs. For example, an SGD was used effectively to teach a student with ASD to spell words (Schlosser, Blischak, Belfiore, Bartley, & Barnett, 1998). Sigafoos et al. (2004) used SGDs to repair communicative breakdowns with two adolescent students with ASDs. In addition, several studies have also addressed the use of SGDs to teach requesting to individuals with ASDs (Brady, 2000; Durand, 1999; Sigafoos & Drasgow, 2001; Son, Sigafoos, O'Reilly, & Lancioni, 2006; Van Acker & Grant, 1995). Chapter 5 in this volume provides an extensive review of the research in this area.

In a rather unique study, Schepis, Reid, Behrmann and Sutton (1998) evaluated the effects of SGD use in increasing communicative interactions with children with ASDs. Four children, ages 3–5 years, participated in a self-contained classroom for children with ASDs. Each child was provided with an SGD with digitized speech output with either four or eight choices; naturalistic teaching procedures were implemented during a snack or play routine. During intervention, all four children displayed an increase in communicative turns, increasing to approximately 2–3 communicative turns per minute compared to baseline rates of 0.2–1.6 turns per minute. The children used the prerecorded vocabulary primarily to request items but also used vocabulary for answering yes/no questions and communicating some social comments such as *please* and *thank you* within the request.

To date, little consideration has been directed toward the design of AAC technologies to maximize effectiveness for children with ASD. Current AAC technologies are designed to reflect the conceptual models of nondisabled adults (Light & Drager, 2002). However, these technologies may not appeal to young children with ASDs and are often difficult to learn. Light and Drager (2002, 2007) argued that AAC systems need to be redesigned to enhance their appeal and reduce learning demands for all young children with significant communication disabilities. The discussion here will focus on these issues specifically for young children with ASDs.

Increasing Appeal

Current AAC technologies may not appeal to young children. Typically, these systems are unifunctional, square in shape, and drab and matte in color (Light, Drager, & Nemser, 2004). If AAC technologies do not appeal to young children, they may not have an initial attraction to encourage use or have sustaining power for continued use.

To date, no research exists to determine what aspects or features of technologies appeal to children with ASDs. Children with ASDs tend to have idiosyncratic patterns of behavior and areas of interest (American Psychiatric Association, 2000). These idiosyncrasies may affect their interest and motivation to use certain AAC tools. Typically developing children seem to prefer and/or respond to features including the integration of multiple functions (e.g., communication, play, humor, entertainment, artistic expression), multiple bright glossy colors, options for customization and change, interesting sound effects, and personalization of the system, among other features (Light, Drager, & Nemser, 2004; Light, Page, Curran, & Pitkin, 2007). It is possible that some children with ASDs would also find these aspects appealing. Other children with ASDs may find them distracting or a source of overstimulation; however, according to Shane et al. (2005), children with ASDs spend more time with media than with other activities and appear to prefer animated characters.

One potential method for enhancing appeal is to incorporate meaningful and motivating activities into AAC technologies. Some research indicates that communication using AAC technologies can be enhanced when motivation is present (Mirenda & Schuler, 1988; Quill, 1995). For some children with ASDs, it appears that technology itself can be a motivating factor, as illustrated in the results of an investigation by Moore and Calvert (2000). In this study, the researchers randomly assigned children with ASDs, ages 3–6 years, to one of two groups to teach vocabulary. One group was assigned to a behavioral treatment group; the second group paralleled the behavioral intervention but also added sensory reinforcement, color, animation, music, and interesting sounds using a computer. They found that children with ASDs in the computer condition were more attentive, more motivated, and learned more vocabulary words than the children with ASDs in the behavioral treatment group. In fact, children were attentive in the computer condition 97% of the time, compared to 62% of the time in the behavioral group. These results demonstrate that, for some children with ASDs, the use of technology can increase the appeal and motivation of a task, as well as the time spent attending to a task.

Decreasing Learning Demands

In addition to being appealing, AAC technologies also must be easy to learn. Evidence suggests that current AAC technologies place a high learning demand on typically developing children in terms of determining how the technologies are used (e.g., system layout, grid or visual scene display) and how vocabulary is organized (Drager et al., 2003). The demands of these aspects of AAC technology use on children with ASDs who have cognitive impairments may be even higher. Learning demands can be reduced by using appropriate designs for all components of systems, including representation of language concepts, layout and organization of concepts, navigation through the system, selection of the concepts, and output (Light & Drager, 2002).

Representation of Language Concepts   Evidence suggests that children with ASDs can learn to understand and use a variety of symbols, including signs and gestures, line drawings that range in levels of abstractness, and traditional orthography (Mirenda, 2005). The commonality among each of these symbol systems is that they are all visual.

It has often been argued that children with ASDs have relatively strong visual-spatial skills. Although there exists little empirical research to support this assertion, strength in this area has been suggested by authors and clinicians in the field (Ogletree & Harn, 2001; Quill, 1997). Given this, it may be appropriate to consider representations for AAC systems that capitalize on this potential strength.

Most existing AAC symbol set representations reflect the perspectives of adults without disabilities. Lund et al. (1998) and Light, Worah, et al. (2007) argued that children's representations of early emerging language concepts are very different from the representations used in many current symbol sets. In both of these studies, drawings of 10 early emerging concepts by typically developing children were compared to traditional AAC symbols of these concepts and differed significantly. The children's representations made extensive use of context; involved experiences familiar to the child; and used entire scenes to depict the concepts rather than isolated parts of objects or events, as do many traditional representations. There is no available research to determine what types of representations children with ASDs might conceptualize.

Organization   The organization and layout of representations either can facilitate or impede the accuracy and efficiency with which a child is able to locate, select, and functionally use concepts for communication (Light & Drager, 2007). Traditionally, representations have been organized in a grid layout with each AAC symbol in a separate row or column, but this approach may be difficult for young children with ASDs. Although visual/spatial skills in general have frequently been cited as strengths, children with ASDs have also been reported to focus attention on specific details rather than the "big picture"regarding visual information/input they receive (Happe & Frith, 2006; Kanner, 1943). In fact, "persistent preoccupation with parts of objects"is one of the diagnostic criteria for autistic disorder in the *Diagnostic and Statistical Manual of Mental Disorders, Fourth Edition, Text Revision* (American Psychiatric Association, 2000). Representations of concepts in grid displays keep items in separate spaces and do not facilitate an understanding of the whole concept, which may increase this tendency toward preoccupation with parts of objects rather than facilitating integration and comprehension of concepts within a context as a whole.

Recent attention has been given to visual scene displays (VSDs) as a representation and organization strategy (Light & Drager, 2007; Shane, 2006). VSDs use pictures to depict a situation, place, or experience. For example, a photograph may be taken of a place or event in the child's life and placed on the AAC system. Language concepts are then placed under hot spots that can be selected to retrieve the concepts (see Figure 9.1). The scene in Figure 9.1 was developed to facilitate a tickle-game interaction; hot spots were available for the child to choose where he would like to be tickled. Selection of these hot spots resulted in speech output labeling each body part to be tickled. Figure 9.1a depicts the VSD as the child would see it, whereas Figure 9b shows the hotspots outlined (this view would never be available for the child's view).

VSDs are an interesting new concept in designing AAC systems and organizing vocabulary for children with ASDs because they focus information within the whole context, rather than isolating vocabulary into detached elements. In this way, VSDs emphasize the relationships between the concepts and vocabulary that relate to the activity or context of the communicative interaction. This is in contrast to traditional organization of AAC systems comprising grid displays, which separate language concepts into separate boxes. VSDs preserve the conceptual and visual relationships among the symbols that occur in life and embed concepts into the contexts in which they occur. For example, a picture of a person would show the nose as significantly smaller than a leg. This proportionality is not preserved in grid displays, in which the nose would be approximately equal in size to the leg and may be placed next to or below the leg.

To date, the only published research that has addressed the effectiveness of VSDs has involved typically developing children as participants. For example, Drager et al. (2003) conducted an investigation demonstrating that typically developing 2½-year-old children learned vocabulary more quickly with a VSD approach to organization than with a grid approach. Shane (2006) has also presented some alternative uses of VSDs for individuals with ASDs, specifically as a context for instruction and a means for organizing information about an event, beyond that which a visual schedule would provide.

A potential advantage of VSDs is that the scenes, by their nature, organize vocabulary schematically. Although semantic organization preferences of young children is somewhat debated (Traylor, 2004; Wilkinson & Rosenquist, 2006), a predominance of literature has demonstrated a schematic preference for organization for typically developing children ages 5 years and younger (e.g., Fallon, Light, &

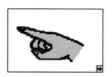

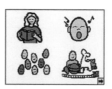

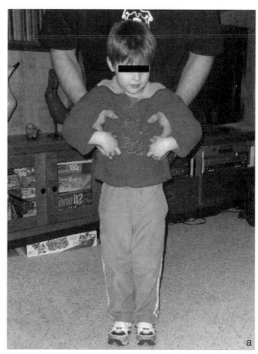

Figure 9.1a. Example of visual scene display for "tickle" activity. (*Note:* Pages are presented in color in the child's system.)

Figure 9.1b.

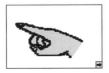

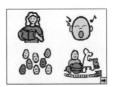

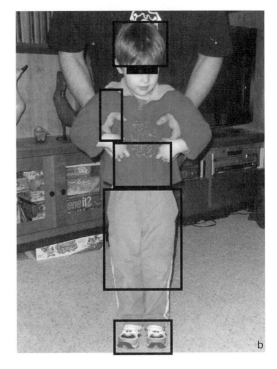

Achenbach, 2003; Lucariello, Kyratzis, & Nelson, 1992; Maaka & Wong, 1994; Nelson, 1996; Sell, 1992). It is interesting to consider the applications of research results obtained with children who are typically developing to children with ASDs. Do children with ASDs think about and organize concepts in a similar fashion to children who are typically developing? Several studies have demonstrated that adolescents with high-functioning ASDs organize vocabulary in ways that are very similar to their typically developing peers (Boucher, 1988; Tager-Flusberg, 1985). However, it is unclear if this would be consistent for young children and for children with ASDs who are unable to use speech to meet their daily communication needs.

It is important to understand the ways that young children with ASDs organize language concepts so that aided AAC system displays can be constructed to match the individual child's internal map of concept organization and facilitate language expression. A preliminary investigation conducted by Wilkinson and Rosenquist (2006) offers a technique designed to provide insight into this issue. These researchers used a modified match-to-sample procedure using picture symbols to evaluate the category structure and semantic organization of individuals with ASDs and limited verbal skills. Their results indicated that, with some instruction provided, a modified match-to-sample task in which multiple answers/selections were allowable can be used to determine how these children organize language concepts. This finding provides a step towards understanding how to design AAC systems that best match how each individual child with ASD thinks about the world, and how and if the semantic organizations of children with ASDs are similar to those that have been suggested for children who are typically developing.

Navigation   Once symbols have been chosen and organized on the system, the next consideration for system design is how the child will locate, or find, the desired symbols (i.e., how the child will navigate through the system). System navigation, particularly for dynamic display systems, requires that children understand that the selections they make will result in additional options. That is, the navigational tools and menu items act as superordinate category labels for the vocabulary items that can be accessed through their selection. For example, a selection of a picture of a slide and monkey bars may link to a page about the playground. It is understood by adults and individuals familiar with the system that these symbols are only superordinate labels that lead to a larger array of similar symbols. However, this means of navigating to a larger array of symbols may be very difficult for children with ASDs to comprehend and use functionally. As children with ASDs often focus on details, they may fail to recognize or understand that the symbol represents a superordinate category label.

As an alternative, Drager et al. (2004) suggested that the representations on the links to additional pages can be smaller versions of the pages themselves. In their study, typically developing 3-year-old children learned vocabulary more quickly (after the initial session) with this type of menu page than with menu pages that contained single symbols representing the themes of the linked pages. Smaller screenshots of the linked pages in a dynamic display menu may assist children with ASDs in deciphering the links. Regardless, a child with ASD who is at the beginning communication stages (i.e., newly symbolic or being provided with a means to communicate symbolically for the first time) may not initially be able to independently navigate between multiple pages. Rather than limiting the number of pages available in this situation, a communication partner can instead scaffold the navigation by helping to locate the desired page (Light & Drager, 2007) until the child has developed the skills to do this independently.

Selection Technique   Once the concepts have been represented appropriately and displayed on the system, the child with ASD will need to select desired vocabulary items. Although some children with ASDs experience difficulties with fine motor skills (Rinehart et al., 2006; Vanvuchelen, Roeyers, & De Weerdt, 2007), the majority are able to use direct selection. However, Rinehart et al. (2006) suggested that many young children with ASDs may have difficulty with motor planning and motor imitation. These potential deficits may affect the child's ability to use a standard keyboard or mouse to control AAC technology, given the level of fine motor control needed.

In addition to these motor demands, use of these external controls requires the cognitive understanding that actions made on the keyboard or mouse will affect the cursor movement on the screen, which is displaced in physical space from the input mechanism. In contrast, touchscreen technology does not impose this cognitive demand because the child's touch on the screen directly impacts the actions on the system. Use of touchscreens may be a way to simplify access to AAC for children with ASDs.

Output   The final component of AAC technologies that may impact learning demands for children with ASDs is the output, which occurs after a selection is made. Output can be in the form of visual (typically, printed) or auditory modalities. Little research addresses output for individuals with ASDs, although there is some evidence that children with intellectual disabilities learn symbols more quickly with the presence of speech output than without it (Koul & Schlosser, 2004; Schlosser et al., 1995).

Research on the output of AAC technologies has been primarily focused on investigating the performance of adults and older children without disabilities using synthesized speech output. Research with young children as participants has demonstrated that children 4–6 years of age perform less accurately with synthesized speech than natural speech (Axmear et al., 2005). Intelligibility of synthesized and digitized speech is particularly low (55%–75%) for single-word messages for child listeners 3–5 years of age (Drager, Clark-Serpentine, Johnson, & Roeser, 2006). It is unclear what advantage speech output might have for individuals with ASDs, who may be more likely to respond to visual than auditory stimuli. However, speech output does allow for more naturalistic interaction with familiar and unfamiliar partners (Mirenda, 2001), although the speech output needs to be intelligible to be effective.

Auditory output may also include nonspeech sounds. Some evidence supports that children with ASDs are more likely to respond to nonsocial auditory stimuli, such as sound effects like toys rattling or music playing, than social stimuli, such as a spoken label or their name (Dawson, Meltzoff, Osterling, Rinaldi, & Brown, 1998).

Summary

For AAC systems to serve as effective tools for communication and vehicles for social interaction, they need to be designed appropriately for children with ASDs. Research is required to determine which factors make AAC systems appealing to children with ASDs to support sustained use. Additionally, many of the aspects of AAC systems—representation, organization, navigation, selection, and output—are based in large part on the conceptual framework of adults without disabilities. Research is required to determine the conceptual development of children with ASDs and to develop design specifications for AAC technologies. AAC systems need to be designed to maximize the skills of the child with ASDs while serving as supports to accommodate the needs of the child.

INTERVENTION TECHNIQUES

AAC technologies that are appropriately designed for children with ASDs can provide the tools for social engagement and communication. However, children with ASDs will also require appropriate interventions to facilitate social interaction. Communication intervention approaches might be described along a continuum from structured behavioral interventions to those that are child-centered and socially pragmatic in nature (Prizant & Wetherby, 1998). At one end, the continuum of intervention methods is anchored with interventions that are based on traditional behavioral principles, and utilize discrete trial and massed practice, direct instructional techniques (e.g., Lovaas, 1977). Teaching methods are highly structured in these interventions and the initial focus is on adult-directed activities. All applied behavioral analysis approaches have their roots in these principles, although many contemporary approaches tend to lie closer to the middle of the continuum (e.g., pivotal response training; Koegel & Johnson, 1989). On the other end of the continuum are social-pragmatic, developmental approaches that place an emphasis on naturally occurring events within a flexible structure and meaningful activities (e.g., the SCERTS®

Model detailed in Chapter 7; Prizant, Wetherby, Rubin, Laurent, & Rydell, 2006).

Although there is some evidence that naturalistic procedures may be beneficial for language learning for speaking children (Camarata, Nelson, & Camarata, 1994; Koegel, Koegel, & Surratt, 1992), there is no evidence to date of the relative efficacy of AAC interventions that lie at different points on the intervention continuum. However, evidence suggests that AAC interventions using a variety of instructional/intervention methods can have a positive effect on the communication skills of young children with ASDs, including interventions using both structured behavioral methods (e.g., Richman, Wacker, & Winborn, 2001) and those using social-pragmatic methods (e.g., Wetherby & Woods, 2006). The most effective strategies will likely depend on an interaction between the individual and the goals of the intervention. In building social interactions, there may be some strength to interventions that are more developmental and socially pragmatic because of the nature of the end goal of social interaction.

COMPONENTS OF A SOCIAL-PRAGMATIC APPROACH TO INTERVENTION

As noted previously, much of the intervention research to date has targeted the communication of needs and wants—specifically, requesting. Limited research exists on interventions designed specifically to promote social interaction for children with ASDs who require AAC. In this section, a social-pragmatic intervention approach, which is designed to address the social interaction difficulties of young children with ASDs who require AAC, will be discussed.

According to Prizant and Wetherby (1998) and Woods and Wetherby (2003), a social-pragmatic intervention approach 1) involves the family and other caregivers, 2) takes place in the natural environment, 3) is embedded into functional and meaningful contexts, and 4) uses communication that is transactional in nature.

Intervention Involves the Family and Other Caregivers

Familiar caregivers play a critical role in social interaction and language learning for children with ASDs (Kaiser, Hancock, & Nietfeld, 2000). Modifications of the caregiver's interaction style have considerable influence on the communication skills of a child with ASD (Koegel, 2000). Parents and caregivers often have a vested interest in the development and well-being of the child and are frequently motivated to carry through such interventions. Research with populations other than those with ASDs has demonstrated that family variables are an important predictor in outcomes for early intervention (Shonkoff, Hauser-Cram, Krauss, & Upshur, 1992). When intervention is not prescribed for designated time periods, but occurs instead throughout the day in natural routines, gains in child communication can be seen at the same time that family stress is reduced (Koegel, Bimbela, & Schreibman, 1996; McConachie & Diggle, 2006; Schreibman, Kaneko, & Koegel, 1991). Regardless of who takes the primary role during intervention sessions when a professional is present, it is the family members who will be in the environment when everyone else leaves. Thus, caregivers need to be involved in the intervention process to provide consistency and continuity.

Intervention Takes Place in the Natural Environment

Woods and Wetherby (2003) described intervention in the natural environment as meeting the following criteria: 1) children learn functional and meaningful skills, 2) learning occurs within daily activities, and 3) caregivers mediate the learning process for the child as it occurs. The natural environment is the context within which social interaction will ultimately take place. Intervention within the natural environment offers a number of advantages by insuring that target skills are relevant, as well as by facilitating spontaneous and generalized use of those skills (Light & Binger, 1998). In addition, the use of people and events that are familiar to the child with ASD will likely promote engagement in these activities. Further, it has been shown that spending more time in active, positive engagement results in better outcomes for young children in need of early intervention (Woods & Wetherby, 2003).

For young children, the natural environment will most often be the home. However, in a review of intervention research with children with ASDs ages 8 years and younger, Wolery and Garfinkle (2002) noted that most studies have occurred in classroom environments, with little attention on families. Similarly, Mirenda (2003) stated that almost no research has been conducted into the use of AAC technologies in home or community settings.

Intervention Is Embedded into
Functional and Meaningful Contexts

In social interactions, the individuals involved must sustain the interaction through the active engagement or involvement of both participants (Light, Parsons, & Drager, 2002). This is in significant contrast to interactions involving communication of needs and wants, in which the focus of the interaction is not on the people but rather on the target object or action (Light, 1988). Too often, AAC interventions take place during daily routines such as snack or meal times. Although it is important to have the skills to regulate the behavior of others, such as in requesting, these contexts do not easily support social interaction. Rather, interactions must by sustained over several turns within meaningful, motivating contexts to maintain active engagement of participants. According to Watson, Lanter, McComish, and Poston Roy (2004), the strategy of engaging in motivating activities that are meaningful to the child is important to facilitate language and communication development in young children with ASDs. There is also some evidence that the choice of activity or vocabulary has a direct influence on intervention outcomes (Koegel, O'Dell & Koegel, 1987).

Meaningful contexts are those that occur in the natural environment, take place with familiar people, and involve activities that are motivating. Meaningful contexts should provide natural cues for interaction to indicate opportunities for communication. Individuals who do not recognize natural cues may have difficulty generalizing skills (Halle, 1987).

Communication Is Transactional in Nature

Communication is a reciprocal process and is transactional in nature (McLean, 1990; McLean & Snyder-McLean, 1978; Wetherby & Prizant, 2000). From this perspective, communication development depends upon interactions between a child and a communicative partner. These reciprocal interactions are characterized by a series of actions and responses. The response of the communication partner is dependent on the context in which the interaction (the communication) occurs and the type of behavior (the action) produced by the child. Within a transactional framework, communication can be seen as a dynamic process in which the child, communication partner, and environment equally influence the nature and outcome of the interaction (Sameroff & Chandler, 1975). When communication is conceptualized in this way, intervention to remediate any breakdowns in this process must focus on the behaviors of the child and his or her caregivers, as well as the environment in which the interaction takes place. Interventions should assist caregivers in learning to use strategies that support the child's communication, such as clearly marking turn opportunities, providing models of communicative behavior, and using natural consequences.

Clearly Marking Turn Opportunities   Opportunities for communication can be marked through an expectant delay (i.e., focus attention on the child with an air of expectancy and wait; Halle, Marshall, & Spradlin, 1979; Kozleski, 1991). Once an opportunity has been marked, it is important to wait for the child to take a turn using any means available. It has been reported that parents of children with ASDs are more directive and controlling than parents of typically developing children (Kasari, Sigman, Mundy, & Yirmiya, 1988; Siller & Sigman, 2002). Additionally, the use of an expectant delay is difficult for some parents to learn and to use consistently (Elder, Valcante, Won, & Zylis, 2003). However, when provided with expectant delays by their parents, children with ASDs have been reported to increase communicative utterances (Seung, Ashwell, Elder, & Valcante, 2006). Using an expectant or time delay has been reported to be facilitative in increasing communication for both speaking and nonverbal children with ASDs (Hwang & Hughes, 2000).

Providing Models of Communicative Behavior   Models provided to the child during interaction can consist of various combinations: speech and signs/gestures, speech and low-tech symbols, or speech and high-tech systems. Visual models serve multiple purposes in an interaction. Using the AAC system shows the child what can be accomplished by using the system and demonstrates to the child that the AAC system is an acceptable form of communication (see Chapter 8; Romski & Sevcik, 1996). These visual models may facilitate comprehension for children who have difficulty with spoken words alone. In interventions to build social interaction, models also demonstrate to the child appropriate play and social interaction skills, as well as provide opportunities for the child to learn new language concepts (Binger & Light, 2007; Drager, Postal, et al., 2006).

Several AAC instructional techniques use modeling as one of a number of other strategies (see Chapter 8). These include aided language stimulation (Goossens', 1989; Goossens', Crain, & Elder, 1992; Elder & Goossens', 1994), the System for Augmenting Language (Romski and Sevcik, 1996; Sevcik, Romski, Watkins, & Deffebach, 1995), natural aided language (Cafiero, 1998, 2001), and aided language modeling (Drager, Postal, et al., 2006). With the exception of published accounts of aided language stimulation, each of the instructional techniques has been demonstrated to be effective with children with ASDs. Although they differ in many ways, all of the specific intervention strategies contained two common components of augmenting the message and providing a model of expansion. In addition, all can be implemented during opportunities that arise out of the natural context.

Providing Natural Consequences   Reciprocity is inherent in social interactions, so the actions of the communication partner are as important as the skills of the child with ASD. Contingent responding has been shown consistently in the research to be beneficial to the development of language and communication for young children with developmental disabilities, including children with ASD (Siller & Sigman, 2002; Warren, Yoder, Gazdag, Kim, & Jones, 1993; Watson, 1998; Yoder, Kaiser, Alpert, & Fischer, 1993; Yoder & Warren, 1998). Facilitators can respond to all attempts at communication, either through unaided or aided means, by responding to what is thought to be the child's communicative intent and/or expanding upon the child's message and modeling a more sophisticated communicative form. Siller and Sigman (2002), for example, found that language outcomes for preschool children with ASDs (measured 10 and 16 years later) were positively associated with the amount of time that parents talked about their child's current focus of attention (without directing the child's behavior).

Summary

Although little evidence exists that one specific intervention approach is more effective in increasing social interaction than another, social pragmatic approaches offer considerable promise in that they place an emphasis on reciprocal interpersonal interactions as the context for enhancing communicative competence (Prizant & Wetherby, 1998). Hence, this emphasis may be important in an approach to increase social interactions. The components of this approach—including intervention in the natural environment, intervention embedded into functional and meaningful daily routines, an emphasis on the transactional nature of communication, and the involvement of family and other caregivers—may also enhance social interaction of children with ASDs who require AAC.

CLINICAL IMPLICATIONS
FOR PRACTICE: A CASE STUDY

Given the potential benefits of both AAC technologies for children with ASDs and a social-pragmatic approach to intervention, Drager et al. (2005) conducted a preliminary investigation of the effects of a social-pragmatic approach to AAC intervention using AAC technologies on the social interaction and communication of four preschoolers with ASDs. Three children had a diagnosis of autism and one child had a diagnosis of pervasive developmental disorder-not otherwise specified.

The intervention was designed to address the goals of increasing the children's participation and social engagement, as well as the range and breadth of semantic concepts. The focus of the intervention was to facilitate sustained social interaction. Although requesting and other behavior regulation acts also serve an important purpose, these were not the primary goals of the intervention. The children, all boys, were 3–5 years of age at the beginning of the intervention. The data for one of these children are presented here to illustrate the use of AAC technologies to build social communication for children with ASDs.

Participant

Wes (not his real name) was 39 months of age at the beginning of the intervention and was diagnosed with autism. Wes used two signs with some regularity: MORE and FINISHED. He attended preschool in a self-contained autism support classroom, four mornings a week. Wes had access to approximately 10 Picture Communication Symbols (PCS) at the preschool to request items, such as toys or snacks, but only used them with a great deal of prompting.

Wes's gross and fine motor skills were functional. He was an active, mobile child who frequently engaged in high-energy activities, such as chase and trampoline jumping. He was able to isolate his index finger to point when prompted (although his spontaneous pointing was inconsistent) and thus was a candidate for direct selection with an aided system. He could approximate his two signs (MORE and FINISHED) with fair accuracy, such that they were readily recognizable. His vision and hearing were within normal limits, although Wes appeared to be hypersensitive to loud sounds.

Other than the two manual signs, the PCS, and some challenging behaviors, Wes did not have other means of expression. Wes's parents completed the MacArthur Communicative Development Inventory: Words and Gestures (Fenson et al., 1993) at the beginning of the study. They indicated that he responded to some commands, such as *No no, Come here*, and *Let's go bye-bye*. He did not respond to his name or react to comments such as *There's mommy/daddy*. In addition, Wes appeared to understand some basic animal sounds and names, vehicles, toys, food and drink, clothing, some body parts, furniture and rooms, household items, some people, and some action words. He understood very few descriptive words (*bad, good, sleepy,* and *tired* were the exceptions) and no pronouns, question words, or prepositions. He also demonstrated very few communicative gestures (such as showing behaviors or shaking head) and did not participate in any common games or routines.

Baseline

Wes was observed three times for 15 minutes each while he interacted with his parents before intervention was initiated. During these observations, Wes averaged approximately 2 turns each session (using the sign MORE) or an average of 0.13 turns per minute, which was significantly below the rate expected for children his age (Paul, 2001).

Intervention

The intervention was implemented with the following steps (derived from Light & Drager, 2005): 1) identify meaningful contexts for communication and motivating activities; 2) develop appropriate AAC systems; 3) accommodate joint attention demands through positioning of the child, partner, and AAC system; 4) identify and mark opportunities for communication; 5) model use of the multimodal AAC system along with speech; 6) respond to communication attempts; and 7) introduce new contexts as appropriate. Intervention sessions took place approximately once a week for about 30 minutes, in his home with one or both parents.

Meaningful and motivating activities were determined by observing Wes's choices of activities during free time and by parent report. The intervention targeted sustained social activities. The following activities were developed: 1) familiar books were scanned into the SGD with hot spots of the text; 2) familiar songs were recorded into the SGD with representations that corresponded to the key vocabulary words; and 3) familiar activities, such as the tickle game, and familiar toys, such as a marble tower, were incorporated. As Wes became more competent with these activities, new activities were introduced. Books, songs, and play activities that were not familiar to him were introduced as well over time. New activities were introduced approximately every 1–2 weeks (i.e., sessions).

To decrease the demands on Wes to shift attention between himself, the communication partner, the AAC technology, and the ongoing activity, the interventionist sat directly in front of Wes, holding the SGD directly in front of him just below the interventionist's face and placing the system within the same line of sight as the partner. For familiar activities (e.g., the tickle game or toy play), several opportunities for Wes to engage the communication partner were presented. Wes was able to make several choices, such as who could take the next turn, whether mom or dad should tickle him, and where on his body he wanted to be tickled. At the beginning of the intervention, Wes's parents were not confident that he would participate without an external reinforcer, so at various intervals, Wes was given the choice of continuing to participate or have a small food item. This choice was gradually faded out.

The representations on the SGD were primarily digital photographs of Wes engaged in the activity or of scanned familiar books and song images. The organization utilized VSDs. For example, for the tickle game, Wes could choose this activity by selecting a smaller picture of himself being tickled from the menu page. Once selected, the same picture would then fill the screen, and hotspots on the page would be available for him to indicate which body part was to be tickled (e.g., leg, tummy, foot). As Wes gained competence, the displays were gradually changed to a hybrid display, where the VSD was accompanied by other selections in a grid format (such as a picture of mom and a picture of dad to choose who does the tickling).

Many of the symbols available on the SGD were also presented to Wes as nonelectronic symbols. These were approximately 2 inches by 2 inches in size and were cut out for easy use during activities. Wes appeared to be more motivated to use the computer-based system than the available nonelectronic symbols. Throughout the intervention, several new signs were modeled with Wes.

Results

Each baseline and intervention session was videotaped. A representative sample of 15 minutes was chosen for each session. Results are shown in Figure 9.2, which represents sessions over 1 year of intervention. Upon

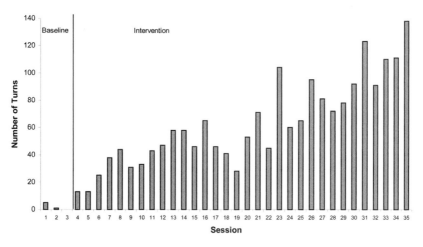

Figure 9.2.   Number of communicative turns expressed by Wes in 15-minute interactions at baseline and intervention. (*Note:* Wes did not take any communicative turns during session 3 of baseline.)

initial introduction to the AAC systems, Wes's turn taking increased to 13 turns in the 15-minute session from a rate of 2 turns in 15 minutes at baseline (a 6-fold increase). Over the next year (to the age of 4 years 3 months), Wes averaged 63 turns per 15-minute session (an average of 4.2 turns per minute, more than 30 times the rate during baseline), with a maximum of 138 turns (9.2 turns per minute). In comparison, by 24 months of age, typically developing children are interacting at a rate of approximately 7.5 turns per minute during free play (Paul, 2001). Wes made substantial gains during the course of the 1-year intervention, although his average rates did not reach the rates of typically developing children. The majority of these turns (94%) were accomplished with the aided systems (primarily the SGD), with a smaller percentage (6%) using signs.

At baseline, Wes expressed a very limited range of intents; he communicated only for behavior regulation (specifically, requests for more or protests). During intervention, Wes learned to express a wider range of intents. Intents were categorized using the taxonomy presented by Wetherby, Cain, Yonclas, and Walker (1988) into communicative functions of behavior regulation, social interaction, and joint attention. Throughout the year of intervention, Wes used all three types of communicative functions. Specifically, he used behavior regulation

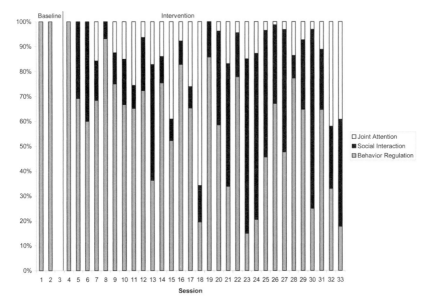

Figure 9.3. Percent of Wes's turns that expressed joint attention, social interaction, and behavior regulation for each session during baseline and intervention. (*Note:* Wes did not take any communicative turns during session 3 of baseline.)

messages 55% of the time, consisting primarily of requests for objects, requests for actions, and occasional protests. He expressed social inter- action messages 30% of the time, all of which were to participate in social routines. He used joint attention messages 15% of the time, pri- marily to comment on objects or events.

Figure 9.3 shows the relative proportion of each communicative function for each session. At baseline, Wes communicated only behav- ior regulation messages. At the beginning of the intervention, Wes communicated more behavior regulation messages as well. Over the course of the intervention, he demonstrated an increase in social inter- action and joint attention messages. In comparison, typically develop- ing children at the one-word stage use somewhat fewer behavior regulation acts (approximately 42% of the time, compared with Wes's 55%), fewer social interaction acts (approximately 19% of the time, compared with Wes's 30%), and significantly more joint attention acts (approximately 39% of the time, compared with Wes's 15%) (Wetherby et al., 1988).

Turns were also coded for semantic relations, based on the taxon- omy described by Retherford, Schwartz, and Chapman (1981). Although during baseline observations, Wes used only one concept (*more*, a recurrence), he quickly began to express a variety of semantic relations, including actions, affirmations, agents, attributes, entities, negations, objects, quantifiers, recurrence, social interjections, as well as lines from a book or song. Semantic relations that were used more frequently than others included objects (i.e., a person or thing that received the force of an action), attributes (i.e., an adjectival description of the size, shape, or quality of an object or person), entities (i.e., the use of an appropriate label for a person or object in the absence of any action on it), and recurrence (i.e., a request for or comment on an additional instance or amount). These relations tended to be more con- crete than agents (i.e., the performer, animate or inanimate, of an action) and actions (i.e., a perceivable movement or activity engaged in by an agent).

Wes primarily used one concept per turn, both during baseline and intervention. After approximately 9 months of intervention, Wes began combining concepts to produce novel utterances. These combinations were either using the SGD, signs, or a combination of SGD plus sign. For example, during the first session that Wes began combining symbols he signed MORE and used the SGD to request *apple*. A few intervention sessions later, Wes used the SGD to combine *mom* and *tummy* to indicate that he wanted his mother to tickle him on the stomach. He also began to use the navigation tools on the computer- based system (*main menu, go back*) without direct instruction after approximately 6 months of intervention that included partner modeling of navigation.

Discussion

The current evidence is based on a single case study and generalization of these results is limited. However, although the evidence presented in this case study is preliminary, the results of the intervention are promising. AAC technologies with appropriate AAC system design and interventions with a focus on social engagement can have a positive impact on the social interaction of young children with ASDs. It is possible to demonstrate an increase in social interaction through the implementation of effective intervention principles designed to address these goals.

It will be important for any intervention for children with ASDs who require AAC to focus on the core deficits of the disorder. An emphasis needs to be placed on the social aspects of communication. Although it is important for individuals with ASD to be able to request and reject, these are not the only functions that are necessary for the development of communicative competence.

FUTURE RESEARCH

There remains a need to investigate AAC interventions to enhance social interaction with individuals with ASDs. There are many unanswered questions involving AAC systems and AAC interventions. Future research will be critical to improve the designs of AAC systems, especially AAC technologies, to accommodate the characteristic needs and skills of children with ASDs. It will be important to enhance appeal and decrease the learning demands for children with ASDs. It is also critical to investigate techniques to redesign AAC technologies to provide a dynamic social context to support social interaction and learning. Future research is needed to determine the impact of these designs on social interaction, language development, and effective communication.

Additionally, future research is required to investigate appropriate AAC interventions to maximize social engagement and language development for children with ASDs. Although the case study presented here and other pilot results present some preliminary data on this intervention, the current evidence of effectiveness is limited. Also, only a social-pragmatic approach was implemented in the case study. Future research is required to determine the relative effectiveness on social interaction of various intervention techniques along the continuum of behavioral to social-pragmatic approaches.

Because ASDs are characterized by a large degree of heterogeneity, it will also be important to determine which techniques are most effective for individual characteristics of children and under what conditions. Finally, future translational work is required to ensure appropriate research to practice. It is important to identify effective evidence-based interventions with children with ASD to maximize social interaction.

SUMMARY

Children with ASDs frequently have difficulty with the social aspects of communication. AAC technologies have the potential to address the core deficit of social interaction for children with ASDs. To date, AAC approaches have largely focused on the communication of needs and wants; less attention has been paid to the development of social interaction skills. AAC approaches to date have also focused on unaided and low-tech aided systems. This chapter has considered the use of AAC technologies as a means to enhance social interaction with individuals with ASDs. Future research is urgently required to investigate AAC systems and interventions to increase social interaction.

REFERENCES

American Psychiatric Association. (2000). *Diagnostic and statistical manual of mental disorders* (4th ed., Text rev.). Washington, DC: American Psychiatric Association.

Astington, J.W., & Baird, J.A. (2005). Introduction: Why language matters. In J.W. Astington & J.A. Baird (Eds.), *Why language matters for Theory of Mind* (pp. 3–25). New York: Oxford University Press.

Axmear, E., Reichle, J., Alamsaputra, M., Kohnert, K., Drager, K., & Sellnow, K. (2005). Synthesized speech intelligibility in sentences: A comparison of monolingual English speaking and bilingual children. *Language, Speech, and Hearing Services in Schools, 36,* 244–250.

Binger, C., & Light, J.C. (2007). The effect of aided AAC modeling on the expression of multi-symbol messages by preschoolers who use AAC. *Augmentative and Alternative Communication, 23,* 30–43.

Bondy, A.S., & Frost, L.A. (1994). The picture exchange communication system. *Focus on Autistic Behavior, 9,* 1–19.

Boucher, J. (1988). Word fluency in high-functioning autistic children. *Journal of Autism and Developmental Disorders, 18,* 637–645.

Brady, N.C. (2000). Improved comprehension of object names following voice output communication aid use: Two case studies. *Augmentative and Alternative Communication, 16,* 197–204.

Cafiero, J. (1998). Communication power for individuals with autism. *Focus on Autism and Other Developmental Disabilities, 13,* 113–121.

Cafiero, J. (2001) The effect of an augmentative communication intervention on the communication, behavior, and academic program of an adolescent with autism. *Focus on Autism and Other Developmental Disabilities, 16,* 179–193.

Camarata, S.N., Nelson, K.E., & Camarata, M.N. (1994). Comparison of conversational-recasting and imitative procedures for training grammatical structures in children with specific language impairment. *Journal of Speech and Hearing Research, 37,* 1414–1423.

Dawson, G., Meltzoff, A.N., Osterling, J., Rinaldi, J., & Brown, E. (1998). Children with autism fail to orient to naturally occurring social stimuli. *Journal of Autism and Developmental Disorders, 28,* 479–485.

Drager, K., Light, J.C., Angert, E., Finke, E., Johnson, J., Larson, H., Shemeley, K., & Venzon, L. (2005, November). *AAC & interactive play: Language learning in children with autism.* Seminar presented at the Annual Conference of the American Speech-Language and Hearing Association, San Diego.

Drager, K., Light, J.C., Carlson, R., D'Silva, K., Larsson, B., Pitkin, L., & Stopper, G. (2004). Learning of dynamic display AAC technologies by typically developing 3-year-olds: Effect of different layouts and menu approaches. *Journal of Speech Language Hearing Research, 47,* 1133–1148.

Drager, K.D.R., Clark-Serpentine, E.A., Johnson, K.E., & Roeser, J.L. (2006). Accuracy of repetition of digitized and synthesized speech for young children in background noise. *American Journal of Speech-Language Pathology, 15,* 155–164.

Drager, K.D.R., Light, J.C., Curran Speltz, J., Fallon, K.A., & Jeffries, L.Z. (2003). The performance of typically developing 2$\frac{1}{2}$-year-olds on dynamic display AAC technologies with different system layouts and language organizations. *Journal of Speech Language Hearing Research, 46,* 298–312.

Drager, K.D.R., Postal, V.J., Carrolus, L., Castellano, M., Gagliano, C., & Glynn, J. (2006). The effect of aided language modeling on symbol comprehension and production in two preschoolers with autism. *American Journal of Speech-Language Pathology, 15,* 112–125.

Durand, V.M. (1999). Functional communication training using assistive devices: Recruiting natural communities of reinforcement. *Journal of Applied Behavior Analysis, 32,* 247–268.

Elder, J.H., Valcante, G., Won, D., & Zylis, R. (2003). Effects of in-home training for culturally diverse fathers of children with autism. *Issues in Mental Health Nursing, 24,* 273–295.

Elder, P., & Goosens', C. (1994). *Engineering training environments for interactive augmentative communication: Strategies for adolescents and adults who are moderately/severely developmentally delayed.* Birmingham, AL: Southeast Augmentative Communication Conference Publications.

Fallon, K.A., Light, J.C., & Achenbach, A. (2003). The semantic organization patterns of young children: Implications for augmentative and alternative communication. *Augmentative and Alternative Communication, 19,* 74–85.

Fenson, L., Dale, P.S., Reznick, J.S., Thal, D., Bates, E., Hartung, J.P., Pethick, S., & Reilly, J.S. (1993). *The MacArthur Communicative Development Inventories: User's guide and technical manual.* San Diego: Singular Publishing Group.

Goosens', C. (1989). Aided communication intervention before assessment: A case study of a child with cerebral palsy. *Augmentative and Alternative Communication, 5,* 14–26.

Goosens', C., Crain, S., & Elder, P. (1992). *Engineering the preschool environment for interactive symbolic communication 18 months to 5 years developmentally.* Birmingham, AL: Southeast Augmentative Communication Publications.

Halle, J.W. (1987). Teaching language in the natural environment: An analysis of spontaneity. *Journal of The Association for Persons with Severe Handicaps, 12,* 28–37.

Halle, J.W., Marshall, A.M., & Spradlin, J.E. (1979). Time delay: A technique to increase language use and facilitate generalization in retarded children. *Journal of Applied Behavior Analysis, 12,* 431–439.

Happe, F., & Frith, U. (2006). The weak coherence account: Detail-focused cognitive style in autism spectrum disorders. *Journal of Autism and Developmental Disorders, 36,* 5–25.

Hwang, B., & Hughes, C. (2000). The effects of social interactive training on early social communicative skills of children with autism. *Journal of Autism and Developmental Disorders, 30,* 331–343.

Kaiser, A.P., Hancock, T.B., & Nietfeld, J.P. (2000). The effects of parent-implemented enhanced milieu teaching on the social communication of children who have autism. *Early Education and Development, 11,* 423–446.

Kanner, L. (1943). Autistic disturbances of affective contact. *Nervous Child, 2,* 217–250.

Kasari, C., Sigman, M., Mundy, P., & Yirmiya, N. (1988). Caregiver interactions with autistic children. *Journal of Abnormal Child Psychology, 16,* 45–56.

Koegel, L.K. (2000). Interventions to facilitate communication in autism. *Journal of Autism and Developmental Disorders, 30,* 383–391.

Koegel, R.L., Bimbela, A., & Schreibman, L. (1996). Collateral effects of parent training on family interactions. *Journal of Autism and Developmental Disorders, 26,* 347–359.

Koegel, R.L., & Johnson, J. (1989). Motivating language use in autistic children. In G. Dawson, *Autism, nature, diagnosis, and treatment* (pp. 310–325). New York: Guilford Press.

Koegel, R.L., Koegel, L.K., & Surratt, A. (1992). Language intervention and disruptive behavior in preschool children with autism. *Journal of Autism and Developmental Disorders, 22,* 141–153.

Koegel, R.L., O'Dell, M.C., & Koegel, L.K. (1987). A natural language teaching paradigm for nonverbal autistic children. *Journal of Autism and Developmental Disorders, 17,* 187–200.

Koul, R.K., & Schlosser, R.W. (2004). Effects of synthetic speech output in the learning of graphic symbols of varied iconicity. *Disability and Rehabilitation: An International Multidisciplinary Journal, 26,* 1278–1285.

Kozleski, E.B. (1991). Expectant delay procedure for teaching requests. *Augmentative and Alternative Communication, 7,* 11–19.

Light, J.C. (1988). Interaction involving individuals using augmentative and alternative communication systems: State of the art and future directions. *Augmentative and Alternative Communication, 4,* 66–82.

Light, J.C., & Binger, C. (1998). *Building communicative competence with individuals who use augmentative and alternative communication.* Baltimore: Paul H. Brookes Publishing Co.

Light, J.C., & Drager, K. (2002). Improving the design of augmentative and alternative communication technologies for young children. *Assistive Technology, 14,* 17–32.

Light, J.C., & Drager, K. (2005, November). *Maximizing language development for young children who require AAC.* Seminar presented at the Annual Conference of the American Speech-Language-Hearing Association, San Diego.

Light, J.C., & Drager, K. (2007). AAC technologies for young children with complex communication needs: State of the science and future research directions. *Augmentative and Alternative Communication, 23,* 204–216.

Light, J.C., Drager, K.D.R., & Nemser, J.G. (2004). Enhancing the appeal of AAC technologies for young children: Lessons from the toy manufacturers. *Augmentative and Alternative Communication, 20,* 137–149.

Light, J.C., Page, R., Curran, J., & Pitkin, L. (2007). Children's designs of assistive technologies for young children with complex communication needs. *Augmentative and Alternative Communication, 23,* 274–287.

Light, J.C., Parsons, A.R., & Drager, K.D.R. (2002). "There's more to life than cookies": Developing interactions for social closeness with beginning communicators who require augmentative and alternative communication. In D.R. Beukelman & J. Reichle (Series Eds.) & J. Reichle, D.R. Beukelman, & J.C. Light (Vol. Eds.), *Augmentative and alternative communication series. Exemplary practices for beginning communicators: Implications for AAC* (pp. 187–218). Baltimore: Paul H. Brookes Publishing Co.

Light, J.C., Roberts, B., DiMarco, R., & Greiner, N. (1998). Augmentative and alternative communication to support receptive and expressive communication for people with autism. *Journal of Communication Disorders, 31,* 153–180.

Light, J.C., Worah, S., Drager, K., Bowker, A., Burki, B., D'Silva, K., et al. (2007). *Graphic representations of early emerging language concepts by young children from different cultural backgrounds: Implications for AAC symbols.* Manuscript in preparation.

Lord, C., Risi, S., & Pickles, A. (2004). Trajectory of language development in autistic spectrum disorders. In M.L. Rice & S.F. Warren (Eds.), *Developmental language disorders: From phenotypes to etiologies* (pp. 1–38). Mahwah, NJ: Lawrence Erlbaum Associates.

Lovaas, O. (1977). *The autistic child: Language development through behavior modification.* New York: Irvington.

Lucariello, J., Kyratzis, A., & Nelson., K. (1992). Taxonomic knowledge: What kind and when. *Child Development, 63,* 978–998.

Lund, S., Millar, D., Herman, M., Hinds, A., & Light, J.C. (1998, November). *Children's pictorial representations of early emerging concepts: Implications for AAC.* Poster presented at the American Speech-Language-Hearing Association Annual Convention, San Antonio, TX.

Maaka, M., & Wong, E. (1994, April). *Semantic memory in young children: The script-based categorization of early words*. Paper presentation at the annual meeting of the American Educational Research Association, New Orleans, LA.

McConachie, H., & Diggle, T. (2006). Parent implemented early intervention for young children with autism spectrum disorder: A systematic review. *Journal of Evaluation in Clinical Practice, 13*, 120–129.

McLean, J.E., & Snyder-McLean, L.K. (1978). *A transactional approach to early language training*. Columbus, OH: Charles E. Merrill.

McLean, L.K. (1990). Communication development in the first two years of life: A transactional process. *Zero to Three Bulletin, 11*, 13–19.

Mirenda, P. (2001). Autism, augmentative communication, and assistive technology: What do we really know? *Focus on Autism and Other Developmental Disabilities, 16*, 141–151.

Mirenda, P. (2003). Toward functional augmentative and alternative communication for students with autism: Manual signs, graphic symbols, and voice output communication aids. *Language, Speech, and Hearing Services in Schools, 34*, 203–216.

Mirenda, P. (2005, November). *AAC for individuals with autism: From symbol wars to EBP*. Short course presented at the annual convention of the American Speech-Language-Hearing Association, San Diego.

Mirenda, P., & Schuler, A.L. (1988). Augmenting communication for persons with autism: Issues and strategies. *Topics in Language Disorders, 9*, 24–43.

Moore, M., & Calvert, S. (2000). Brief report: SGDbulary acquisition for children with autism: Teacher or computer instruction. *Journal of Autism and Developmental Disorders, 30*, 359–362.

Mundy, P., & Stella, J. (2000). Joint attention, social orienting, and nonverbal communication in autism. In S.F. Warren & J. Reichle (Series Eds.) & A.M. Wetherby & B.M. Prizant (Vol. Eds.), *Communication and language intervention series: Vol. 9. Autism spectrum disorders: A transactional developmental perspective* (pp. 55–77). Baltimore: Paul H. Brookes Publishing Co.

National Research Council. (2001). In C. Lord & J.P. McGee (Eds.), *Educating children with autism*. Committee on Educational Interventions for Children with Autism. Division of Behavioral and Social Sciences and Education. Washington, DC: National Academies Press.

Nelson, K. (1996). *Language in cognitive development: Emergence of the mediated mind*. New York: Cambridge University Press.

Ogletree, B.T., & Harn, W.E. (2001). Augmentative and alternative communication for persons with autism: History, issues, and unanswered questions. *Focus on Autism and Other Developmental Disorders, 16*, 138–140.

Paul, R. (2001). *Language disorders from infancy through adolescence: Assessment and intervention* (2nd ed.). St. Louis, MO: Mosby.

Prizant, B.M., & Wetherby, A.M. (1998). Understanding the continuum of discrete-trial traditional behavioral to social-pragmatic developmental approaches in communication enhancement for young children with autism/PDD. *Seminars in Speech and Language, 19*, 329–353.

Prizant, B.M., Wetherby, A.M., Rubin, E., Laurent, A.C., & Rydell, P.J. (2006). *The SCERTS® Model: A comprehensive educational approach for children with autism spectrum disorders.* Vol. 1: Assessment. Baltimore: Paul H. Brookes Publishing Co.

Quill, K.A. (1995). Visually cued instruction for children with autism and pervasive developmental disorders. *Focus on Autistic Behavior, 10,* 10–20.

Quill, K.A. (1997). Instructional considerations for young children with autism: The rationale for visually cued instruction. *Journal of Autism and Developmental Disorders, 27,* 697–714.

Retherford, K.S., Schwartz, B.C., & Chapman, R.S. (1981). Semantic roles and residual grammatical categories in mother and child speech: Who tunes into whom? *Journal of Child Language, 8,* 583–608.

Richman, D.M., Wacker, D.P., & Winborn, L. (2001). Response efficiency during functional communication training: Effects of effort on response allocation. *Journal of Applied Behavior Analysis, 34,* 73–76.

Rinehart, N.J., Bellgrove, M.A., Tonge, B.J., Brereton, A.V., Howells-Rankin, D., & Bradshaw, J.L. (2006). An examination of movement kinematics in young people with high-functioning autism and Asperger's disorder: Further evidence for a motor planning deficit. *Journal of Autism and Developmental Disorders, 36,* 757–767.

Romski, M.A., & Sevcik, R.A. (1996). *Breaking the speech barrier: Language development through augmented means.* Baltimore: Paul H. Brookes Publishing Co.

Sameroff, A.J., & Chandler, M.J. (1975). Reproductive risk and the continuum of caretaking casualty. In F. Horowitz (Ed.), *Review of child development research* (Vol. 4, pp. 187–244). Chicago: University of Chicago Press.

Schepis, M.M., Reid, D.H., Behrmann, M.M., & Sutton, K.A. (1998). Increasing communicative interactions of young children with autism using a voice output communication aid and naturalistic teaching. *Journal of Applied Behavior Analysis, 31,* 561–578.

Schlosser, R.W., Belfiore, P.J., Nigam, R., Blischak, D., & Hetzroni, O. (1995). The effects of speech output technology in the learning of graphic symbols. *Journal of Applied Behavior Analysis, 28,* 537–549.

Schlosser, R.W., Blischak, D.M., Belfiore, P.J., Bartley, C., & Barnett, N. (1998). The effects of synthetic speech output and orthographic feedback on spelling in a student with autism: A preliminary study. *Journal of Autism and Developmental Disorders, 28,* 319–329.

Schreibman, L., Kaneko, W.M., & Koegel, R.L. (1991). Positive affect of parents of autistic children: A comparison across two teaching techniques. *Behavior Therapy, 22,* 479–490.

Sell, M. (1992). The development of children's knowledge structures: Events, slots, and taxonomies. *Journal of Child Language, 19,* 659–676.

Seung, H.K., Ashwell, S., Elder, J.H., & Valcante, G. (2006). Verbal communication outcomes in children with autism after in-home father training. *Journal of Intellectual Disability Research, 50,* 139–150.

Sevcik, R.A., Romski, M.A., Watkins, R., & Deffebach, K. (1995). Adult partner-augmented communication input to youth with mental retardation using the System for Augmenting Language (SAL). *Journal of Speech and Hearing Research, 38,* 902–912.

Shane, H. (2006). Using visual scene displays to improve communication and communication instruction in persons with autism spectrum disorders. *Perspectives on Augmentative and Alternative Communication, 15,* 7–13.

Shane, H.C., Sorce, J., Fleisch Cordeiro, R., Duggan, M., & Weiss-Kapp, S. (2005, November). *Video technology for language instruction for children with ASD.* Paper presented at the American Speech-Language-Hearing Association Annual Convention, San Diego.

Shonkoff, J.P., Hauser-Cram, P., Krauss, M.W., & Upshur, C.C. (1992). Development of infants with disabilities and their families: Implications for theory and service delivery. *Monographs of the Society for Research in Child Development, 57,* v-153.

Sigafoos, J., & Drasgow, E. (2001). Conditional use of aided and unaided AAC: A review and clinical case demonstration. *Focus on Autism and Other Developmental Disabilities, 16,* 152–161.

Sigafoos, J., Drasgow, E., Halle, J.W., O'Reilly, M., Seely-York, S., Edrisinha, C., & Andrews, A. (2004). Teaching SGD use as a communicative repair strategy. *Journal of Autism and Developmental Disorders, 34,* 411–422.

Siller, M., & Sigman, M. (2002). The behaviors of parents of children with autism predict the subsequent development of their children's communication. *Journal of Autism and Developmental Disorders, 32,* 77–89.

Son, S., Sigafoos, J., O'Reilly, M., & Lancioni, G. (2006). Comparing two types of augmentative and alternative communication systems for children with autism. *Pediatric Rehabilitation, 9,* 389–395.

Stone, W.L., Ousley, O.Y., Yoder, P.J., Hogan, K.L., & Hepburn, S.L. (1997). Nonverbal communication in two- and three-year-old children in autism. *Journal of Autism and Developmental Disorders, 27,* 677–696.

Stromer, R., Kimball, J.W., Kinney, E.M., & Taylor, B.A. (2006). Activity schedules, computer technology, and teaching children with autism spectrum disorders. *Focus on Autism and Other Developmental Disabilities, 21,* 14–24.

Tager-Flusberg, H. (1985). The conceptual basis for referential word meaning in children with autism. *Child Development, 56,* 1167–1178.

Tager-Flusberg, H. (1996). Brief report: Current theory and research on language and communication in autism. *Journal of Autism and Developmental Disorders, 27,* 169–172.

Traylor, V.S. (2004). The effect of taxonomic and thematic organization on typically developing preschoolers' matching in a dynamic display. *Dissertation Abstracts International, 64,* 6050.

Van Acker, R., & Grant, S. (1995). An effective computer-based requesting system for persons with Rett syndrome. *Journal of Childhood Communication Disorders, 16,* 31–38.

Vanvuchelen, M., Roeyers, H., & De Weerdt, W. (2007). Nature of motor imitation problems in school-aged boys with autism: A motor or a cognitive problem? *Autism, 11,* 225–240.

Warren, S.F., Yoder, P.J., Gazdag, G.E., Kim, K., & Jones, H.A. (1993). Facilitating prelinguistic communication skills in young children with developmental delay. *Journal of Speech and Hearing Research, 36,* 83–97.

Watson, L.R. (1998). Following the child's lead: mothers' interactions with children with autism. *Journal of Autism and Developmental Disorders, 28,* 51–59.

Watson, L.R., Lanter, E., McComish, C., & Poston Roy, V. (2004). Enhancing the communication development of toddlers with autism spectrum disorders. *Journal of Cognitive and Behavioral Psychotherapies, 4,* 179–201.

Wetherby, A.M., Cain, D.H., Yonclas, D.G., & Walker, V.G. (1988). Analysis of intentional communication of normal children from the prelinguistic to the multiword stage. *Journal of Speech and Hearing Research, 31,* 240–252.

Wetherby, A.M., & Prizant, B.M. (Vol. Eds.). (2000). *Autism spectrum disorders: A transactional developmental perspective.* In S.F. Warren & J. Reichle (Series Eds.), *Communication and language intervention series: Vol. 9.* Baltimore: Paul H. Brookes Publishing Co.

Wetherby, A.M., Prizant, B.M., & Schuler, A.L. (2000). Understanding the nature of communication and language impairments. In S.F. Warren & J. Reichle (Series Eds.) & A.M. Wetherby & B.M. Prizant (Vol. Eds.), *Communication and language intervention series: Vol. 9. Autism spectrum disorders: A transactional developmental perspective* (pp. 109–142). Baltimore: Paul H. Brookes Publishing Co.

Wetherby, A.M., & Woods, J.J. (2006). Early social interaction project for children with autism spectrum disorders beginning in the second year of life: A preliminary study. *Topics in Early Childhood Special Education, 26,* 67–82.

Wilkinson, K.M., & Rosenquist, C. (2006). Demonstration of a method for assessing semantic organization and category membership in individuals with autism spectrum disorders and receptive SGDbulary limitations. *Augmentative and Alternative Communication, 22,* 242–257.

Wolery, M., & Garfinkel, A.N. (2002). Measures in intervention research with young children who have autism. *Journal of Autism and Developmental Disorders, 32,* 463–478.

Woods, J.J., & Wetherby, A.M. (2003). Early identification of and intervention for infants and toddlers who are at risk for autism spectrum disorder. *Language, Speech, and Hearing Services in Schools, 34,* 180–193.

Yoder, P.J., Kaiser, A.P., Alpert, C., & Fischer, R. (1993). Following the child's lead when teaching nouns to preschoolers with mental retardation. *Journal of Speech and Hearing Research, 36,* 158–167.

Yoder, P.J., & Warren, S.F. (1998). Maternal responsivity predicts the prelinguistic communication intervention that facilitates generalized intentional communication. *Journal of Speech, Language, and Hearing Research, 41,* 1207–1219.

10

The Picture Exchange Communication System

Clinical and Research Applications

ANDY BONDY AND LORI FROST

The Picture Exchange Communication System (PECS) was developed in 1985 by the authors in response to our difficulty in successfully using a variety of communication training programs with young students with autism spectrum disorders (ASD). We had been using traditional speech training protocols but were frustrated by the failure of many of our young students to develop speech imitation skills. In addition, we were concerned with the length of time needed to teach functional speech to children who learned speech imitation.

We taught several children sign language but were troubled by the limited number of communicative partners these children had, given the idiosyncratic signs they were using because of their fine motor limitations. When we attempted to teach picture-point systems, we found that either the children did not initiate communicative exchanges by directly interacting with a communicative partner or that they had many competing hand movements, which made their messages difficult to interpret. For example, some students could not isolate their index fingers to point to a picture. These children often slapped their communication books, making contact with several pictures at the same time; it was then up to a communication partner to interpret their messages. Other children would point to a picture but look away from the pictures and the teacher, which was also difficult to interpret because we were unsure whether or not the child was communicating intentionally. In addition, it appeared to us that these picture-based systems taught students to direct their actions to a picture rather than another person, thus ignoring the social aspects that are integral to communication.

Originally, PECS was developed for use with preschool-age children with ASDs who exhibited little or no functional or socially acceptable speech. These are children who do not speak at all, speak only in a "self-stimulatory" manner, speak only when prompted to do so, or are extremely echolalic. Their communicative difficulties are socially related: they do not routinely approach others to communicate, actively avoid interaction with others, or only communicate in response to direct cues to do so. Over the years, we have recognized that many children in addition to those with ASDs also have difficulty acquiring speech. We now teach PECS to children and adults with a variety of diagnoses or educational classifications.

The PECS training protocol (Frost & Bondy, 2002) is based on research and practice in the principles of applied behavior analysis. Distinct teaching, reinforcement, error correction, and generalization strategies are essential for teaching each skill. The PECS training protocol also closely parallels typical language development in that it first teaches the child how to communicate and the basic rules of communication. Children using PECS learn to communicate first with single pictures (or three-dimensional objects; see Ganz, Cook, Corbin-Newsome, Bourgeois, & Flores, 2005) and then choose among two or more pictures. Finally, the children combine pictures to produce a variety of grammatical structures, semantic relationships, and communicative functions.

PECS AND VERBAL BEHAVIOR

An important theoretical underpinning for PECS was provided by the analysis of language provided in B.F. Skinner's seminal book, *Verbal Behavior* (1957). In this book, Skinner presented a perspective on language based on a functional analysis of fundamental units. Each of these units—or verbal operants—is defined by observable behaviors or aspects of the environment, in terms of both antecedents and consequences.

Skinner defined verbal behavior as any behavior that is reinforced through the mediation of other people. Central to his analysis is the recognition that verbal operants are defined functionally and are not related to issues of modality. Thus, within Skinner's analysis, *verbal* does not mean *vocal*. Any behavior that can affect someone else can come to serve verbal functions, including the use of pictures or objects, as in PECS.

Verbal behavior is observed when one person does something to another person, who then provides some type of reinforcer that is either concrete or social in nature. For example, a mand specifies its own reinforcer and is preceded by some type of motivational operation (rather than by specific stimuli in the environment). Such actions are similar to requests—com*mands* or de*mands*. A tact is controlled by specific aspects of the environment (including things that may happen within us) but results in social reinforcement. Intraverbals are controlled by preceding verbal behaviors (i.e., those that are initially produced someone else), but the form of the intraverbal is not the same of the form of the prior verbal stimulus (e.g., on hearing *Two, four, six…*, one responds with *eight*). Intraverbals are reinforced by social consequences. The analysis of such units and their various combinations is crucial for planning conceptually sound lessons involving the acquisition of various aspects of language (Bondy, Tincani, & Frost, 2004).

In this chapter, we will first describe the phase structure of PECS before noting several factors that have guided its development. We will then describe several ways that PECS can be used for vocabulary expansion and increasing the complexity of the structure of language. Finally, we will review research pertaining to PECS and its associated benefits and discuss implications for future research.

THE PECS PROTOCOL

The PECS protocol is divided into six distinct training phases. All students begin at Phase I, which teaches the basic principle of communication. All that is necessary to begin PECS is a reinforcer assessment (Frost & Bondy, 2002). Once the teacher has identified potential rewards (i.e., items for which the learner persistently reaches), PECS can begin immediately.

Phase I: Teaching the Communicative Exchange

Phase I begins by teaching the child the physical behavior that will be communicative. We broadly describe this phase as teaching the child to request (i.e., to mand, within Skinner's framework). No picture discrimination is required prior to beginning PECS or during this initial phase. One teacher (called the communicative partner) shows the child a desired item. The child is physically assisted (from behind by a second teacher called the physical prompter) to give a picture of that item to the communicative partner. Upon receipt of the picture, the communicative partner immediately labels the item requested (e.g., *Oh, you want a cookie*) and gives the child the item. There is no vocal prompting prior to the exchange; hence, the response is not under the additional control of the speech of the communicative partner. The communicative partner does not show an open hand until the child reaches for the reward or the picture; this method avoids having the hand function as a controlling stimulus for the picture exchange. No vocal imitation is prompted or expected of the child at this point. The physical prompts delivered by the physical prompter to teach the child to pick up, extend, and exchange the picture are faded using a backward-chaining format. Thus, the physical prompt that is faded last involves picking up the picture.

Phase II: Teaching Persistence

After a few trials of independently exchanging pictures for objects while the communicative partner is within arm's reach, Phase II begins. For the majority of students who demonstrate motivation to access reinforcers, this typically occurs within the first training session. Phase II teaches the student to be persistent across various obstacles, such as increasing distances to the communicative partner and/or the communication book. The communicative partner begins to move farther from the child to teach the child to seek out the communicative partner wherever he or she may be located in the environment. In addition, very early in training, other people take on the role of the communicative partner so that the child does not learn to associate the picture exchange solely with one person. A final aspect of this early phase of training is teaching the child to move to the picture and then find the communicative partner. This contingency enhances searching for the picture even if the picture is neither near the desired object nor near the listener. At the successful completion of this aspect of training, the child can find his communication book with a single picture on it, pick it up, take it to someone who controls access to a desired object, and hand the picture to that person to receive the object.

O'Neill (1990) suggested that learners should be taught to request a communicative partner's attention before learning to request particular items or actions. PECS does not require such prerequisite training because giving the picture to the teacher functions in a similar manner to the request for attention noted by O'Neill (1990). However, during the initial exchanges between child and adult, most children are looking at the hand of the teacher rather than at the teacher's eyes when they approach with their picture. To establish the importance of eye contact as a critical feature of the communicative partner, teachers are advised to sit with their head (and thus eyes) cast downward as the child approaches with a picture. The physical prompter physically guides the child to touch the teacher's shoulders or to gently lift the teacher's face prior to extending the picture. This step can be added only after the exchange is established during Phase II. This training sequence essentially teaches the child that eye contact with the communicative partner is important to set the occasion for the exchange. Thus, rather than the traditional approach of teaching the child that it is important for the child to look at the teacher's eyes when asked to do so (e.g., *Look at me*), PECS teaches that it is important to make the teacher look at the child.

Phase III: Discrimination Training

In Phases I and II, only a single picture is available in each situation during which a particular reinforcer is most likely to be effective. Phase III introduces the skill of discriminating between pictures. A variety of techniques can be used to develop discrimination. One such strategy is to use pairs of pictures in which one picture is of a highly desired item or matches a specific context, whereas the other picture is of an item that is undesired or that does not fit the immediate context. For example, a child might like a toy car but not care to play with a sock. The teacher would show the child both items while providing pictures of each. If the child hands over the picture of the toy car, he is given the car; conversely, if he gives the teacher the picture of the sock, he receives that item instead. If the latter occurs, the child is very likely to reject the sock. At this point, the teacher proceeds to implement a specific error correction strategy to promote selection of the correct picture. The context associated with particular items also can be used to emphasize the reinforcing value of one particular item within a paired choice (Frost & Bondy, 2002).

During Phase III, the correspondence between what a child asks for using a picture and what he or she selects when presented with two options is also tested. We do this because, given equally reinforcing choices, we cannot anticipate which item the child may want on a particular trial. Thus, the second part of discrimination training involves saying *Go ahead*, *Take it*, or *Show me* upon receipt of a picture from the child. Naming the requested item is avoided because the purpose of the correspondence check is to determine whether or not the child understands the relationship between the picture—not the verbal label—and the item. If the child reaches for the item requested with the picture, he or she is allowed immediate access. However, if the child selects an item that does not correspond with the picture, an error correction strategy is used. As correct performance is maintained, the number of pairs of items and corresponding symbols is varied across the day and the size of the picture array is gradually expanded.

Phase IV: Teaching *I Want* Sentences

When typically developing children begin to use single-word utterances, they use words to request, comment, and label. Their adult communicative partners discriminate between these functions by hearing differences in the inflections (or intonation patterns) that accompany single words. Thus, *Ball?* is understood as a request, whereas *Ball* (perhaps accompanied by a point) is understood as a comment or label. However, when a child uses only a single picture to communicate, it is often difficult for the communicative partner to know whether the child is using it to make a request or a comment.

It is important to develop an equivalent strategy for intonation at this phase of PECS training, allowing children to clarify the function of pictures they select. Thus, in Phase IV, the child is taught to construct the sentence *I want [desired item]* with two distinct pictures. The *I want* symbol is a single picture. The use of this symbol is taught in a backward-chaining format, with the symbol initially being placed upon a removable strip, called the "sentence strip," by the teacher (for more details, see Frost & Bondy, 2002).

Phase V: Teaching a Response to *What Do You Want?*

The purpose of Phase V is to bring the child's request under the influence of words spoken by someone else—that is, the child is taught to respond to simple questions. Within Skinner's analysis, this step involves the introduction of an intraverbal because the form of the child's response is not related to the form of the question. This step is accomplished by asking *What do you want?* while simultaneously pointing to the *I want* symbol, then introducing a progressive delayed-prompt strategy to remove the gestural prompt. The form of the response—using the sentence strip to create *I want [desired item]*—was taught in Phase IV and is already available within the child's repertoire. However, the use of the question by the teacher brings the response partially under the control of this verbal stimulus as well. By the end of Phase V, the child can use symbols to both spontaneously request and respond to a question with a request. These two skills set the stage for the next stage of training.

Phase VI: Teaching Use of Additional Sentence Starters

During Phase VI, the teacher introduces new sentence starters to the communication display. These units include *I see, I have, I hear,* and so forth. With a minimally desired object in sight, the teacher asks "What do you see?" while simultaneously touching the *I see* card. This gestural prompt, established in the previous phase of training, is likely to be sufficiently effective so that the child picks up the sentence starter symbol and places it on the sentence strip. The child is then likely to place the picture of the stimulus item on the sentence strip and give it to the communicative partner. Upon its receipt, the communicative partner reads back "I see the ball" or something similar; however, the ball is not given to the child. Thus, this phase introduces the use of a tact (i.e., label), although it is still related to the intraverbal control of the teacher's question.

To develop spontaneous comments, the teacher's question must be eliminated. A variety of procedures can be used to accomplish this. For example, the communicative partner makes a general statement such as "Look!" or "Wow!" while displaying an item. Over subsequent trials, the communicative partner then fades the statement and replaces it with a nonvocal prompt such as an arched eyebrow or an expectant look. As long as comments are produced solely in response to the actions of the communicative partner (whether vocal or nonvocal), a spontaneous comment has not been established. Thus, the goal of Phase VI is to establish a pure tact that is produced spontaneously.

PECS STRATEGIES FOR VOCABULARY EXPANSION

The PECS protocol can also be expanded to teach additional language forms, including those related to attributes such as color, size, shape, texture, and location; body parts; and verbs. In this section, we describe basic strategies for expanding learners' vocabularies in one or more of these ways.

Teaching Attributes

Many students with ASDs have very idiosyncratic preferences. When offered a bucket of blocks, they might systematically pull out only the big blocks, the long blocks, the triangular blocks, or the green blocks. By such selective response to aspects of objects (or events), students indicate their awareness about features that can be thought of as attributes or properties of the object or event. The student who picks out green blocks may never have had a single lesson aimed at teaching colors; yet, he is clearly responsive to color differentiation. In such situations, the student's ability to make requests with PECS is used to teach him or her to use attributes that refine or clarify the request. That is, we rely on a child's differential responses to a particular feature before we address that feature within a communication lesson.

Many teachers believe that students must learn these attributional concepts receptively prior to using them productively within a PECS request. We are not aware of any supportive research for this claim. Furthermore, two recent studies have demonstrated that children can learn to discriminate pictures without prior demonstration of receptive match-to-sample skills (Dyer, Sulzer-Azaroff, & Bondy, 2006; Peterson, Bondy, Glassberg, & Neef, 2002). In each case, matching-to-sample improved after the acquisition of discrimination skills within Phase III. Given this, there is no evidence that a student must be able to respond to the direction "Touch yellow" before he can learn to ask for something yellow. If a student always reaches for the yellow juice at lunch and always protests when offered red juice, we can reasonably conclude that the student sees and recognizes color differences. Touching yellow in response to "Touch yellow" or asking for a yellow block are both ways a student can demonstrate communication skills about colors.

Another factor to consider is the motivation associated with these different skills. For example, when a child asks for the yellow candy, he gets the yellow candy; however, when he successfully responds to "Touch the yellow paper," he receives only praise, not the paper. Especially for children with ASDs, asking for *yellow* is likely to be far more motivating than pleasing someone else by correctly responding to an instruction.

The critical first step in teaching attributes is to first identify when a particular attribute is important to the student. If the student does not care which color cookie he gets, he is not going to be motivated to learn how to communicate about cookie colors. Thus, we start by surveying the student's current vocabulary and determining whether a particular size, color, shape, or other aspect is highly reinforcing. We include information from the correspondence checks conducted during Phase III as one component of this survey. For example, perhaps the student took only the biggest chips when offered a bowl of potato chips or selected only green markers when offered an array of markers. Perhaps a student is known to prefer a specific texture of peanut butter (crunchy versus smooth), a specific temperature of a drink (cold versus warm), or a particular shape of cookie. If so, the preference is a good indication that color, texture, temperature, and/or shape are important to the child within a specific context. Because we know that he or she is motivated to seek items with a specific attribute, we begin teaching that attribute in the context of requesting.

The first step is to create a lesson involving materials for which a particular attribute is important. For example, perhaps a student has shown a preference for orange nail polish and a distinct dislike of blue nail polish. Initially, we would arrange the communication display so that the only pictures available are *I want, orange,* and *nail polish.* When the student constructs a sentence strip with *I want nail polish,* we use a forward-chaining strategy and physically prompt her to put the *orange* symbol on the strip, between *want* and *nail polish,* as depicted in Figure 10.1.

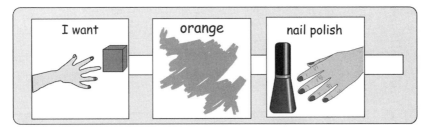

Figure 10.1.   PECS sentence strip to ask for a specific color of nail polish.

Once the student is constructing and exchanging the three-picture sentence strip independently, we begin teaching discrimination between two color symbols using the same strategy as in the basic Phase III: discrimination between a highly preferred and a nonpreferred attribute. Because the student does not like blue nail polish, those two symbols are included on the front of the communication board and the student must use the *orange* symbol to get orange nail polish. If there are two or more colors that the student prefers at different times, the teaching strategy is the same as the correspondence checks conducted in Phase III. Once the student has constructed and exchanged the sentence strip, the communicative partner conducts a correspondence check to assess correct use of the color symbol. Rather than naming the color when reading the sentence strip, the communicative partner tells the student "Get it" or "Go ahead." If the student reaches for the color that she requested, she is allowed access. If the student reaches for a color that is different than the one requested, the communicative partner conducts an error correction. We have taught a variety of attributes within the requesting function of PECS, as displayed in Table 10.1.

An even more sophisticated communication skill occurs when a child requests an item that varies along several dimensions. For example, while building a block tower, a student might want a specific color of block to add next, as well as one of a specific size. Asking for a *big block* might result in access to the wrong color, whereas asking for a *blue block* might result in access to the wrong size. Asking for a *big, blue block*, however, results in access to the perfect block. Perhaps there are two *big red* blocks—one triangular block and one rectangle block. In this case, the student must ask for the *big, red, triangular block*. Perhaps the student is an expert tower builder and not only wants big, red, triangular blocks, but also wants more than one at a time and must ask for *three big, red, triangular blocks*.

The teaching strategy for this multiconcept request would involve having materials on hand that involve discriminating between *all* of

Table 10.1. Concepts and sample materials for teaching attributes using Picture Communication Symbols

Concept	Materials		Example
Colors	Skittles Fruit rolls Licorice Starburst Markers Paint Juice	Cookies Crackers Lipstick Nail polish Shoes Clothing	I want — orange — nail polish
Size (e.g., big/little, long/short)	Food Miniature toys Pencils Licorice strands		I want — long — pencil
Shapes	Cookies Crackers Cookie cutters Blocks Parquetry blocks		I want — triangle — cookie cutter
Body parts	Mr. Potato Head Band Aid where? Massager where? Lotion where? Ink stamps where? Brushing where? Temporary tattoos where?		I want — lotion — arm
Position (e.g., in, on, under, behind, first, second, near, far)	Any "generic" reinforcer for which one exemplar is nonpreferred and one is preferred. The preferred item is put in the target location.		I want — middle — cookie
Textures	Salty versus unsalted pretzels Sand versus regular paper Ridged versus smooth potato chips		I want — rough — chips

the targeted variables. For example, we might first teach a student to ask for *egg* because we have filled several plastic eggs with a favorite item such as a candy. Once the student can ask for *egg*, we begin varying which egg has the candy so that one egg is full and the rest are empty or contain a nonpreferred item such as paper. We place the candy in the egg in front of the student so that he or she can see where it goes. Initially, we teach the student to ask for a specific color or size of egg; eventually, we vary both characteristics so that the student must track both color and size to request the egg containing the candy. We may even combine two colors (e.g., blue plus orange) to make a complete egg and teach the student to use *and* in his request (e.g., *I want the big blue-and-orange egg*). Figure 10.2 displays the materials required to teach such a multicomponent request.

Teaching Verbs

We view teaching verbs in a manner that is similar to our approach to attributes. Children in language-training programs typically are exposed to "verb training" that requires them to label pictures or comment on the actions of others. For children with ASDs who do not enjoy these activities, we teach them to request a particular action for an item they like or an action they enjoy seeing someone perform. For example, we may teach a student to request *I want [to] kick [the] ball.* Using the correspondence check procedures described previously, after we say "Go ahead," we watch closely to determine that the student is about to kick as opposed to throw the ball. If he or she kicks, we allow it. If he or she starts to throw the ball, we block this action and conduct an error correction. Similarly, we worked with one student who loved ordering

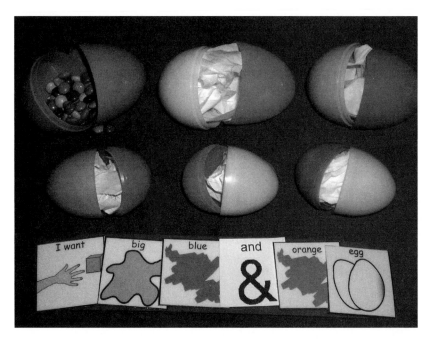

Figure 10.2. Materials and pictures used to teach the multidimensional request, "I want the big blue-and-orange egg."

her teacher, Meg, to perform specific actions. She would request, for example, *I want Meg [to] cry* or *I want Meg [to] dance.*

Generative Use of PECS

A very important skill to teach any student using an augmentative and alternative communication (AAC) system is what to do in response to an offer of an item for which he or she has no picture. In such situations, we wait and see which picture(s) the student uses to ask for the item. Many students will come up with interesting (and often novel) ways of describing what they want. For example, when a group of preschool children are offered a pink iced toaster pastry but none of the students has the corresponding picture, they may instead request *I want rectangle cookie, I want flat cake,* or *I want pink rectangle.* Such requests reflect the children's creative and versatile use of language.

Marckel, Neef, and Ferreri (2006) taught two young boys with autism to solve problems (i.e., improvise) by using descriptors (such as functions, colors, and shapes) to request desired items for which specific pictures were unavailable. The results of this multiple-baseline, across-descriptors study showed that PECS instruction increased the number of improvised requests. These skills generalized to novel items and across settings and listeners in the natural environment.

Teaching Use of a *HELP* Symbol

A functional assessment of problem behaviors such as aggression or tantrums often suggests that such behaviors are maintained by escape or avoidance (see Chapter 12). For situations in which problem behavior is exhibited in reaction to task difficulty (e.g., a bottle that will not open, a lace that will not tie, a toy that does not work properly, a pen that does not write), a symbol representing *help* may be used to request assistance.

The HELP symbol can be taught just like any other symbol within PECS, with the simple modification of having the communicative partner provide help rather than a tangible item or activity as the reinforcer. Similarly, for situations in which task demands are high, a symbol representing *break* can be taught in the same way, so that the student is able to request a short time away from the situation. Use of a *break* card implies that the child will return to the activity after a period of time rather than abandon it altogether. The basic strategies within the PECS protocol can be used to teach the appropriate use of the *break* card as well.

PECS AS AN
AUGMENTATIVE COMMUNICATION SYSTEM

Most interventionists recognize that a child who is not speaking can learn how to communicate using AAC strategies such as PECS or sign language. However, we believe that the use of AAC to teach speaking children more complex communication and language skills is largely unrecognized and underutilized. Several potential ways to use PECS with speaking children are described this section. Many of these were originally suggested in the PECS Manual (Frost & Bondy, 2002) based on our clinical experiences and await independent research verification.

Children Who Talk But Do Not Initiate

Communicative behavior involves two people: a communicator and a listener or receiver of the message. Children must learn to assume both roles. Some children with ASDs who are able to speak are quite adept at the listener or responder role and can answer questions such as *What do you want?* or *What is this?* However, many of these children do not learn to take the initiative in conversation; rather, they usually wait for others to approach them or to begin an interaction. This lack of spontaneity can lead to frustration on the part of the child and is often viewed negatively by the people with whom he or she interacts.

One strategy for teaching initiation is to have children use a symbol to begin an interaction. Within PECS, we advise using a second person to provide physical prompts that can be quickly faded rather than having the communicative partner both entice the interaction and provide prompts as well. Prompts that are paired with the interaction are more likely to lead to prompt dependency. In our experience, once children who can speak (but do not initiate) learn how to communicate spontaneously with PECS and put pictures together to make simple sentences, they almost always discontinue using pictures and instead use their speech to initiate interactions.

Children Who Have Echolalia

Some children may have a high degree of echolalia—that is, they can repeat words and phrases and may answer direct questions, but usually only after repeating the question. PECS has been used successfully with such children. We have observed them putting picture sentences together rather than repeating a communicative partner's question, then saying the answer out loud while exchanging the sentence. We have used this strategy for as little as a few weeks before noticing that many children learn when to use spoken words as a result. It appears that PECS gives these children another way to rehearse or to "buy time" before answering the question and thus circumvents their echolalic responding (for other examples, see Frost, 2003).

Children Whose Speech Is Unintelligible

Some children require more time than others to develop intelligible speech. They might have sound substitutions or distortions (i.e., artic- ulation disorders) or they might combine sounds into words inappro- priately using simplification strategies (i.e., phonological disorders). A subset of these children use unusual speech production patterns due to motoric difficulties, which make executing and coordinating the movements necessary for connected speech difficult (i.e., developmen- tal apraxia of speech). Some children with these difficulties might use gestures to augment their speech. However, many children with ASDs do not readily develop an effective gestural repertoire and thus are at risk for developing inappropriate behaviors when their spoken com- municative attempts are not understood.

Communication interventions for this group of children should include a combination of techniques directed at improving spoken communication and providing an effective and quickly learned means of communicating with an alternative modality. These children often learn quite quickly to interact with a variety of communicative part- ners using PECS; the children can then expand these interactions as they learn to combine pictures to formulate specific grammatical struc- tures. Often, these students gradually discontinue the use of PECS as they acquire more intelligible speech (Frost, Daly, & Bondy, 1997).

PECS RESEARCH REVIEW

We reported the first description of PECS and its general impact on a group of 85 preschoolers with ASDs within a public school program (Bondy & Frost, 1994). Of the 66 children who began using PECS prior to age 5 years and who used PECS for at least 1 year, 39 children were able to use speech as their sole communication modality, whereas 25 others used speech plus PECS. Of this mixed-modality group, the great majority ultimately relied on speech as their sole modality, but only after several additional years in the school program. A very small subset of children acquired some speech but not to the extent that it was their sole communicative modality; some of this group switched from PECS to speech-generating devices (SGDs) to accommodate their growing symbolic vocabulary needs. Five students acquired skills within PECS but did not develop speech; these children also displayed severe global developmental delays as well as ASDs.

The pace of publications regarding PECS has grown substantially in the past few years. Between the initial description in 1994 and the year 2000, only three additional publications described case or group implementation of PECS. However, from 2001–2004, there were 12 publications; since 2005, more than 18 additional studies have been added to this body of work. The fact that we were not the authors or designers of any of these studies demonstrates the robust appeal of PECS. Further evidence of the general positive impact of PECS is that 13 publications thus far have originated outside of the United States.

Of the 33 publications regarding PECS that were available when this chapter was written, 11 involved case studies, 12 involved small groups of 10 or fewer participants, and 10 involved groups of 10 or more. The original publication about PECS involved preschool children with ASDs who were under the age of 5 years when the system was introduced (Bondy & Frost, 1994). Of the other publications, 11 involved preschoolers, 24 involved children in elementary to high school (with several overlapping with preschoolers), and 3 involved adults (Chambers & Rehfeldt, 2003; Rehfeldt & Root, 2005; Stoner et al., 2006). For the studies wherein disabilities were specified, individuals with ASDs were the focus of 23 publications, whereas 7 studies involved individuals with global developmental disabilities (including Bock, Stoner, Beck, Hanley, & Prochnow, 2005; Chambers & Rehfeldt, 2003; Rehfeldt & Root, 2005; Stoner et al., 2006), including cerebral palsy (Almeida, Piza, & LaMonica, 2005), blindness (Lund & Troha, 2007), and deafness (Okalidou & Malandraki, 2007).

Across this age range and diversity of disability issues, PECS has been highly successful with regard to the development of functional communication skills. In a summary of research regarding PECS and SGDs, Lancioni et al. (2007) noted that, of the 173 individuals involved in PECS-related publications, there was substantial progress in all but three cases.

PECS and Reductions in Problem Behavior

In our description of PECS (Bondy & Frost, 1994), we noted broad improvements in speech development and concomitant improvements in problem behavior, which included global reductions in specific targets as well as reductions in key characteristics in autism (as measured by the Aberrant Behavior Checklist; Krug, Arick, & Almond, 1980). Since that time, six other research publications have also noted reductions in problem behavior targets (Anderson, Moore, & Bourne, 2007; Charlop-Christy, Carpenter, Le, LeBlanc, & Kelley, 2002; Frea, Arnold, & Vittimberga, 2001; Okalidou & Malandraki, 2007; Webb, Baker, & Bondy, 2005; Yokoyama, Naoi, & Yamamoto, 2006).

For the most part, these changes have been correlational, although a few studies have documented these changes empirically. For example, Charlop-Christy et al. (2002) noted a series of behavior targets (including tantrums, grabbing, out-of-seat behavior, and disruptive behaviors) for three children with ASDs in both academic and play settings. They noted an overall reduction of 70% of problem behaviors across behaviors and settings, with complete elimination of four targets following PECS training. In a 3-year long-term follow up report on one of these children, Kern, Gallagher, Starosta, Hickman, and George (2006) noted that teaching the child to use a *break* card within his PECS system was one component of an effective overall behavioral strategy.

PECS and Improvements in Play and Social Interaction Skills

A number of studies have examined correlations between PECS use and improvements in play and other social interaction skills. These include play during free time (Anderson et al., 2007), increased interactions with teachers (Carr & Felce, 2007), improved toy play and joint attention during free play situations (Charlop-Christy et al., 2002), improvements in social interactions with peers at school (Kravits, Kamps, & Kemmerer, 2002), improved social approach behaviors with parents at home (Okalidou & Malandraki, 2007), increased social approach and play behaviors among preschoolers (Schwartz, Garfinkle, & Bauer, 1998) and increased peer interactions during story time (Webb et al., 2005).

As an example, Carr and Felce (2007) found substantial improvements in spontaneous communication after only 15 hours of PECS training within a school setting. They also noted additional changes in the interaction patterns between students and their teachers, including an "increased responsiveness by adults and children to each other's communications and in a decreased tendency by adults to communicate with the children in a way that did not allow them sufficient opportunity to respond" (p. 732). Carr and Felce noted that aspects of Phase II within the PECS protocol appeared particularly effective in teaching children to be persistent communicators with a number of different partners. Of interest is their observation that, following PECS training, teachers decreased their preemptive communications to the children and increased the number of available opportunities for child initiations. They also noted that the children were more responsive to the teacher's communicative attempts.

PECS and Natural Speech Development

In our description of 66 preschoolers with ASDs who began to use PECS prior to age 5 years and used the system for more than 1 year, a total of 88% were able to use speech as either their sole strategy (59%) or in combination with PECS (29%; Bondy & Frost, 1994). For children who used PECS for less than 1 year, the proportion of children using speech was considerably lower. For a subset of seven preschoolers who developed speech as their sole communicative modality and whose mean age upon entry into the program was 3.5 years, the average time to their first spoken word was 5.4 months and the average time to the point when their spoken words matched the number of pictures they used was 11.3 months. At that time, they used a mean of 71.3 pictures to communicate.

The pattern of speech development for these children typically showed steady growth in the size of their picture vocabularies, followed by a period of gradual growth of speech, and then a period of rapid speech development coinciding with a gradual reduction of the use of pictures. Again, it should be pointed out that there was no experimental design used across these children; rather, these were descriptive outcomes for preschoolers who entered the Delaware Autism Program over a 5-year period.

Of the other publications on PECS, 11 have specifically addressed the issue of speech development (see Chapter 6 for more information on this topic). Of particular interest are some factors that relate to the specific aspects of the PECS protocol. Ganz and Simpson (2004) used a within-subjects design for three children with ASDs or other developmental disabilities, ages 3–7 years. All three children learned PECS through Phase IV (simple sentence structure) within 2 months and demonstrated substantial increases in speech production as well as the mean lengths of their spoken utterances—of which there was a dramatic increase once Phase IV was introduced. That is, once the sentence structure and the delayed-prompt strategy were introduced within PECS, an increase in speech use was noted for all three children. Tincani, Crozier, and Alazetta (2006) also noted this effect of Phase IV for one of two school-age children. Furthermore, they empirically demonstrated that for this child, the explicit reinforcement strategy built into Phase IV controlled the increase in vocalizations. That is, when reinforcement was withheld for vocalizing, speech output substantially decreased.

Carr and Felce (2006) provided further clarification on the impact of PECS on speech by noting an increase in speech production in 5 of 24 preschool children who were taught PECS only through Phase III (symbol discrimination). Taken together, it appears that there is a modest but reliable impact of PECS on speech production through Phase III but a more robust increase following the introduction of Phase IV.

Comparison of PECS and Other Communication Interventions

Recently, a few studies comparing the use of PECS to other AAC or communication interventions have appeared in the literature. These include comparison of PECS and manual signing, SGDs, and a prelinguistic communication intervention. We review this small body of research in this section.

PECS and Sign Language   Only two studies to date have compared the use of PECS to sign language. These comparisons have looked at rates of vocabulary acquisition and potential effects on speech production. Furthermore, these studies examined the impact of PECS only through Phase III—prior to the point in the protocol that is most noted for having an impact on speech. In one case study (Adkins & Axelrod, 2002), the authors noted greater improvements in functional communication with PECS than with manual signs. However, Tincani (2004) reported that one student developed a picture repertoire faster than a sign repertoire, whereas another student showed a reversed effect. In this study, the total number of signs and pictures was quite small in both cases.

PECS and Speech-Generating Devices   A few studies have also compared the use of PECS and SGDs. Bock et al. (2005), using an alternating treatment design for preschoolers with developmental delays, showed that the children acquired initiation skills with both PECS and SGDs and that some children showed preferences for one or the other. As noted earlier, Lancioni et al. (2007) reviewed 15 years of literature on PECS and SGD use, although very few of these studies involved direct comparisons. They noted that both PECS and SGDs can support functional communication and do not appear to interfere with the development of speech. One study included in Lancioni et al. (Son, Sigafoos, O'Reilly, & Lancioni, 2006) illustrates some of the difficulties in conducting comparison studies. In this publication, the authors compared SGD use with a strategy they referred to as "picture exchange." Properly, they did not refer to PECS in the study because their teaching strategy was radically different from the PECS protocol.

PECS and Responsive Education and Prelinguistic Milieu Teaching Yoder and Stone (2006a, 2006b) compared PECS training with an intervention approach called Responsive Education and Prelinguistic Milieu Teaching (RPMT). RPMT focuses on teaching parents how to play with and talk to their children in ways that should facilitate the development of language. In this study, preschool children were randomly assigned to two intervention groups: 19 in the PECS condition and 17 in RPMT. After 6 months of training, children in the PECS group demonstrated greater increases in the frequency of nonimitative words and the number of different nonimitative words produced compared to the children in the RPMT group. No information regarding child-specific patterns was provided. The authors also noted that, after a 6-month follow-up period, children who initially had no interest in objects showed an equivalent increase in word production as did the children in the PECS group. Further research is needed to clarify whether conditions prior to or within the follow-up period had an impact on the children involved in the study.

RESEARCH IMPLICATIONS

PECS was developed within a program serving children with ASDs, but it is becoming increasingly clear that it is not an "autism-specific" strategy. Over the past decade, there are increasing reports of effective PECS use by individuals with a variety of disabilities. It is hoped that these reports will expand, as will efforts to examine a broader range of ages for PECS users. Furthermore, although the reports of collateral changes with regard to decreases in problem behavior as well as increases in speech production and social approach behaviors are encouraging, more research is necessary to clarify these effects.

Another area for ongoing research involves separating PECS as a way to teach picture and symbol use from the effectiveness of specific teaching strategies that are built into the PECS protocol. For example, several studies have used one or more elements of the PECS protocol to teach the use of other AAC modalities (e.g., manual signing by Adkins & Axelrod, 2002, and Tincani, 2004; SGD use by Bock et al., 2005). These elements included using a two-person prompt strategy, starting the protocol with requesting but without a prerequisite array of discrimination skills, and promoting generalization before beginning discrimination training. Furthermore, several error-correction strategies that are described in the PECS protocol require independent research to support efficacy. In short, PECS may be effective with some individuals not simply because of the specific AAC modality involved but because of the effective teaching strategies that are built into the protocol. This issue has implications for AAC instruction in general and requires additional research.

Fidelity of PECS Implementation

A second edition of the PECS Manual was issued in 2002 (Frost & Bondy, 2002). The revision contained much more detailed information about strategies and instructional options, as well as a clearer specification of protocol fidelity and how it can be measured. We have also developed a PECS certification process (Frost & Sulzer-Azaroff, 2007) that helps to assure the quality with which people implement the phases within PECS. This process involves answering standard multiple-choice and short-essay questions to assess knowledge about PECS, but primarily relies on videotaped or live behavioral samples of the instructor implementing key strategies within PECS. Thus, those identified as being "Certified PECS Implementers" have demonstrated their understanding of the contents of the protocol, as well as their ability to implement specific teaching skills with PECS clients.

We believe that these standards should be maintained in research involving the PECS protocol to assure the quality of the implementation. Several published studies have included statements such as "the protocol provided within the PECS manual was followed," but do not provide specific information regarding implementation fidelity. A notable exception to this was offered by Yoder and Stone (2006a), who did measure fidelity to the PECS protocol using a rating scale that they developed. Hopefully, this issue will be addressed more consistently in future studies.

Assessing the Effectiveness of PECS

A related issue concerns how the success of PECS is assessed. For example, we believe that the primary aim of PECS is to teach functional communication, whereas a secondary effect is its impact on speech development. Thus, if a child successfully learns Phases I–VI of PECS and has a substantial vocabulary (i.e., 80 or more pictures) but does not acquire speech independent of PECS use, we would not view the situation as a failure—and certainly, the child did not fail at anything.

The acquisition of speech is a complex process that requires considerable time and opportunity for practice and use. Hart and Risley (1999) estimated that a typical 3-year-old child has heard 1.5 million utterances prior to learning to talk—an enormous expenditure of effort to acquire functional speech. Given this, it is unlikely that substantial changes in speech production (or understanding) will occur concurrent with PECS acquisition during the first year of use.

In light of this, we do not believe that PECS effectiveness is appropriately assessed using measures that are removed from those directly involved with functional communication. For example, Howlin, Gordon, Pasco, Wade, and Charman (2007) used a randomized clinical trial to assess the impact of PECS training on the performance of school-age children in the United Kingdom (mean age, 6.8 years). Appropriately, one of the outcome measures included the students' rate of communicative initiations; there was a substantial positive effect in this regard following PECS training. No other direct measures of PECS use were recorded (e.g., the number of pictures used, number of phases completed, the complexity of sentence structures produced). Rather, the children were tested after 5 months of PECS training with various standardized language tests, both receptive and productive, and no substantial improvements were noted. While it is important to look for such potential side effects of PECS, we hope that future research will continue to focus on direct measures of PECS use rather than on potential ancillary benefits.

CONCLUSION

We have described the protocol that has been used to teach the use of PECS. Over the past two decades, the effectiveness of PECS has been demonstrated by both its worldwide popularity and a growing body of ongoing research supporting its use. Clinical observations and research using both single-subject and small-group designs have demonstrated numerous positive side effects of PECS use, including promoting speech acquisition and complexity, social approach behaviors, and reductions in problem behaviors. PECS was developed for young children with ASDs but has since been shown to be effective with learners of any age who experience a variety of communication difficulties.

We hope that future research will continue to refine the basic teaching strategies within the standard PECS protocol and that a variety of efficient and effective strategies can be identified to help skills within each of the phases of PECS. We anticipate that research will continue to identify issues that relate to promoting secondary gains with regard to speech (or other AAC modalities), social interactions, and behavior management issues. Finally, we look forward to continued research that addresses how best to help professionals, paraprofessionals, and parents teach PECS to those who will most benefit from its use.

REFERENCES

Adkins, T., & Axelrod, S. (2002). Topography- versus selection-based responding: Comparison of mand acquisition in each modality. *The Behavior Analyst Today, 2,* 259–266.

Almeida, M., Piza, M., & LaMonica, D. (2005). Adaptações do sistema de comunicação por troca de figuras no contexto escolar [Adaptation of the Picture Exchange Communication System in a school context]. *Pró-Fono Revista de Atualização Científica, 17,* 233–240.

Anderson, A., Moore, D., & Bourne, T. (2007). Functional communication and other concomitant behavior changes following PECS training: A case study. *Behavior Change, 24,* 1–8.

Bock, S.J., Stoner, J.B., Beck, A.R., Hanley, L., & Prochnow, J. (2005). Increasing functional communication in non-speaking preschool children: Comparison of PECS and VOCA. *Education and Training in Developmental Disabilities, 40,* 264–278.

Bondy, A., & Frost, L. (1994). The Picture Exchange Communication System. *Focus on Autistic Behavior, 9,* 1–19.

Bondy, A., Tincani, M., & Frost, L. (2004). Multiply controlled verbal operants: An analysis and extension to the Picture Exchange Communication System. *The Behavior Analyst, 27,* 247–261.

Carr, D., & Felce, J. (2006). Increase in production of spoken words in some children with autism after PECS teaching to Phase III. *Journal of Autism and Developmental Disabilities, 37,* 780–787.

Carr, D., & Felce, J. (2007). The effects PECS teaching to Phase III on the communicative interactions between children with autism and their teachers. *Journal of Autism and Developmental Disabilities, 37,* 724–737.

Chambers, M., & Rehfeldt, R. (2003). Assessing the acquisition and generalization of two mand forms with adults with severe developmental disabilities. *Research in Developmental Disabilities, 24,* 265–280.

Charlop-Christy, M.H., Carpenter, M., Le, L., LeBlanc, L., & Kelley, K. (2002). Using the Picture Exchange Communication System (PECS) with children with autism: Assessment of PECS acquisition, speech, social-communicative behavior, and problem behaviors. *Journal of Applied Behavior Analysis, 35,* 213–231.

Dyer, K., Sulzer-Azaroff, B., & Bondy, A. (2006). *Teaching picture discrimination to children with autism: "Traditional match-to-sample" training vs. "naturalistic PECS" training.* Paper presented at the annual Association for Behavior Analysis convention, Atlanta, GA.

Frea, W., Arnold, C., & Vittimberga, G. (2001). A demonstration of the effects of augmentative communication on the extreme aggressive behavior of a child with autism within an integrated preschool setting. *Journal of Positive Behavior Intervention, 3,* 194–198.

Frost, L. (2003). Effective ways to use PECS with verbal children. *Autism/Asperger Digest, 31,* 24–25.

Frost, L., & Bondy, A. (2002). *Picture Exchange Communication System training manual* (2nd ed.). Newark, DE: Pyramid Education Products.

Frost, L., Daly, M., & Bondy, A. (1997). *Speech features with and without access to PECS for children with autism.* Paper presented at meeting of the New Jersey Center for Outreach and Services for the Autism Community, Inc. (COSAC), Long Beach, NJ.

Frost, L., & Sulzer-Azaroff, B. (2007). PECS certification. Retrieved June 4, 2008, from http://www.pecs.com/Certification.htm

Ganz, J., & Simpson, R. (2004). Effects on communicative requesting and speech development of the Picture Exchange Communication System in children with characteristics of autism. *Journal of Autism and Developmental Disabilities, 34,* 395–409.

Ganz, J.B., Cook, K.E., Corbin-Newsome, J., Bourgeois, B., & Flores, M. (2005). Variations on the use of a pictorial alternative communication system with a child with autism and developmental delays. *TEACHING Exceptional Children Plus, 1,* Article 3.

Hart, B., & Risley, T.R. (1999). *The social world of children learning to talk.* Baltimore: Paul H. Brookes Publishing Co.

Howlin, P., Gordon, R.K., Pasco, G., Wade, A., & Charman, T. (2007). The effectiveness of Picture Exchange Communication System (PECS) training for teachers of children with autism: A pragmatic, group randomised controlled trial. *Journal of Child Psychology and Psychiatry, 48,* 473–481.

Kern, L., Gallagher, P., Starosta, K., Hickman, W., & George, M. (2006). Longitudinal outcomes of functional behavioral assessment–based intervention. *Journal of Positive Behavior Interventions, 8,* 67–78.

Kravits, T.R., Kamps, D.M., & Kemmerer, K. (2002). Brief report: Increasing communication skills for an elementary-aged student with autism using the Picture Exchange Communication System. *Journal of Autism and Developmental Disorders, 32,* 225–230.

Krug, D.A., Arick, J.R., & Almond, P.J. (1980). Behavior checklist for identifying severely handicapped individuals with high levels of autistic behavior. *Journal of Child Psychology and Psychiatry, 21,* 221–229.

Lancioni, G., O'Reilly, M., Cuvo, A., Singh, N., Sigafoos, J., & Didden, R. (2007). PECS and VOCAs to enable students with developmental disabilities to make requests: An overview of the literature. *Research in Developmental Disabilities, 28,* 468–488.

Lund, S.K., & Troha, J.M. (2007). Teaching young people who are blind and have autism to make requests using a variation on the Picture Exchange Communication System with tactile symbols: A preliminary investigation. *Journal of Autism Developmental Disorders, 38,* 719–730.

Marckel, J.M., Neef, N.A., & Ferreri, S.J. (2006). A preliminary analysis of teaching improvisation with the Picture Exchange Communication System to children with autism. *Journal of Applied Behavior Analysis, 39,* 109–115.

Okalidou, A., & Malandraki, G. (2007). The application of PECS in children with autism and deafness: A case study. *Focus on Autism and Other Developmental Disabilities, 22,* 23–32.

O'Neill, R. (1990). Establishing verbal repertoires: Toward the application of general case analysis and programming. *The Analysis of Verbal Behavior, 8,* 113–126.

Peterson, S., Bondy, A., Glassberg, M., & Neef, N. (2002, May). *The relationship of match-to-sample to visual discrimination skills utilized within PECS.* Paper presented at the annual Association for Behavior Analysis convention, Toronto.

Rehfeldt, R., & Root, S. (2005). Establishing derived requesting skills in adults with severe developmental disabilities. *Journal of Applied Behavior Analysis, 38,* 101–105.

Schwartz, I.S., Garfinkle, A.N., & Bauer, J. (1998). Communicative outcomes for young children with disabilities. *Topics in Early Childhood Special Education, 18,* 144–159.

Skinner, B.F. (1957). *Verbal behavior.* Englewood Cliffs, NJ: Prentice Hall.

Son, S-H., Sigafoos, J., O'Reilly, M., & Lancioni, G.E. (2006). Comparing two types of augmentative and alternative communication systems for children with autism. *Pediatric Rehabilitation, 9,* 389–395.

Stoner, J., Beck, A., Bock, S., Hickey, K., Kosuwan, K., & Thompson, J. (2006). The effectiveness of the Picture Exchange Communication System with nonspeaking adults. *Remedial and Special Education, 27,* 154–165.

Tincani, M. (2004). Comparing the Picture Exchange Communication System and sign language training for children with autism. *Focus on Autism and Other Developmental Studies, 19,* 152–163.

Tincani, M., Crozier, S., & Alazetta, L. (2006). The Picture Exchange Communication System: Effects on manding and speech development for school-aged children with autism. *Education and Training in Developmental Disabilities, 41,* 177–184.

Webb, T., Baker, S., & Bondy, A. (2005). Picture Exchange Communication System. In L. Wankoff (Ed.), *Innovative methods in language intervention* (pp. 111–139). Austin, TX: PRO-ED.

Yoder, P., & Stone, W. (2006a). Randomized comparison of two communication interventions for preschoolers with autism spectrum disorders. *Journal of Consulting and Clinical Psychology, 74,* 426–435.

Yoder, P., & Stone, W. (2006b). Randomized comparison of the effect of two prelinguistic communication interventions on the acquisition of spoken communication in preschoolers with ASD. *Journal of Speech, Language, and Hearing Research, 49,* 698–711.

Yokoyama, K., Naoi, N., & Yamamoto, J. (2006). Teaching verbal behavior using the Picture Exchange Communication System (PECS) with children with autistic spectrum disorder. *Japanese Journal of Special Education, 43,* 485–503.

11

A Picture Is Worth a Thousand Words

Using Visual Supports for Augmented Input with Individuals with Autism Spectrum Disorders

PAT MIRENDA AND KENNETH E. BROWN

It is well established that most individuals with autism spectrum disorders (ASDs) are strong visual learners (Grandin, 1995; Hodgdon, 1995, 1996). In addition, the results of some research suggest a possible advantage of pictures over words in access to semantics for these individuals (Kamio & Toichi, 2000). Thus, use of the visual medium for instruction may facilitate the ability of individuals with ASDs to make sense of and provide order to the complex social world in which they live, work, go to school, and play (Quill, 1995a).

Visual supports are instructional aids that are designed to enhance comprehension and learning through the presentation of graphic media such as photographs, symbols, or line drawings. The underlying concept is the use of graphic media to facilitate learning and understanding. In so doing, visual support strategies appear to alleviate at least some of the confusion, anxiety, and frustration that many individuals with ASDs experience when they encounter unexpected events. Such strategies may also facilitate their abilities to understand social situations and cause-and-effect relationships, and to learn new skills and alternative behaviors. The end result is often a reduction in problem behaviors that are used to escape from confusing and/or novel situations.

Wood, Lasker, Siegel-Causey, Beukelman, and Ball (1998), in their presentation of an input framework for augmentative and alternative communication (AAC), referred to visual supports as strategies for "augmenting the message"—that is, assisting an individual to receive and make meaning of information more accurately and efficiently. A few studies have shown that individuals with ASDs appear to process and use information more efficiently when it is presented in visual plus verbal rather than verbal-only form (e.g., Brown & Mirenda, 2006; Forsey, Raining-Bird, & Bedrosian, 1995; Peterson, Bondy, Vincent, & Finnegan, 1995). For example, Vaughn and Horner (1995) described a situation that arose at mealtimes with Karl, a young man with ASD. Sometimes, food choices were presented to Karl verbally (i.e., "Do you want cereal or an egg for breakfast?"), while at other times they were presented both verbally and with their corresponding photographs. With verbal-only choices, Karl accepted around two-thirds of the foods he chose and exhibited frequent disruptive and aggressive behaviors. When both verbal and photographic choices were provided, Karl's acceptance rate for the foods he chose increased to 85%–100% and there were many days on which he exhibited no problem behaviors at mealtime. The authors hypothesized that the photographs clarified the choices that were available to Karl in a visual modality that he understood more accurately than verbal speech alone.

From Wood et al.'s (1998) perspective, visual supports can be understood as AAC input techniques that are designed to increase an individual's comprehension of verbally conveyed messages, environmental expectations, and/or upcoming events. Shane and Weiss-Kapp (2008) referred to these goals in the context of the Visual Immersion Program, a comprehensive visual language approach designed specifically for individuals with ASDs. The Visual Immersion Program is comprised of the visual expression mode, in which visual supports are used for expressive communication; the visual instructional mode, in which visual supports are used to enhance comprehension; and the visual organizational mode, in which visual supports are used to represent the organization of an activity, routine, or schedule. In this context, the visual supports examined in this chapter are examples of strategies in both the visual expression mode and the visual organizational mode.

This chapter begins with the most well-researched visual support strategies: between-activity schedules, within-activity schedules, and visually augmented Social Stories. Then, the more limited research is examined, including strategies for video-enhanced activity schedules, contingency maps, Power Cards, rule scripts and charts, and cognitive picture rehearsal scripts.

BETWEEN-ACTIVITY SCHEDULES

It has long been noted by researchers and clinicians that individuals with ASDs often excel in highly structured environments (Dawson &

Osterling, 1997; Quill, 1995a, 1995b). Early research focused on providing such individuals with a high degree of consistency and stability with regard to schedules, activities, staffing patterns, and physical space (Schopler, Brehm, Kinsgourne, & Reichler, 1971). Although this research concluded that positive behavior and learning outcomes could be achieved through a high degree of consistency (Olley, 1987), maintaining such consistency within real-world situations is extremely difficult for parents, teachers, and others to achieve. As a result, recent studies have attempted to uncover *why* individuals with ASDs seem to excel in highly structured environments (Flannery & Horner, 1994). This research has led to an understanding that predictability is an important feature of such environments; many persons with ASDs seem to prefer environments and activities that afford the ability to predict future events accurately (Flannery & O'Neill, 1995). Because family, school, and community life is often impossible to arrange consistently from day to day, strategies are needed to help individuals with ASDs better understand and predict their ever-changing routines and schedules.

Between-activity schedules are interventions that represent a sequence of planned activities using some type of symbol. They originally came from the work of Stillman and Battle (1984) and other practitioners supporting individuals with deafblindness who used objects arranged in a "calendar box" to represent various activities. Others have referred to them as schedule systems (Mesibov, Browder, & Kirkland, 2002) or timetables and diaries (Bloomberg, 1996). Regardless, these visual supports were developed to provide individuals with ASDs with increased predictability and understanding regarding upcoming events. Often, these individuals are verbally informed about upcoming events; however, they may not comprehend the language used to describe the event sequence. Visual aids in the form of between-activity schedules may be used to augment the verbal message and enhance understanding. Typically, object or picture symbols or written words are presented in sequential order to inform individuals of their scheduled activities across time. The entire schedule may be depicted with a problematic transition point and upcoming activity highlighted or single objects, pictures, or words may be presented to indicate the next activity in a sequence. Regardless, between-activity schedules ensure that salient cues related to transitions are provided. Figure 11.1 provides an example of a between-activity schedule using object symbols that was designed for a preschooler with ASD to inform her of upcoming activities in her preschool classroom.

There is a growing body of research supporting the use of between-activity schedules for individuals with ASDs. Table 11.1 presents

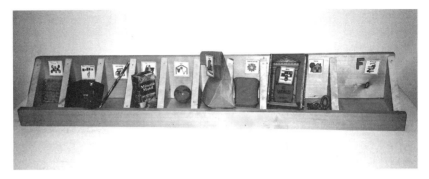

Figure 11.1.   Between-activity schedule using real-object symbols depicting the preschool routine for a young child with ASD.

examples of these studies, including information about the participants, settings, problem behaviors, schedule types and symbols used,
and outcome measures for each study. Only studies with experimental
designs that had the potential to demonstrate a functional relationship
between the independent and dependent variable(s) were included
in Table 11.1.

A study by Dooley, Wilczenski, and Torem (2001) exemplifies the
use of a between-activity schedule. The authors developed the
schedule for use in a special education preschool to reduce tantrums
and the aggressive behavior of a 3-year-old boy diagnosed with pervasive developmental disorder. The authors first performed a functional
behavior assessment, consistent with the procedures recommended by
O'Neill et al. (1997). Information obtained from the functional behavior
assessment indicated that the boy's behavior occurred in response to
teacher-prompted transitions; it was maintained by both escape from
the demands of the new activity and teacher attention that was provided during the tantrums. To better support the child through transitions, a picture-based schedule system was developed, in which
line-drawing symbols were presented sequentially on a schedule
board. The boy was taught to review the schedule at the beginning of
each day, and then proceed through his day by 1) removing the first
activity symbol, 2) locating and matching the activity symbol to the
actual activity, 3) engaging in the activity, 4) recognizing and
responding appropriately to the transition cue of flickering lights or
activity completion, 5) depositing the completed activity symbol in a
container, and 6) returning to the schedule to get the next activity symbol. Within 3 days of implementing the schedule system, the boy's
compliance with transition cues had dramatically increased and his
problem behavior had reduced to near-zero levels. These results
remained stable for the rest of the school year and generalized to both

Table 11.1. Between-activity schedule articles involving participants with ASDs

Authors	Participants (age in years, diagnosis)	Setting	Problem behavior/ context	Type of schedule and symbols used	Outcome
Arntzen, Gilde, & Pedersen (1998)	Girl (14, autism)	Classroom and kitchen of residential treatment center	Prompt dependent/ during leisure and self-care activities	Photographs in binder (plus within-activity schedule)	GSI on-task behavior
Bryan & Gast (2000)	Alan (8, autism); Tim (8, autism); Jack (8, autism); Jenny (8, autism)	Pull-out resource classroom	Off-task behavior/ language arts	Line drawings in small photo album, one photo per page	ISI in on-task and on-schedule behavior to near-100% levels
Clarke, Dunlap, & Vaughn (1999)	John (10, Asperger syndrome)	Family home, during morning routine	Disruptive, tantrum, off-task behavior/ during verbal demands	Pictures and word labels attached to a sheet (plus within-activity schedule)	ISR-PB to near-zero levels, ISR in time to complete routine, ISI in on-task behavior to near-100% levels, anecdotal GEN
Dettmer, Simpson, Myles, & Ganz (2000)	Jeff (32 months, autism, ID); Josh (5, PDD)	Community outings (Jeff); in-home 1:1 program (Josh)	Noncompliance/transitions between activities	Line drawing attached to sheet (plus timer and written within-activity schedule for Josh)	ISR-PB to 30% of baseline, anecdotal GEN
Dooley, Wilczenski, & Torem (2001)	Chris (3, PDD)	Half-day segregated special education preschool	Disruptive and aggressive behavior/classroom activity changes	Line drawings sequenced on one page	ISR-PB to near-zero levels; ISI in transition compliance, anecdotal FU and GEN to end of school year

(Continued)

307

Table 11.1. *(Continued)*

Authors	Participants (age in years, diagnosis)	Setting	Problem behavior/ context	Type of schedule and symbols used	Outcome
Flannery & Horner (1994)	Aviv (16, autism, mild cerebral palsy, ID)	Self-contained special education classroom	Property destruction and aggression/instructional sessions with unpredicted sequence and duration	Page with printed sequence of activities (plus timer)	ISR-PB to near-zero levels; anecdotal GEN
Krantz, MacDuff, & McClannahan (1993)	Jack (8, autism); Jay (6, autism); Mike (7, autism)	Family home	Disruptive and aggressive behavior/transitions (reported for only one participant)	Photograph schedule in three-ring binder, 1 photo per page	ISR-PB to near-zero levels, ISI in on-task behavior to near-90% levels
MacDuff, Krantz, & McClannahan (1993)	Mike (9, autism); Walter (9, autism); Steve (11, autism); Roy (14, autism)	Community-based teaching-family model group home	Off-task behavior/unstructured leisure and homework activities	Photograph schedule in three-ring binder, 1 photo per page	ISI-PB on-task and on-schedule behavior to near-100% levels
Morrison, Sainato, BenChaaban, & Endo (2002)	Ned (4, autism); Kelly (5, autism); Michael (3, autism); Janet (5, autism)	Integrated pre-school classroom	On-task behavior/chosen activities in four play areas of classroom	Photograph schedule on a clipboard, with matching photos on toy bins in classroom	ISI for on-task behavior with schedules only and when correspondence training added
Newman et al. (1995)	Scott (14, autism, ID); Peter (16, autism, ID); Alex (17, autism, ID)	After-school program in a public school	Prompt dependence/unattended activities	List of sequenced activities and time (plus timer)	GSI independent identification of transition to near-75% and 85% for Scott and Peter, variable improvement for Alex, 1-month FU

| Schmit, Alper, Raschke, & Ryndak (2000) | Alex (6, autism) | Segregated early childhood special education class | Disruptive and aggressive behavior/transitions and physical guidance | Photograph cueing of upcoming activity during transition | ISR-PB to near-zero levels for two environments, GSR-PB to near-zero levels for one environment |
| Watanabe & Sturmey (2003) | Mark (22, autism); Bob (40, autism); Nick (30, autism) | Adult services program | Off-task behavior/ structured tasks | Written schedule task schedule of participant's chosen activities | ISI for on-task behavior from 19%–41% in baseline to 59%–77% during FU |

Key: ASD, autism spectrum disorder; FU, follow-up; GEN, generalization of strategy and results to novel environment/situation; GSI, gradual and sustained increase; GSR-PB, gradual and sustained reduction in identified problem behavior; ISI, immediate and substantial increase; ISR-PB, immediate and substantial reduction in identified problem behavior; ID, intellectual disability.

the community and the boy's home following his family's implementation of the schedule system.

The positive results obtained by Dooley et al. (2001) are consistently demonstrated in the between-activity schedule studies presented in Table 11.1. Between-activity schedules have been effectively employed across a range of environments, including family homes, community settings, child-care settings, segregated classrooms, and integrated classrooms. These interventions have produced positive behavioral outcomes for children with ASDs across a range of ages, from toddlers (e.g., Dettmer, Simpson, Myles, & Ganz, 2000) to adolescents and adults (e.g., Newman et al., 1995; Watanabe & Sturmey, 2003). Children with ASDs appear to benefit from between-activity schedules regardless of their level of presumed cognitive ability.

Positive outcomes from the studies to date have included 1) increased ability to make independent transitions between activities and decreased prompt dependency; 2) increased on-task behavior and decreased off-task behavior; 3) increased transition compliance; 4) increased speed of task completion; and 5) decreased disruptive, aggressive behavior, stereotypic, and/or destructive behavior. Although this breadth of change is impressive, the speed and magnitude of change is even more so. Across the majority of studies, substantial behavioral changes were reported to be immediate, dramatic, and stable over time. It seems that, in many cases, between-activity schedules provided a means through which the researchers were able to enhance participants' understanding and ability to predict upcoming events and changes, while simultaneously alleviating the distress and problem behaviors associated with unpredictability and uncertainty.

WITHIN-ACTIVITY SCHEDULES

Within-activity schedules (also known as activity schedules; see McClannahan & Krantz, 1999) pictorially represent a sequence of steps within an activity or task. Although within-activity schedules are similar to between-activity schedules in form, they differ considerably in their function and focus. Between-activity schedules typically span several hours within a day and, as noted previously, are usually intended to enhance predictability and reduce problem behavior associated with changes or transitions from one activity to the next. In contrast, the focus of within-activity schedules is on *one* activity rather than several in a sequence. The goal of within-activity schedules is to increase an individual's ability to perform a single activity without assistance, by depicting the series of discrete steps or skills that are required in sequential order. The individual is taught to refer to the within-activity

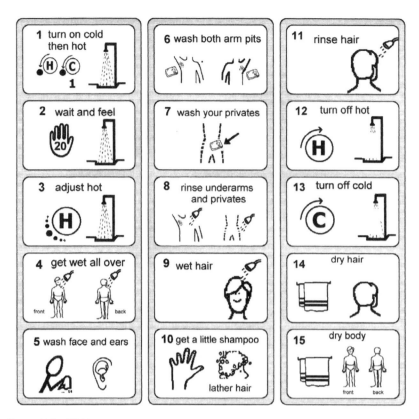

Figure 11.2. Within-activity schedule for showering that was created for an adolescent with ASD. (From Brown, K.E. [2004]. *Effectiveness of functional equivalence training plus contingency mapping with a child with autism.* Unpublished master's thesis. University of British Columbia, Vancouver; reprinted with permission.)

schedule after completing each step in the sequence and to use the pictures as reminders of the steps that follow. Figure 11.2 depicts a within-activity schedule for taking a shower that was created for an adolescent with autism (Brown, 2004). Prior to his use of the schedule, this young man required constant assistance in the form of verbal and physical prompting to complete the task. However, by using the within-activity schedule, he was able to shower independently.

The first published example of the use of a within-activity schedule for children with ASDs was provided by Hall, McClannahan, and Krantz (1995). Three children enrolled in integrated classrooms participated in this study; one was diagnosed with hyperactivity, one had fragile X syndrome, and the third child, Larry, was diagnosed with ASD. Larry was extremely dependent on adult assistance to complete tasks such as writing. He was therefore presented with the steps of a writing activity from initiation to completion in sequential order, using photographs in a small photo album. For example, the photos depicted 1) Larry engaged in the activity immediately prior to writing, 2) Larry going to his desk, 3) Larry taking out his pencil case, 4) Larry finding his pencil in the case, 5) Larry removing his pencil from the case, and so forth. Larry's classroom assistant was instructed in the use of the within-activity schedule and encouraged to resist using verbal and gestural prompts to guide Larry through the writing task. Results indicated that Larry's independence and successful completion of the tasks increased dramatically when the within-activity schedule was provided and both verbal and gestural prompts were removed.

As can be seen in Table 11.2, several additional studies have also shown within-activity schedules to be effective in promoting independence across a wide array of tasks, including meal preparation (Arntzen, Gilde, & Pedersen, 1998), occupational tasks (Copeland & Hughes, 2000), and educational tasks (Dettmer et al., 2000). This research demonstrates that such schedules may be effectively employed to teach individuals with ASDs to engage independently in a variety of new tasks. Only studies with experimental designs that had the potential to demonstrate a functional relationship between the independent and dependent variable(s) were included in Table 11.2.

VISUALLY AUGMENTED SOCIAL STORIES

The Social Story intervention is designed to encourage appropriate social behavior through the use of short narratives that describe social situations in terms of their relevant cues, other people's perspectives, and appropriate responses (Gray, 2000; Gray & Garand, 1993). The narratives are meant to be used proactively with individuals with ASDs to explain upcoming events, so that misinterpretations, confusion, and unpredictability do not lead to inappropriate behavior. Carol Gray, the developer of Social Stories, now adds pictures to written text, as exemplified in *My Social Stories Book* (Gray & White, 2002). Typically, pictures are used to facilitate participants' comprehension and retention of the information presented within the Social Story. Table 11.3 displays examples of visually supported Social Stories with experimental designs, along with participant information, settings, target behaviors, concurrent interventions, and outcomes.

A typical example of a Social Story intervention that used visual supports was reported by Lorimer, Simpson, Myles, and Ganz (2002). For this study, the participant was a 5-year-old boy with ASD who participated in an early childhood special education classroom in which he demonstrated tantrums (i.e., screaming, hitting, kicking, and throwing

Table 11.2. Within-activity schedule articles involving participants with ASDs

Authors	Participants (age in years, diagnosis)	Setting	Problem behavior/context	Type of schedule and symbols used	Outcome
Arntzen et al. (1998)	Girl (14, autism)	Classroom and kitchen of residential treatment center	Prompt dependent/during leisure and self-care activities	Photographs in binder (plus between-activity schedule)	GSI on-task behavior and near 100% independence in tasks
Clarke et al. (1999)	John (10, Asperger syndrome)	Family home, during dressing routine	Off-task, disruptive, tantrum behavior/during verbal prompts	Pictures and word labels attached to a sheet (plus between-activity schedule)	ISR-PB to near-zero levels, ISR in time to complete routine, ISI in on-task behavior to near-100% levels, anecdotal GEN
Copeland & Hughes (2000)	Charles (15, autism)	Employment training: faculty lounge	Prompt dependent/cleaning routine	Small photo album	ISI in independent completion of task (near 100%)
Dettmer et al. (2000)	Josh (5, PDD)	In-home one-to-one program	Noncompliance/transitions between activities	Line drawing and written words attached to sheet (plus timer and between-activity schedule)	ISR-PB to 30% of baseline, anecdotal GEN
Hall et al. (1995)	Larry (7, autism)	Regular integrated classroom	Off-task and prompt dependent/initiating writing	Small photo album	GSI in independent initiation of activities

(Continued)

Table 11.2. (Continued)

Authors	Participants (age in years, diagnosis)	Setting	Problem behavior/context	Type of schedule and symbols used	Outcome
Massey & Wheeler (2000)	Karl (4, autism)	Integrated preschool classroom	Task engagement; aggression, destructive behavior; tantrums, noncompliance, stereotypy/work, leisure, and lunch (GEN)	Color photos attached to a manila folder or cardboard	ISI in task engagement for work and lunch (GEN), with ISR-PB as well; GI in task engagement but slight increase in PB for leisure
Pierce & Schreibman (1994)	Jon (8, autism); Howard (9, autism); Robby (6, autism)	Clinic and home settings	On-task and inappropriate behavior/three daily living tasks per child	Small photo album for each task	ISI for on-task behavior to near-100% and GSR-PB; GEN to home for all but one task; good results at 2-month FU

Key: ASD, autism spectrum disorder; FU, follow-up; GEN, generalization of strategy and results to novel environment/situation; GSI, gradual and sustained increase; GSR-PB, gradual and sustained reduction in identified problem behavior; ISI, immediate and substantial increase; ISR-PB, immediate (within 3 sessions/days) and substantial reduction in identified problem behavior.

objects). Lorimer and colleagues first conducted a functional behavior assessment using the Motivation Assessment Scale (Durand & Crimmins, 1992). Data from the Motivation Assessment Scale suggested that the boy's problem behavior served to gain attention and tangible reinforcement; direct observations confirmed this assessment. In addition, the observations suggested that the boy consistently attempted to communicate his wants and needs prior to engaging in problem behaviors through ineffective and somewhat inappropriate verbalizations (e.g., he would repeatedly yell, "Stop talking!" "Listen to me!" or "You are too loud!").

Following the functional behavior assessment, the authors developed a Social Story intervention designed to teach the boy to raise his hand or say "Excuse me" to gain the attention of an adult, and then wait his turn to talk. His Social Story also contained several suggestions of activities he could do if he had to wait, including watching a video, listening to an audio book, looking at a book, or playing a game. Because the boy was a pre-reader, line drawings were paired with the written text and the Social Story was read to him. Figure 11.3 depicts the boy's visually augmented Social Story.

An A-B-A-B design was used to evaluate the success of the intervention. Immediately following implementation of the Social Story, the boy's inappropriate verbalizations reduced dramatically and his tantrums reduced to near-zero levels. This effect was repeated after the second baseline condition. The authors therefore concluded that the visually augmented Social Story was effective in reducing both the pre-tantrum and tantrum behavior.

Various symbol sets have been employed with Social Stories, including line drawings, photographs, and full-motion videotapes. In addition, it appears that visually augmented Social Stories can be used to remediate a variety of behaviors across a range of situations. The majority of studies in Table 11.3 reported significant reductions in problem behavior and/or increases in appropriate behavior. Nonetheless, several other reviews of the Social Story research have raised concerns about the methodological rigor of many of the existing studies and have called for more focused analyses of both the experimental and practical significance of changes that result from the application of this intervention (Ali & Frederickson, 2006; Sansosti, Powell-Smith, & Kincaid, 2004; Rust & Smith, 2006).

VISUAL SUPPORTS WITH A LIMITED RESEARCH BASE

Although within-activity schedules, between-activity schedules, and visually augmented Social Stories comprise the most well-researched

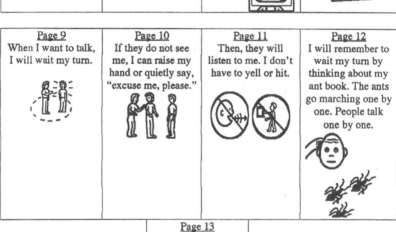

Page 1 Adults like to talk.	Page 2 Sometimes they talk to each other.	Page 3 Sometimes they talk to my brother.	Page 4 Sometimes they talk on the phone.
Page 5 Sometimes they talk to me.	Page 6 When adults are talking to someone else, I can probably **?**	Page 7 watch a video, listen to a book tape	Page 8 look at a book, or play a quiet game.

Page 9 When I want to talk, I will wait my turn.	Page 10 If they do not see me, I can raise my hand or quietly say, "excuse me, please."	Page 11 Then, they will listen to me. I don't have to yell or hit.	Page 12 I will remember to wait my turn by thinking about my ant book. The ants go marching one by one. People talk one by one.

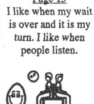

Page 13
I like when my wait
is over and it is my
turn. I like when
people listen.

Figure 11.3. "Talking with Adults" Social Story. (From Lorimer, P.A., Simpson, R.L., Myles, B.S., & Ganz J.B. [2002]. The use of Social Stories as a preventative behavioral intervention in a home setting with a child with autism. *Journal of Positive Behavior Interventions, 4,* 56; reprinted with permission.)

Table 11.3. Visually augmented social story articles involving participants with ASDs

Authors	Participants (age in years, diagnosis)	Setting	Target behavior(s)/context(s)	Concurrent interventions	Symbol set	Outcome
Agosta, Graetz, Mastropieri, & Scruggs (2004)	Robert (6, autism)	Self-contained classroom	Screaming, yelling, crying, humming/ group circle time activity	Tangible reinforcement system for quiet sitting	Text and PCS	Marginal decrease in problem behavior and slight increase in quiet sitting
Barry & Burlew (2004)	Holly (7, autism); Aaron (8, autism)	Self-contained special education classroom	Appropriate play skills, independent choice making, sharing and talking to peers/learning centers in classroom	Teacher prompts, corrective feedback, and reinforcement of target behaviors	Text read to each student, with photographs	GSI in choice making for both children; GI for appropriate play for Holly, less increase for Aaron
Crozier & Tincani (2007)	Thomas (3, autism); Daniel (3, autism); James (5, autism)	Integrated preschool classrooms	Sitting appropriately/circle time (Thomas); talking to peers/snack time (Daniel); appropriate peer play and hitting, grabbing, yelling, pushing/block center (James)	Comprehension questions asked after each story reading; prompts to talk to peers added for Daniel after session 10	Text read to participants with color symbols	ISI in appropriate sitting and play for Thomas and James; ISR-PB in grabbing, and so forth, for James; ISI in talking to peers when prompts added for Daniel; good FU at 2 and 3 weeks for Thomas only

(Continued)

Table 11.3. *(Continued)*

Authors	Participants (age in years, diagnosis)	Setting	Target behavior(s)/ context(s)	Concurrent interventions	Symbol set	Outcome
Hagiwara & Myles (1999)	Participant 1 (7, autism); participant 2 (9, autism); participant 3 (7, autism)	General education classroom and resource room	Noncompliance with hand washing/ before snack and meal; off-task behavior/during academic activity in resource room or integrated classroom	Task analysis of hand washing (during intervention)	Computer presentation of story with text, photos, video, and audio narration	Marginal increase in hand washing and on-task behavior
Kuoch & Mirenda (2003)	Andrew (3, autism); Henry (5, autism); Neil (6, PDD-NOS)	Home (Andrew), summer pre-school (Henry), summer school (Neil)	Aggression, crying, yelling/when asked to share toy (Andrew); inappropriate vocalizations, regurgitation, touching genitals/ during meal times (Henry); cheating, inappropriate and negative comments/ when playing games with peers (Neil)	No other intervention	Text and PCS or cartoon pictures	ISR-PB to near-zero levels for Henry and Neil; ISR-PB for Andrew
Kuttler, Myles, & Carlson (1998)	Jon (12, autism, fragile X, and intermittent explosive disorder)	Segregated class-room	Precursors to tantrum (inappropriate vocalizations and dropping to floor/in class during unexpected transitions, wait time, and free time	Token reinforcement	Text read to participant and PCS	ISR to near-zero levels across environments

Study	Participants	Setting	Target behavior	Other intervention	Social Story format	Outcome
Lorimer et al. (2002)	Gregg (5, autism)	Self-contained special education classroom	Pretantrum interruptions and tantrum/ when preferred activity not scheduled and when preferred adult attending to others	Mini-schedule, timer and emotion worksheet (during both baseline and intervention)	Text read to participant with PCS	ISR-PB to near-zero levels
Quilty (2007)	Ben (6, autism); Sarah (10, autism); Adam (10, autism)	Autism resource room (Ben, Sarah); general education classrooms (Adam)	Repetitive requests to go home/seatwork (Ben); aggression/ computer time (Sarah); "silly" behaviors (e.g., laughing, falling to floor, tickling)/gym, art, music (Adam)	No other interventions reported	Text and photographs	GSR-PB; maintained for all at 6-week FU and for Ben and Sarah at 9-week FU
Reynhout & Carter (2007)	Adam (8, autism)	Self-contained special education classroom	Tapping hands on any surface/reading activity	Teacher verbal prompts to look at the story	Text and photographs	Slight reduction in problem behavior from 63% to 41% of intervals
Thiemann & Goldstein (2001)	Greg (7, autism); John (8, autism); Casey (6, autism); Ivan (12, autism)	Integrated small-group room in library	Impaired communication skills/in small-group training session with peers	Visual cuing, video feedback	Text and PCS or photographs	ISI communication skills taught, maintenance generally demonstrated; minimal generalization to new environment

Key: ASD, autism spectrum disorder; PCS, Picture Communication Symbol; FU, follow-up; GSI, gradual sustained increase; GSR-PB, gradual sustained reduction in identified problem behavior; ISI, immediate substantial increase; ISR-PB, immediate (within 3 sessions/days) substantial reduction in identified problem behavior; PDD-NOS, pervasive developmental disorder-not otherwise specified.

visual support strategies for children with ASDs, a number of other strategies also exist. These strategies include video-enhanced activity schedules, Power Cards, contingency maps, rule scripts/charts, and cognitive picture rehearsal scripts.

Video-Enhanced Activity Schedules

Stromer, Kimball, Kinney, and Taylor (2006) noted the "natural goodness of fit between activity schedules and computers, because the latter can pair static visual support with additional instructional stimuli such as audio and video recordings" (p. 14). Such video-enhanced activity schedules have received considerable research attention over the past few years with participants with ASDs. Using Microsoft PowerPoint (Rehfeldt, Kinney, Root, & Stromer, 2004), video-enhanced activity schedules combine the pictorial aspects of within-activity schedules with embedded video clips depicting someone performing selected steps of the target routine.

Although none of the video-enhanced activity schedule studies to date have involved individuals who use AAC to communicate, the intervention does fit within the framework of augmented input (Wood et al., 1998) in that video-enhanced activity schedules enhance the meaning, salience, and/or comprehension of instruction through the use of graphic media. Figure 11.4 depicts a video-enhanced activity schedule designed for a 6-year-old girl with ASD to teach her independent play (listening to a book on tape), sociodramatic play (engaging in dialogue with puppets), and peer play skills (asking a peer to play Ring Around the Rosy) in her private day-school classroom (Stromer et al., 2006).

Another video-enhanced activity schedule application was described by Dauphin, Kinney, and Stromer (2004) with a 3-year-old boy with ASD who was learning to engage in sociodramatic play. His within-activity video-enhanced activity schedule consisted of photos and video models illustrating toys with which to play, how to play with each of them, and what to say about them. Individual PowerPoint slides were constructed to depict each step of the toy play routine, with "cue-to-play" slides inserted after each instructional sequence to provide the boy with opportunities to play with each toy as depicted. After 10 practice sessions, the boy played with each of the target toys and imitated the target phrases with 100% accuracy; he also demonstrated a high degree of generalization to six novel toys and phrases. Subsequently, the child was able to transfer learning to a conventional pictorial schedule using only photographs of the toy play routine. Video-enhanced activity schedules have also been used effectively

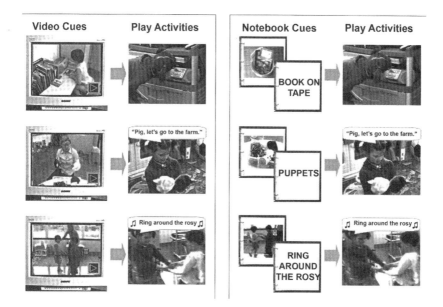

Figure 11.4. Segments of a video-enhanced activity schedule with video and photographic cues for (a) listening to a book on tape, (b) playing with puppets, and (c) playing Ring Around the Rosy. The photos in the right-hand column show the child with ASD engaged in the scheduled activities. (From Stromer, R., Kimball, J., Kinney, E., & Taylor, B. [2006]. Activity schedules, computer technology, and teaching children with autism spectrum disorders. *Focus on Autism and Other Developmental Disabilities, 21,* 18; reprinted with permission of Sage Publications.)

with children with ASDs to teach peer play initiation skills (Kimball, Kinney, Taylor, & Stromer, 2004); independent schedule following (Kalaigian, Kinney, Taylor, Stromer, & Spinnato, 2002); generative spelling skills (Kinney, Vedora, & Stromer, 2003); and basic counting skills (Vedora, Bergstrom, Kinney, & Stromer, 2001).

Power Card Strategy

The Power Card Strategy is "a visually based strategy used to connect an appropriate behavior or social skill to an individual's special interest" (Keeling, Myles, Gagnon, & Simpson, 2003, p. 104). The strategy consists of a personalized script that is read to the individual prior to an event that is problematic and that describes 1) the individual's hero or special interest model (e.g., Homer Simpson, dinosaurs) with relevant pictures or other graphics, 2) the problem behavior or situation, 3) the hero/model attempting a solution to the problem behavior or situation using a 3–5 step strategy that results in a successful outcome, and (d) a recommendation that the individual try to use the same strategy that was used successfully by the hero/model (Gagnon, 2001).

In the only published study to date, Keeling et al. (2003) used a multiple-baseline design to assess the use of the Power Card Strategy with a 10-year-old girl with ASDs who demonstrated poor sportsmanship behaviors (i.e., whining and screaming) when she lost a game or academic contest at school. The girl was fascinated with the Powerpuff Girls. Therefore, she was provided with a 3-inch by 5-inch power card that had a picture of the Powerpuff Girls on one side and a simple story describing how they behave when they win or lose a game or contest on the other (e.g., "The Powerpuff Girls want everyone to have fun playing games… If you win a game you can: smile, give a high five, or say *Yay!* If you lose a game, you can: take a deep breath, say *Good job!* to your friend, or say *Maybe next time*," [p. 106]). The card was accompanied by a brief script that the girl read prior to each game session, as well as a scorecard on which she monitored the players and who won or lost each game. Results indicated that the girl's whining and screaming were eliminated across three sequential activities following introduction of the Power Card Strategy. While the relative contribution of the pictorial depiction of Nancy's special interest model and the script were not assessed, this appears to be a visual support strategy that holds promise, at least for some individuals with ASDs and problem behavior.

Contingency Maps

Contingency maps are graphic (i.e., pictorial) representations of environment–behavior–consequence relationships (Brown, 2004; Brown & Miranda, 2006). The aim of a contingency map is to make the contingencies that govern both inappropriate (i.e., problem) and appropriate (i.e., alternative) behavior transparent to the learner by graphically depicting both current and alternative antecedent–behavior–consequence pathways. As such, contingency maps represent all the following components, as well as the relationships between them: 1) the common antecedent that precedes both the problem and the alternative behavior, 2) depictions of both the problem and alternative behaviors, 3) the functional reinforcer that will be provided contingent on alternative behavior(s), and 4) the consequence that will be provided contingent on problem behavior(s).

Brown (2004) described a clinical example of the use of a contingency map with a 5-year-old boy with ASD who attended kindergarten in his small suburban school. Although the boy's verbal skills were beginning to emerge, his primary mode of communication was through gestures and problem behaviors such as tantrums (i.e., screaming, crying, hitting, and running away). His tantrum behavior was most problematic at school; it often resulted in the boy being removed from class and placed in a time-out chair for a short period of time.

A functional behavior assessment (O'Neill et al., 1997) revealed that the boy's tantrums occurred primarily in response to specific types of noises—including crying children, sirens, loud motorcycles, and loud kitchen appliances—and that they served the function of allowing him to escape from the noise. Following the assessment, the boy's support team agreed to teach him that, when he was confronted with an aversive noise, he should cover his ears and point to the closest door to ask to leave the environment. Unfortunately, although the support plan appeared to be technically sound and was vigorously supported by the boy's team, this intervention failed to produce meaningful change. The boy continued to engage in tantrums whenever he encountered specific types of noise.

Because many members of the child's team believed him to be a strong visual learner, a decision was made to depict the antecedent–behavior–consequence contingencies of his support plan using a contingency map, as shown in Figure 11.5. Using the pictures on the contingency map, the boy's educational assistant explained to him that, if he heard a loud noise, he should put his hands over his ears and ask to leave by pointing to the door. She also explained that if he asked to leave, he would be allowed to move to a quiet place. On the other hand, she told him that if he encountered loud noise and had a tantrum, he would no longer be removed to get away from the noise. The contingency map

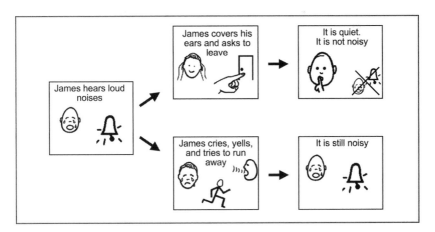

Figure 11.5. Contingency map to explain the contingencies for the alternative behaviors (covering ears and pointing to the door) and problem behaviors (crying, yelling, running away). (From Brown, K.E. [2004]. *Effectiveness of functional equivalence training plus contingency mapping with a child with autism.* Unpublished master's thesis. University of British Columbia, Vancouver; adapted with permission.)

was presented to the boy throughout the day before every major transition at school, with a brief explanation. Within a few days, his problem behavior was reduced to near-zero levels and he began to place his hands over his ears and gesture to leave without prompting. It seemed that the contingency map helped the boy to learn the new behavior–environment contingency and to understand the advantage of engaging in the alternative behaviors of covering his ears and pointing.

In a subsequent investigation, Brown and Mirenda (2006) provided an empirical demonstration of the effectiveness of contingency maps with a 13-year-old boy with ASD and extreme prompt dependency at school. When the boy completed an assigned task, he never informed the teacher that he had done so; thus, he often sat unoccupied for long periods of time until someone noticed that he had finished. He never engaged in the alternative behavior of showing the teacher his completed work when he was provided with verbal information about his problem behavior, the desired alternative, and the respective consequences (e.g., "If you finish your work and don't bring it to your teacher, you will not get a treat [i.e., his choice of a preferred snack item]. If you finish your work and show it to your teacher, you will get a treat."). However, when the same verbal information was paired with pictorial depictions of the contingencies, the boy immediately began to engage in the alternative behavior of showing his work to the teacher, across three classroom routines. The authors suggested that "[c]ontingency mapping adds a new alternative to the existing repertoire of visual support strategies in the form of an intervention that can be used to teach individuals why and under what conditions they should engage in an alternative replacement behavior" (p. 161).

Rule Scripts/Charts and Cognitive Picture Rehearsal

A visual support strategy that is similar to a contingency map has been referred to as a rule script (Mirenda, MacGregor, & Kelly-Keough, 2002) or rule chart (Hodgdon, 1995). Rule scripts depict problem situations and their associated social rules; they may be used to rehearse, clarify, prompt, and review rules during target activities. Mirenda et al. (2002) provided an clinical example of twin girls with pervasive developmental disorders and profound deafness who were provided with a simple pictorial script that informed them of the rules for watching television in the morning at home (i.e., TV was not allowed during school mornings, but was allowed during weekend mornings). Anecdotally, Mirenda et al. reported that within 2 weeks of implementing the rule script, the twins' tantrums that were associated with being denied access to television on school mornings were reduced to near-zero levels.

Hodgdon (1995, 1999) offered a number of additional clinical examples and postulated that the power of rule scripts to promote behavior change is related to 1) the authority many children appear to grant visual aids, 2) the ability of rule scripts to clarify the behavioral expectations held by adults, and 3) the fact that visual depictions of events may serve to increase consistency both within and between caregivers. Additional research is needed to establish the effectiveness of rule scripts empirically and to clarify the factors that may enhance their effectiveness.

A final visual support strategy is cognitive picture rehearsal, an "instructional strategy that uses repeated practice of a sequence of behaviors by presenting the sequence to the child in the form of pictures and an accompanying script" (Groden & LeVasseur, 1995, p. 288). Cognitive picture rehearsal is an imagery-based procedure that is used in conjunction with progressive relaxation training (Cautela & Groden, 1978) and is based on the notion that covert events, such as imagining, follow the same behavioral laws as observable behaviors (Cautela, 1979). Thus, the manipulation of imagined events that follow imagined actions can be used to change both overt and covert behavior. Groden and LeVasseur (1995) proposed that pictures could be used to facilitate the imagery process and referred to this procedure as *cognitive picture rehearsal*.

Similar to contingency mapping, cognitive picture rehearsal requires the sequential presentation of photographs or line drawings depicting antecedents, alternative behavior(s), and positive consequences related to a problem behavior. However, cognitive picture rehearsal differs significantly from contingency mapping in that no actual consequences are manipulated in the real world; also, cognitive picture rehearsal usually does not include depictions of either the problem behavior or its consequences. Figure 11.6 depicts a cognitive picture rehearsal script for a youngster who became upset when he made an error on a class assignment (Groden & LeVasseur, 1995). The script was designed to teach him a coping statement that he could use when he became upset and incorporated the use of a relaxation procedure the child was learning to use to reduce stress.

Despite the lack of empirical evidence supporting this technique, the anecdotal evidence provided by its authors (Cautela & Kearney, 1993; Groden & LeVasseur, 1995) and the existence of empirical support for covert conditioning with other populations (Mirenda, 1986) suggest that it may be useful as a visual support strategy under some circumstances. Again, research is needed to examine its effectiveness and clarify the circumstances in which it might be appropriate.

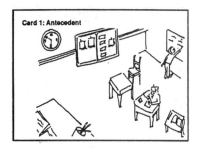

You're at your desk working on addition.

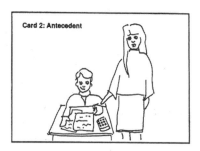

The teacher looks at your paper and says, "Tom, check the last problem. That's not the right answer."

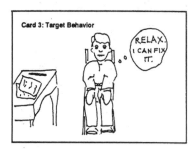

You take a deep breath, relax your arms. You breathe out slowly and say, "No big deal, I can fix it."

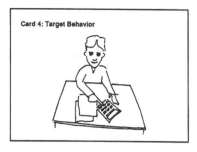

You use your calculator and do the problem again.

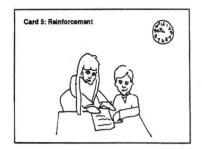

Now you have the right answer; you feel good about that. You tell the teacher.

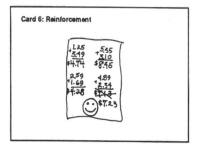

She smiles and puts a sticker on your paper. You're happy. You can't wait to show Mom when you get home today.

Figure 11.6. Cognitive picture rehearsal script designed for a child who became upset when he made a mistake in class. (From QUILL. Teaching Children with Autism, IE; © 1996 Delmar Learning, a part of Cengage Learning, Inc. Reproduced by permission. www.cengage.com/permissions)

SUMMARY AND RESEARCH IMPLICATIONS

Frequently, visual support strategies are used with individuals with ASDs who engage in problem behavior of one type or another. Thus, the likelihood of obtaining a positive outcome with the use of visual supports is greatly enhanced by first conducting a functional behavior assessment (Bopp, Brown, & Mirenda, 2004). In addition to identifying the function and context of problem behavior, functional behavior assessment can help to establish the type of visual support that is needed. For example, individuals who require high levels of predictability may benefit from between-activity schedules that enable them to predict upcoming events and then transition successfully from one activity/context to the next. Those who struggle with independent performance may require step-by-step within-activity schedules that enable them to complete specific tasks that are currently associated with problem behaviors. Individuals with poor understanding of social events and expectations may benefit from visually augmented Social Stories that employ a specific style and format to describe a situation, skill, or concept in terms of relevant social cues, other peoples' perspectives, and appropriate behavior responses.

When teaching new social or academic skills is the main concern, video-enhanced activity schedules may be appropriate. Individuals with special interests may be motivated to engage in appropriate behavior through the use of Power Cards, whereas contingency maps appear to be especially useful as an adjunct to teaching alternative behaviors (including those that are communicative in nature) to replace problem behavior. Finally, rule scripts/charts may be used to clarify the social rules that are associated with specific contexts and cognitive picture rehearsal can be used in conjunction with imagery and relaxation techniques to teach self-control and self-management skills.

Despite the availability of numerous types of visual supports for individuals with ASDs, little is known about how to match specific learner characteristics to specific strategies. In fact, clinical decisions about the use of visual supports often appear to be made arbitrarily. For example, no information was provided in any of the studies summarized in Tables 11.1–11.3 about how the researchers selected the type of symbol used in the intervention (e.g., object, photograph, line drawing, written words). This implies that a systematic symbol assessment procedure was not used to make this determination, despite the fact that this is a common practice among AAC clinicians (Beukelman & Mirenda, 2005). Similarly, little information is available about the language comprehension or literacy requirements of strategies such as Social Stories and Power Cards, or about the extent to which the addition of pictures to these interventions actually enhances their effectiveness. Research that seeks to explore how to use visual support strategies most effectively with individuals with specific skill profiles is needed to clarify issues such as these.

REFERENCES

Agosta, E., Graetz, J., Mastropieri, M., & Scruggs, T. (2004). Teacher–researcher partnerships to improve social behavior through Social Stories. *Intervention in School and Clinic, 39,* 276–287.

Ali, S., & Frederickson, N. (2006). Investigating the evidence base of Social Stories. *Educational Psychology in Practice, 22,* 355–377.

Arntzen, E., Gilde, K., & Pedersen, E. (1998). Generalized schedule following in a youth with autism. *Scandinavian Journal of Behavior Therapy, 27,* 135–141.

Barry, L., & Burlew, S. (2004). Using Social Stories to teach choice and play skills to children with autism. *Focus on Autism and Other Developmental Disabilities, 19,* 45–51.

Beukelman, D.R., & Mirenda, P. (2005). *Augmentative and alternative communication: Supporting children and adults with complex communication needs* (3rd ed.). Baltimore: Paul H. Brookes Publishing Co.

Bloomberg, K. (1996). *PrAACtically speaking information and resource booklet.* Melbourne, Victoria, Australia: Yooralla Society of Victoria, Functional Communication Outreach Service.

Bopp, K., Brown, K., & Mirenda, P. (2004). Speech-language pathologists' roles in the delivery of positive behavior support for individuals with developmental disabilities. *American Journal of Speech-Language Pathology, 13,* 5–19.

Brown, K.E. (2004). *Effectiveness of functional equivalence training plus contingency mapping with a child with autism.* Unpublished master's thesis. University of British Columbia, Vancouver.

Brown, K., & Mirenda, P. (2006). Contingency mapping: A novel visual support strategy as an adjunct to functional equivalence training. *Journal of Positive Behavior Interventions, 8,* 155–164.

Bryan, L.C., & Gast, D.L. (2000). Teaching on-task and on-schedule behaviors to high-functioning children with autism via picture activity schedules. *Journal of Autism and Developmental Disorders, 30,* 553–567.

Cautela, J.R. (1979). Covert conditioning: Assumptions and procedures. In D. Upper & J.R. Cautela (Eds.), *Covert conditioning* (pp. 3–16). New York: Pergamon.

Cautela, J., & Groden, J. (1978). *Relaxation: A comprehensive manual for adults, children, and children with special needs.* Champaign, IL: Research Press.

Cautela, J.R., & Kearney, A.J. (1993). *The covert conditioning casebook.* Pacific Grove, CA: Brooks/Cole.

Clarke, S., Dunlap, G., & Vaughn, B. (1999). Family-centered, assessment-based intervention to improve behavior during an early morning routine. *Journal of Positive Behavior Interventions, 1,* 235–241.

Copeland, S.R., & Hughes, C. (2000). Acquisition of a picture prompt strategy to increase independent performance. *Education and Training in Mental Retardation and Developmental Disabilities, 35,* 294–305.

Crozier, S., & Tincani, M. (2007). Effects of Social Stories on prosocial behavior of preschool children with autism spectrum disorders. *Journal of Autism and Developmental Disorders, 27,* 1803–1814.

Dauphin, M., Kinney, E., & Stromer, R. (2004). Using video-enhanced activity schedules and matrix training to teach sociodramatic play to a child with autism. *Journal of Positive Behavior Interventions, 6,* 238–250.

Dawson, G., & Osterling, J. (1997). Early intervention in autism. In M.J. Guralnick (Ed.), *The effectiveness of early intervention* (pp. 307–326). Baltimore: Paul H. Brookes Publishing Co.

Dettmer, S., Simpson, R.L., Myles, B.S., & Ganz, J.B. (2000). The use of visual supports to facilitate transitions of students with autism. *Focus on Autism and Other Developmental Disabilities, 15,* 163–169.

Dooley, P., Wilczenski, F.L., & Torem, C. (2001). Using an activity schedule to smooth school transitions. *Journal of Positive Behavior Interventions, 3,* 57–61.

Durand, V.M., & Crimmins D.B. (1992). *The Motivation Assessment Scale (MAS) administration guide.* Topeka, KS: Monaco & Associates.

Flannery, K.B., & Horner, R.H. (1994). The relationship between predictability and problem behavior for students with severe disabilities. *Journal of Behavior Education, 4,* 157–176.

Flannery, K.B., & O'Neill, R.E. (1995). Including predictability in functional assessment and individual program development. *Education and Treatment of Children, 18,* 499–502.

Forsey, J., Raining-Bird, K., & Bedrosian, J. (1996). The effects of typed and spoken modality combinations on the language performance of adults with autism. *Journal of Autism and Developmental Disorders, 26,* 643–649.

Gagnon, E. (2001). *Power Cards: Using special interests to motivate children and youth with Asperger syndrome and autism.* Shawnee Mission, KS: Autism Asperger Publishing Company.

Grandin, T. (1995). The learning style of people with autism: An autobiography. In K.A. Quill (Ed.), *Teaching children with autism: Strategies to enhance communication and socialization* (pp. 33–52). New York: Delmar.

Gray, C.A. (2000). *Writing Social Stories with Carol Gray* [videotape and workbook]. Arlington, TX: Future Horizons.

Gray, C.A., & Garand, J.D. (1993). Social Stories: Improving responses of students with autism with accurate social information. *Focus on Autistic Behavior, 8,* 1–10.

Gray, C., & White, A. (2002). *My Social Stories book.* Philadelphia: Jessica Kingsley.

Groden, J., & LeVasseur, P. (1995). Cognitive picture rehearsal: A system to teach self-control. In K.A. Quill (Ed.), *Teaching children with autism: Strategies to enhance communication and socialization* (pp. 287–305). New York: Delmar.

Hagiwara, T., & Myles, B.S. (1999). A multimedia Social Story intervention: Teaching skills to children with autism. *Focus on Autism and Other Developmental Disabilities, 14,* 82–95.

Hall, L.J., McClannahan, L.E., & Krantz, P.J. (1995). Promoting independence in integrated classrooms by teaching aides to use activity schedules and decreased prompts. *Education and Training in Mental Retardation and Developmental Disabilities, 30,* 208–217.

Hodgdon, L. (1995). Solving social-behavioral problems through the use of visually supported communication. In K.A. Quill (Ed.), *Teaching children with autism: Strategies to enhance communication and socialization* (pp. 265–285). New York: Delmar.

Hodgdon, L. (1996). *Visual strategies for improving communication.* Troy, MI: QuirkRoberts.

Hodgdon, L. (1999). *Solving behavior problems in autism: Improving communication with visual strategies.* Troy, MI: QuirkRoberts.

Kalaigian, K., Kinney, E., Taylor, B., Stromer, R., & Spinnato, D. (2002, May). *Computer-mediated activity schedules: Promoting play and social interaction in a preschooler with autism.* Paper presented at the Association for Behavior Analysis International annual conference, Toronto.

Kamio, Y., & Toichi, M. (2000). Dual access to semantics in autism: Is pictorial access superior to verbal access? *Journal of Child Psychology and Psychiatry, 41,* 859–867.

Keeling, K., Myles, B.S., Gagnon, E., & Simpson, R. (2003). Using the power card strategy to teach sportsmanship skills to a child with autism. *Focus on Autism and Other Developmental Disabilities, 18,* 103–109.

Kimball, J., Kinney, E., Taylor, B., & Stromer, R. (2004). Video enhanced activity schedules for children with autism: A promising package for teaching social skills. *Education and Treatment of Children, 27,* 280–298.

Kinney, E., Vedora, J., & Stromer, R. (2003). Computer-presented video models to teach generative spelling to a child with autism spectrum disorder. *Journal of Positive Behavior Interventions, 5,* 22–29.

Krantz, P.J., MacDuff, M.T., & McClannahan, L.E. (1993). Programming participation in family activities for children with autism: Parents' use of photographic activity schedules. *Journal of Applied Behavior Analysis, 26,* 137–138.

Kuoch, H., & Mirenda, P. (2003). Social Story interventions for young children with autism spectrum disorders. *Focus on Autism and Other Developmental Disabilities, 18,* 219–227.

Kuttler, S., Myles, B.S., & Carlson, J.K. (1998). The use of Social Stories to reduce precursors to tantrum behavior in a student with autism. *Focus on Autism and Other Developmental Disabilities, 13,* 176–182.

Lorimer, P.A., Simpson, R.L., Myles, B.S., & Ganz J.B. (2002). The use of Social Stories as a preventative behavioral intervention in a home setting with a child with autism. *Journal of Positive Behavior Interventions, 4,* 53–60.

MacDuff, G.S., Krantz, P.J., & McClannahan, L.E. (1993). Teaching children with autism to use photographic activity schedules: Maintenance and generalization of complex response chains. *Journal of Applied Behavior Analysis, 26,* 89–97.

Massey, N.G., & Wheeler, J. (2000). Acquisition and generalization of activity schedules and their effects on task engagement in a young girl with autism in an inclusive preschool classroom. *Education and Training in Mental Retardation and Developmental Disabilities, 35,* 326–335.

McClannahan, L.E., & Krantz, P.J. (1999). *Activity schedules for children with autism: Teaching independent behavior.* Bethesda, MD: Woodbine House.

Mesibov, G., Browder, D., & Kirkland, C. (2002). Using individualized schedules as a component of positive behavioral support for students with developmental disabilities. *Journal of Positive Behavior Interventions, 4,* 73–79.

Mirenda, P. (1986). Covert conditioning. In G.W. LaVigna & A.M. Donnellan (Eds.), *Alternatives to punishment: Solving behavior problems with non-aversive strategies* (pp. 157–167). New York: Irvington.

Mirenda, P., MacGregor, T., & Kelly-Keough, S. (2002). Teaching communication skills for behavioral support in the context of family life. In J.M. Lucyshyn, G. Dunlap, & R.W. Albin (Eds.), *Families and positive behavior support: Addressing problem behavior in family contexts* (pp. 185–207). Baltimore: Paul H. Brookes Publishing Co.

Morrison, R., Sainato, D., BenChaaban, D., & Endo, S. (2002). Increasing play skills of children with autism using activity schedules and correspondence training. *Journal of Early Intervention, 25,* 58–72.

Newman, B., Buffington, D.M., O'Grady, M.A., McDonald, M.E., Poulson, C.L., & Hemmes, N.S. (1995). Self-management of schedule following in three teenagers with autism. *Behavior Disorders, 20,* 190–196.

O'Neill, R.E., Horner, R.H., Albin, R.W., Sprague, J.R., Storey, K., & Newton, J.S. (1997). *Functional assessment and program development for problem behavior: A practical handbook* (2nd ed.). Pacific Grove, CA: Brooks/Cole.

Olley, J.G. (1987). Classroom structure and autism. In D.J. Cohen & A.M. Donnellan (Eds.), *Handbook of autism and pervasive developmental disorders* (pp. 411–417). New York: John Wiley & Sons.

Peterson, S., Bondy, A., Vincent, Y., & Finnegan, C. (1995). Effects of altering communicative input for students with autism and no speech: Two case studies. *Augmentative and Alternative Communication, 11,* 93–100.

Pierce, K., & Schreibman, L. (1994). Teaching daily living skills to children with autism in unsupervised setting through pictorial self-management. *Journal of Applied Behavior Analysis, 27,* 471–481.

Quill, K.A. (1995a). Visually cued instruction for children with autism and pervasive developmental disorders. *Focus on Autistic Behavior, 10,* 10–20.

Quill, K.A. (1995b). *Teaching children with autism: Strategies to enhance communication and socialization.* New York: Delmar.

Quilty, K. (2007). Teaching paraprofessionals how to write and implement Social Stories for students with autism spectrum disorders. *Remedial and Special Education, 28,* 182–189.

Rehfeldt, R.A., Kinney, E., Root, S., & Stromer, R. (2004). Creating activity schedules using Microsoft PowerPoint. *Journal of Applied Behavior Analysis, 37,* 115–128.

Reynhout, G., & Carter, M. (2007). Social Story efficacy with a child with autism spectrum disorder and moderate intellectual disability. *Focus on Autism and Other Developmental Disabilities, 22,* 173–182.

Rust, J., & Smith, A. (2006). How should the effectiveness of Social Stories to modify the behaviour of children on the autistic spectrum be tested? *Autism: An International Journal of Research and Practice, 10,* 125–138.

Sansosti, F.J., Powell-Smith, K.A., & Kincaid, D. (2004). A research synthesis of Social Story interventions for children with autism spectrum disorders. *Focus on Autism and Other Development Disabilities, 19,* 194–204.

Schmit, J., Alper, S., Raschke, D., & Ryndak, D. (2000). Effects of using a photographic cueing package during routine school transitions with a child who has autism. *Mental Retardation, 38,* 131–137.

Schopler, E., Brehm, S.S., Kinsgourne, M., & Reichler, R.J. (1971). Effect of treatment structure on development in autistic children. *Archives of General Psychiatry, 24,* 415–421.

Shane, H., & Weiss-Kapp, S. (2008). *Visual language in autism.* San Diego: Plural Publishing.

Stillman, R., & Battle, C. (1984). Developing prelanguage communication in the severely handicapped: An interpretation of the Van Dijk method. *Seminars in Speech and Language, 5,* 159–170.

Stromer, R., Kimball, J., Kinney, E., & Taylor, B. (2006). Activity schedules, computer technology, and teaching children with autism spectrum disorders. *Focus on Autism and Other Developmental Disabilities, 21,* 14–24.

Thiemann, K.S., & Goldstein, H. (2001). Social Stories, written text cues, and video feedback: Effects on social communication of children with autism. *Journal of Applied Behavior Analysis, 34,* 425–446.

Vaughn, B., & Horner, R.H. (1995). Effects of concrete versus verbal choice systems on problem behavior. *Augmentative and Alternative Communication, 11,* 89–92.

Vedora, J., Bergstrom, A., Kinney, E.M., & Stromer, R. (2001, October). *Computer-mediated activity schedules for children with autism spectrum disorders: Teaching number and money skills.* Paper presented at the Berkshire Association for Behavior Analysis and Therapy, Amherst, MA.

Watanabe, M., & Sturmey, S. (2003). The effect of choice-making opportunities during activity schedules on task engagement in adults with autism. *Journal of Autism and Developmental Disorders, 33,* 535–538.

Wood, L.A., Lasker, J., Siegel-Causey, E., Beukelman, D.R., & Ball, L. (1998). Input framework for augmentative and alternative communication. *Augmentative and Alternative Communication, 14,* 261–276.

12

Functional Communication Training and Choice-Making Interventions for the Treatment of Problem Behavior in Individuals with Autism Spectrum Disorders

JEFF SIGAFOOS, MARK F. O'REILLY, AND GIULIO E. LANCIONI

Descriptions of individuals with autism spectrum disorders (ASDs) make frequent reference to various types of problem behavior. Kanner (1943), for example, noted a range of problematic behavior in his initial description of 11 children with autism. The problematic behavior patterns that Kanner observed in these children included property destruction, an obsessive insistence on sameness, repetitive speech, screaming, and rage-like temper tantrums. Subsequent reports have described additional forms of problem behavior among individuals with ASDs, including aggression, noncompliance, stereotyped movements, and self-injury (Mancil, 2006). Although not unique to ASDs, data show that these types of behavior problems are at least two to three times more prevalent among individuals with ASDs and other developmental disabilities than in typically developing peers (Einfeld & Tonge, 1996). Given this high prevalence, it is not surprising that a significant amount of research has focused on the assessment and treatment of problem behavior in individuals with ASDs and other developmental disabilities (Matson, Dixon, & Matson, 2005).

In addition to a high prevalence of problem behavior, people with ASDs also present with a range of communication impairments. Osterling, Dawson, and McPartland (2001) noted that approximately 25% of individuals with ASDs fail to acquire any appreciable amount of speech. Other individuals within the autism spectrum may acquire speech but fail to use it in a way that would be considered functional or socially appropriate. For example, the person might simply echo the speech of others or repeat words and phrases heard from television. Even when speech has developed to a considerable degree, many individuals with ASDs maintain rather odd and unusual speech and language characteristics, such as an unusual voice tone and inflection, pronoun reversals, lack of variety in sentence structure, and immature grammar (e.g., simple noun–verb formats). As with problem behavior, the ubiquity of communication disorders in ASDs has stimulated a considerable amount of research into its assessment and treatment (Goldstein, 2002).

In this chapter, we adopt an integrated view of communication disorders and problem behavior. Specifically, we aim to review the use of communication-based interventions for the treatment of problem behavior in individuals with ASDs. Communication-based interventions aim to reduce problem behavior by strengthening communication and choice-making skills (Carr et al., 1994). Support for the logic of this treatment approach is derived from evidence suggesting a possible causal relation between deficits in communication functioning and the emergence of problem behavior in individuals with ASDs and related developmental disabilities.

THE RELATIONSHIP BETWEEN PROBLEM BEHAVIOR AND COMMUNICATION DEFICITS

Researchers have demonstrated several interesting relationships between communication disorders and problem behavior and highlighted the implications of these relations for intervention purposes (Reichle & Wacker, 1993). For example, numerous studies have demonstrated that deficits in expressive and receptive language are associated with an increased prevalence of problem behavior among individuals with developmental disabilities (Beitchman & Peterson, 1986; Chamberlain, Chung, & Jenner, 1993).

In one such study, Sigafoos (2000) assessed 13 preschool children with developmental disabilities. The children's communication skills and the severity of 58 problem behaviors were assessed every 6 months over a 3-year period using standardized measures of early communication development and problem behavior. The results showed a strong inverse relation between communication ability and severity of problem behavior. That is, children with less developed communication skills were rated as having more severe behavior problems and vice versa.

These findings suggest that delayed or impaired communication development may set the stage for the emergence of problem behavior. Problem behavior is perhaps more likely to emerge if the individual has limited communication skills and limited opportunities to experience successful communicative interactions. The data also suggest that the extent of communication impairment may influence the severity of problem behavior in young children with developmental disabilities. However, the data from Sigafoos (2000) and related studies are largely correlational and therefore provide only indirect support for a link between communication deficits and problem behavior.

Bolstering these correlational studies are experimental data suggesting that some problem behaviors may serve a communicative function for individuals with ASDs (Carr & Durand, 1985; Durand, 1986). Along these lines, Iwata, Dorsey, Slifer, Bauman, and Richmond (1982) described an experimental-functional assessment methodology for identifying the reinforcing consequences that maintain problem behavior. Their initial study involved nine children with developmental disabilities and self-injurious behavior. Structured conditions were created and repeated across a number of 10-minute sessions to assess whether the children's self-injury was related to gaining attention, escaping from academic tasks, and/or producing sensory stimulation.

To assess the attention function, the therapist sat nearby but ignored the child until self-injury occurred. Contingent on self-injury, the therapist briefly attended to the child. Some children in the study engaged in high rates of self-injury under this condition, suggesting a possible attention-recruitment function for their behavior. In another (escape) condition, the children were instructed to receptively identify pictures. During this task, each instance of self-injury was followed by brief withdrawal of the instructional demands. Problem behaviors emitted under these conditions could be interpreted as a form of communicative rejecting or protesting. In a third condition, the child was left alone without attention, materials, or any task demands. Several children emitted self-injury in this alone condition, suggesting a possible sensory function for their self-injury. However, as Lovaas (1982) noted, it is often difficult to interpret problem behavior that occurs in the absence of socially mediated consequences. Perhaps these acts functioned to gain sensory stimulation, summon an adult, or communicate boredom (Donnellan, Mirenda, Mesaros, & Fassbender, 1984).

In any event, since Iwata et al.'s (1982) pioneering study, numerous functional assessment studies have shown that problem behavior is often maintained by two types of reinforcement contingencies: 1) positive reinforcement in the form of attention from others or access to preferred tangibles or 2) negative reinforcement in the form of escape from nonpreferred activities or interactions (Iwata et al., 1994). When problem behaviors are maintained by such contingencies, they could be interpreted as intentional communicative acts related to the expression of preferences, wants, and needs (Durand, 1986). More specifically, such problem behaviors could be interpreted as being equivalent to the early emerging communicative functions of recruiting attention; requesting access to preferred objects; and rejecting nonpreferred objects, activities, or interactions. The difference is that unlike typically developing children, who usually acquire a range of conventional responses to achieve these functions (e.g., joint attention skills, directed pointing, speech), individuals with ASDs and substantial communication impairments have substantial deficits in these skills. In the absence of effective intervention to develop appropriate communication skills, problem behaviors are likely to fill the communicative void.

The conceptualization of problem behavior in terms of communicative functions has direct implications for designing interventions to reduce and prevent problem behavior. Indeed, since the early 1980s, a range of communication-based procedures has been empirically validated for the treatment of problem behavior in individuals with ASDs (Carr et al., 1994; Peck Peterson et al., 2005). For the purpose of this chapter, these procedures can be classified into two broad categories: functional communication training and choice-making interventions.

FUNCTIONAL COMMUNICATION TRAINING

Carr and Durand (1985) developed functional communication training (FCT) as a proactive approach for reducing problem behaviors in individuals with developmental disabilities. The FCT approach aims to reduce problem behavior by teaching more appropriate forms of communication. The rationale for this approach is entirely consistent with evidence showing that problem behaviors are often maintained by the same types of socially mediated consequences (i.e., attention, access to preferred objects, escape from nonpreferred activities) that also maintain early emerging communication skills (Sigafoos, Arthur-Kelly, & Butterfield, 2006).

Logically, if problem behaviors are maintained by these types of socially mediated consequences, then they should be treatable by strengthening alternative forms of communication that lead to the same reinforcing consequences for the individual. For example, a nonverbal child might learn to tantrum when hungry if past tantrums were reinforced with food. This scenario might arise if parents attempt to appease the child with candy to stop the tantrum. Following an FCT approach, future tantrums might be made less likely by teaching the child to request preferred foods using manual signs or picture exchange. As another example, an adult with ASD might learn to destroy property to escape from a boring work task. In this case, FCT might focus on teaching the person to request a break from the task on some reasonable schedule.

To test the logic of FCT, Carr and Durand (1985) recruited four children (age 7–14 years) who exhibited problem behavior in the classroom. The children had varying diagnoses (i.e., autism, brain damage, developmental delay with severe hearing impairment) and multiple forms of problem behaviors (e.g., hitting other people, hand biting, screaming). In the first part of the study, the children were exposed to three conditions: 1) a difficult task and frequent adult attention, 2) an easy task with frequent adult attention, or 3) an easy task with reduced levels of attention. Two children (Jim and Eve) showed the highest rates of problem behavior when they were given the difficult task, but each had very little problem behavior in the other conditions. This pattern suggested that their problem behavior functioned as escape responses. The other two children (Tom and Sue), in contrast, engaged in problem behavior more often when attention levels were reduced, suggesting an attention motivation.

In the next phase of the study, the children were taught to use a relevant and an irrelevant communication response when confronted with difficult tasks or reduced adult attention. Because Jim's and Eve's behaviors were related to task difficulty, the relevant response selected for them was to request help with the difficult task by saying, "I don't understand." In response to this statement, the experimenter provided help to enable the child to complete the task. The irrelevant statement selected for Jim and Eve was to recruit attention by asking, "Am I doing good work?" to which the experimenter would respond by interacting socially with the child. In contrast, the relevant response for Tom and Sue was to solicit attention from the experimenter by asking, "Am I doing good work?" This response was considered relevant because their problem behavior appeared to function primarily as a way of gaining attention. The irrelevant response for Tom and Sue was to request help with the task by saying, "I don't understand." This phrase was irrelevant to the function of their problem behavior because it focused on reducing task difficulty, not on gaining attention.

The results confirmed the researchers' predictions in that problem behaviors were reduced in all four cases, but only when the relevant phrase was reinforced. These data therefore suggest that training a relevant communication response was effective in replacing problem behaviors that appeared to function as ways of recruiting attention (Tom and Sue) or escaping from a difficult task (Jim and Eve). The success of the intervention was not due to communication training in general because the irrelevant phrase did not reduce problem behavior.

Following Carr and Durand's (1985) initial study, FCT has been successfully applied to individuals with severe communication impairments that preclude the use of spoken language. Sigafoos and Meikle (1996), for example, evaluated an FCT intervention to replace problem behaviors in two 8-year-old boys with autism, both of whom lacked speech. Because the children had no spoken language, the intervention attempted to replace the children's aggression, self-injury, and disruptive behavior with the use of augmentative and alternative communication (AAC). First, a functional assessment was completed to identify the communicative function of the children's problem behavior. This assessment involved systematically presenting and removing attention, academic tasks, and preferred objects to ascertain the effects of such manipulations on the frequency of problem behavior. High rates of problem behavior when attention was absent versus present, for example, would suggest that the problem behaviors functioned as attention-getting responses. Alternatively, if the highest rates of problem behavior occurred when task demands were present versus absent, then this pattern would suggest an escape function. Finally, if high rates of problem behavior were observed when preferred objects were inaccessible, as compared to when these same objects were accessible, then the problem behaviors could be interpreted as the child's way of requesting access to preferred objects.

The results of this initial assessment phase indicated that these boys' problem behaviors occurred most frequently when attention was temporarily withdrawn and when preferred objects were temporarily inaccessible by being placed out of reach. This suggested that these behaviors served two communicative functions: recruiting attention and requesting access to preferred objects. Based on this analysis, both children were taught to use AAC (i.e., gestures and picture symbols) to both recruit attention from the teacher and request access to preferred objects.

Instruction on the use of AAC to gain attention and request preferred objects occurred under relevant conditions. The relevant conditions for gaining attention were when the teacher was present but not attending to the child. The relevant conditions for requesting access to preferred objects was when preferred objects were in view but temporarily inaccessible because they were placed out of reach. Systematic instructional procedures involving delayed prompting and contingent reinforcement (Duker, Didden, & Sigafoos, 2004) were effective in teaching the two new AAC responses. For both boys, acquisition of the alternative forms for gaining attention and requesting objects was associated with collateral decreases in problem behavior. This study therefore demonstrated the efficacy of using FCT in combination with AAC for multiply determined problem behaviors in children with ASDs who lacked spoken language. Other studies have also shown the viability of FCT when used in combination with AAC (Mirenda, 1997).

Overall, a considerable amount of evidence supports the use of FCT as a treatment for problem behavior in individuals with ASD (Mancil, 2006; Mirenda, 1997). The approach has been successfully applied to various forms of problem behaviors related to a range of communicative functions. The communicative forms that have been taught to replace problem behaviors have included spoken words and phrases, manual signs, picture-based communication systems, and speech-generating devices. From this literature base it appears that successful use of FCT involves three related steps: 1) identifying the communicative function of problem behavior, 2) selecting an appropriate communicative alternative, and 3) implementing systematic instruction to teach the communicative alternative under relevant conditions.

Identifying the Communicative Function of Problem Behavior

A critical first step in planning an FCT intervention is to identify the communicative function, if any, of the presenting problem behavior. Mirenda (1997) emphasized that FCT "requires a thorough assessment to identify the function (or 'message') of the behavior" (p. 207). This is accomplished by undertaking a functional assessment such as that described by Iwata et al. (1982) or related procedures (O'Neill, Horner, Albin, Storey, & Sprague, 1997).

A functional assessment aims to identify the variables that control problem behavior. These variables include the antecedent conditions that set the occasion for the behavior and the reinforcing consequences that maintain the behavior. In a behavior-analytic framework, problem behavior is said to be explained when its controlling variables have been delineated (Skinner, 1988). The results of a functional analysis can therefore often explain problem behavior. Thus, when Sigafoos and Meikle (1996) demonstrated that the problem behaviors exhibited by the two boys in their study were occasioned by certain antecedent conditions (i.e., diverted attention, unavailable preferred objects) and reinforced by specific consequences (i.e., attention from the teacher, access to preferred objects), they had effectively explained the boys' behavior.

Once problem behavior has been explained, it can be useful to interpret the behavior as having a communicative function. A tantrum that is consistently evoked by demands to engage in a nonpreferred task, for example, might be interpreted as a form of communicative protesting. Screaming that begins when the child is denied candy—and stops when candy is obtained—could be interpreted as the child's way of requesting candy. Similarly, if self-injury begins when the teacher moves away, but stops when the teacher approaches and socially inter-acts with the child, then it might be reasonably interpreted as the child's way of recruiting attention.

It is important to note that assigning a communicative function to problem behavior can be difficult and at times even misleading. Durand (1986) cautioned that such interpretations are often best thought of as metaphorical. Such metaphorical interpretations might nonetheless assist clinicians in selecting appropriate intervention targets. Once a problem behavior is interpreted as a form of requesting or rejecting, clinicians can identify alternative and more appropriate ways for the individual to request and reject. Of course, it is not enough to simply interpret problem behavior as communicative. More important than assigning a communicative interpretation to problem behavior is ensuring that the communicative alternative selected for intervention is relevant to the antecedents and consequences that control problem behavior.

Selecting an Appropriate Communicative Alternative

FCT involves teaching new communication skills (e.g., use of picture exchange) that will hopefully replace the person's existing problem behaviors (e.g., tantrums). Clinicians must therefore select for inter-vention a communicative alternative that will function as a good replacement for the problem behavior of concern. Research suggests that two conditions are necessary if the new communication response is to replace the existing problem behavior (Bopp, Brown, & Mirenda, 2004). First, the new response must come to be controlled by the same variables that currently control the individual's problem behaviors. This is why it is necessary to first identify the antecedent conditions that set the occasion for problem behavior and the reinforcing conse-quences that maintain these responses. As demonstrated by Carr and

Durand (1985), the communicative alternative selected for intervention must be relevant to those same antecedents and consequences.

Second, the new communicative response must be more efficient than the problem behavior (see Chapter 13). Efficient, in this context, means that the communicative alternative is easier to perform and will be more quickly and consistently reinforced than the existing problem behavior (Horner & Day, 1991). Clinicians should therefore aim to identify communication alternatives that require minimal physical and cognitive effort (Bopp et al., 2004). If communicative partners are to reinforce quickly and consistently, they must be able to readily interpret the meaning of the new communication response. Manual signs or abstract picture symbols, for example, might prove less efficient in this sense than line drawings, printed words, or speech-generating devices (Durand, 1999; Rotholz, Berkowitz, & Burberry, 1989). Research also shows the importance of simultaneously reducing the efficiency of problem behavior—via concurrent implementation of extinction and punishment procedures—when teaching the selected communicative alternative (Hagopian, Fisher, Sullivan, Acquisto, & LeBlanc, 1998).

Teaching the Communicative Alternative

Teaching new communication skills for the purpose of replacing existing problem behaviors is likely to require systematic instruction (see Chapter 13). A range of systematic instructional procedures has been empirically validated for teaching individuals with ASDs (Snell & Brown, 2006). Fundamental to systematic instruction is implementation of appropriate behavioral teaching procedures, such as stimulus and response prompting, prompt fading, and differential reinforcement (Duker et al., 2004). FCT interventions typically incorporate these types of systematic instructional procedures into the overall intervention program for teaching the communicative alternative. A carefully designed instructional protocol—in which problem behavior is prevented as the communicative alternative is prompted and reinforced—will help ensure more rapid replacement of existing problem behavior by the new communicative alternative.

Along these lines, Martin, Drasgow, Halle, and Brucker (2005) implemented systematic instruction to teach a 10-year-old boy with autism to reject nonpreferred items. Pretreatment observations and assessments indicated that the child used problematic forms of behaviors to reject unwanted objects. Consistent with the logic of FCT, intervention aimed to teach the child a new communication response (i.e., touching a *No thank you* card) to replace his inappropriate forms of rejecting.

To teach the new rejecting response, the teacher offered a nonpreferred object and moved the card within reach. Moving the card within reach served as a stimulus prompt for the child to touch the card. As soon as the child touched the card, the nonpreferred object was removed. Removal of the nonpreferred item functioned as [negative] reinforcement for touching the card. Over successive teaching sessions, the stimulus prompt of moving the card was faded, with the card always remaining within reach. Using these prompting, fading, and reinforcement procedures, the child very quickly learned to touch the *No thank you* card when offered nonpreferred objects instead of engaging in problematic forms of rejecting.

The instructional protocol implemented by Martin et al. (2005) illustrates the general principles of systematic instruction. The protocol involved five main components:

1. Instruction occurred under the same conditions that evoked the problem behavior.

2. The new communicative alternative was prompted and reinforced so as to preempt problem behavior.

3. The use of prompts was faded as the child became more independent in using the new communication response.

4. The new communicative response was reinforced quickly and consistently, every time it occurred. (Reinforcement in this case involved removing the nonpreferred object.)

5. The old problematic forms of rejecting were made less efficient by ensuring that these were no longer reinforced.

In addition to careful use of prompting, prompt fading, and differential reinforcement as illustrated in Martin et al. (2005), instruction to teach the new communicative alternative should occur under the same conditions that currently evoke problem behavior. For example, consider a child who begins to tantrum whenever her father has been talking on the telephone for several minutes. The tantrum could be interpreted as the child's way of trying to regain the father's attention. Following the logic of FCT, the child could be taught to request attention more appropriately, such as by approaching the father and using a speech-generating device to ask how long before he finishes.

To promote functional use of the speech-generating device, instruction should occur under the same conditions that currently set the occasion for tantrums. Therefore, the child should be taught to use the device when her father is talking on the telephone. In addition, the same consequences that maintained tantrums (regaining the father's attention) should be used to reinforce the use of the speech-generating device. The newly acquired communicative alternative is only likely to remain functional for the individual if it eventually occurs without prompting under the same antecedent and motivational conditions that used to set the occasion for problem behavior.

CHOICE-MAKING INTERVENTIONS

The effectiveness of FCT may stem in part from the fact that the new communication skills provide the individual with more efficient ways to exert control, express preferences, and indicate wants and needs. Choice-making interventions represent another and complementary way of enabling individuals to appropriately exert control, express preferences, and indicate wants and needs.

Choice-making interventions aim to increase the individual's choice-making skills and opportunities. These skills and opportunities may or may not involve communication. For example, a person could make a choice between coffee and tea by directly reaching out and taking one of these options. Alternatively, the person might indicate his or her preference by selecting the tea or coffee icon on a speech-generating device to produce a relevant request (e.g., *I would like tea [coffee], please*). Both of these skills can be taught using systematic instructional procedures, but only the latter involves functional communication training per se. Thus, although FCT and choice-making interventions are complementary, they are not necessarily identical in either their aims or foci.

Recall that the main focus of FCT is to teach appropriate communication skills that will serve the same function or purpose as problem behavior. That is, FCT aims to replace problem behavior with functionally equivalent communication skills. As noted by O'Reilly, Cannella, Sigafoos, and Lancioni (2006), choice-making interventions often have a dual focus that includes 1) teaching appropriate choice-making skills that may or may not involve communication and 2) increasing the number and range of opportunities that are available for the individual to make choices, express preferences, and exert control over the environment. If the individual can already make relevant choices, then intervention might consist of incorporating relevant choice-making opportunities into the conditions that currently evoke problem behavior. In contrast, if the individual lacks effective choice making skills, then intervention would initially have to focus on teaching effective choice-making skills. Possible choice-making responses include natural speech, formal or informal gestures, manual signs, picture exchange, or use of a speech-generating device. As with FCT, it is important to select choice-making responses that will be more acceptable and efficient than problem behavior. Although the specific aim or focus may differ, the logic of choice-making interventions is similar to that of FCT. Increasing choice-making skills and opportunities is intended not only to enable greater control and autonomy, but also to reduce the need for problem behavior.

In addition to strengthening efficient choice-making skills, Sigafoos (1998) suggested that any choice-making skills or opportunities targeted for intervention must match the function of the person's problem behaviors. As with the communication skills selected for an FCT intervention, the choice-making skills and opportunities targeted for intervention must be relevant to the variables that control the person's problem behavior. For example, if problem behavior occurs to escape from nonpreferred tasks, the person might be provided with a choice of tasks. Alternatively, if problem behavior is evoked by the presence of certain types of tangible objects, the individual might be provided with frequent opportunities to choose from among an array of tangible objects (Horner & Budd, 1985). As another example, if problem behavior is maintained by attention, the person might be provided with opportunities to choose when and with whom he or she interacts socially.

Providing Opportunities for Choice Making

In some cases, simply providing relevant choice-making opportunities might be sufficient to reduce problem behavior. Bambara, Koger, Katzer, and Davenport (1995) demonstrated the positive impact of creating relevant opportunities for choice making. Their study participant was a 50-year-old man with developmental disabilities who engaged in frequent aggression, yelling, and swearing. His problem behaviors appeared to be escape-motivated in that they occurred most often when he was requested to complete certain household chores (e.g., setting the table, vacuuming the hallway, making juice, taking out the trash).

As a way of increasing opportunities for choice and control, the researchers began offering him more choice over the timing and sequencing of these household tasks. For example, instead of simply asking him to set the table, he was given a choice of tasks (e.g., "Would you like to set the table or make the juice?"). In addition, instead of simply asking him to vacuum, he was given a choice of which room to vacuum (e.g., "Would you like to vacuum this room or that room?"). When these types of choice-making opportunities were incorporated into the daily routine, participation increased and problem behavior decreased.

Unfortunately, it remained somewhat unclear as to why the provision of these choice-making opportunities was effective in reducing problem behavior. One explanation could be that the intervention worked because it increased choice and control. Another plausible explanation is that these types of choices made the household chores less aversive and therefore made escape from these tasks less reinforcing. In any event, subsequent studies have consistently shown that the provision of various types of choices (e.g., choosing reinforcers, choosing materials, choosing what task to do and when) can lead to increased participation and decreased problem behavior in individuals with ASDs and other developmental disabilities (for a review, see Cannella, O'Reilly, & Lancioni, 2005).

The success of choice-making interventions may depend on how the choice-making opportunities are presented to the individual. Individuals with limited receptive language, for example, may do better when choices are presented visually by showing the real objects or pictures of the real objects, rather than verbally by asking "Do you want coffee or tea?" (e.g., Vaughn & Horner, 1995). Furthermore, as mentioned before, the provision of choice-making opportunities is only likely to be effective if the individual has already acquired effective choice making skills. In some cases, such skills may be lacking and will have to be directly taught.

Teaching Choice-Making Skills

Fortunately, the same systematic instructional procedures used in FCT can also be applied to teach effective choice-making skills. To illustrate, Browder, Cooper, and Lim (1998) implemented systematic instructional procedures to teach choice-making skills to three adults with developmental disabilities. The protocol was implemented in the context of assessing their preference for various leisure activities. Each adult was presented with repeated opportunities to choose various activities (e.g., practicing golf, viewing magazines, or attending a social gathering). The trainer initiated choice-making opportunities by presenting a stimulus to signal the availability of the leisure activity. The signal for looking at magazines, for example, involved presenting a subscription card for that magazine. Individuals were prompted to select the stimulus, which was followed by experiencing the associated leisure activity. Over time, prompting was faded as the individuals came to select the stimulus associated with their preferred leisure activities.

For some individuals to make relevant choices, it may be necessary to begin by teaching choice-making skills in the context of fairly basic opportunities. Initially, for example, the choice opportunities might require choosing a preferred snack item, choosing which activity or task to do, or choosing whether to watch television or go outside for a walk. Later, it might be possible to provide the individual with choice opportunities that involve more complicated decisions (e.g., choosing a career, choosing where to live, and choosing with whom to live). As opportunities for choice are expanded, the individual gains increasing control over his or her life. This increased control is not only likely to improve overall quality of life, but it may also eliminate restrictions that can exacerbate problem behavior (Carr et al., 1994).

CLINICAL IMPLICATIONS

The treatment of behavior problems is a major priority in the overall habilitation of individuals with ASDs. In the past 30 years, major advances have occurred in the assessment and treatment of problem behavior. Clinicians working with individuals with ASDs in home, school, clinic, vocational, and community settings should become familiar with these recent developments and advances related to the treatment of problem behavior.

The major assessment advance is the continuing development and refinement of functional assessment methodologies, following the pioneering work of Iwata et al. (1994). Using functional assessment methodologies, clinicians can now often pinpoint specific antecedent conditions that set the occasion for problem behavior and the precise consequences that maintain problem behavior. Current best practice highlights the importance of undertaking a prior functional assessment to identify the influence of a range of possible controlling variables, including attention, access to tangibles, and escape from task demands. Clinicians must therefore gain skills in designing and implementing functional assessments to identify the variables that control problem behavior.

The development of new functional assessment technologies has coincided with conceptual advances in understanding of the communicative bases to problem behavior (Durand, 1986). In many cases, an individual's problem behavior can be interpreted in relation to one or more basic communicative functions. These basic communicative functions include recruiting attention; requesting access to preferred tangibles; and rejecting nonpreferred objects, activities, or interactions. Clinicians must therefore gain skills in interpreting functional assessment data and knowing when it is meaningful to interpret problem behavior from a communicative perspective.

When a communicative interpretation is reasonable in light of the results of reliable and valid functional assessments, the resulting data are used to select appropriate skills to replace problem behavior. There are a number of issues that must be considered when selecting alternative communication and choice-making skills to replace problem behavior. As reviewed in the preceding sections of this chapter, the main issues to consider include social appropriateness, physical and cognitive effort, and understandability.

Advances in treatment include refinements that have greatly extended the generality of communication-based interventions for the treatment of a wide variety of problem behaviors in a range of individuals. Communication-based interventions are in fact among the most effective treatments available for the treatment of problem behaviors in individuals with developmental disabilities (Didden, Duker, & Korzilius, 1997). Clinicians therefore need to learn how to design, implement, and evaluate FCT and choice-making interventions because these will often be the treatments of choice for many individuals with ASDs who present with significant communication impairment and severe behavior problems.

Although FCT (and to a lesser extent, choice-making interventions) has been manualized (Carr et al., 1994; Durand, 1990), clinicians will still face a number of complex decisions when designing, implementing, and evaluating these treatments. Clinicians must not only decide on appropriate replacement skills, but also figure out when and where to implement instruction, what types of prompts to use during instruction, how to fade these prompts, and how to promote generalization and maintenance. Making these types of technical and logistical choices requires a solid understanding of the basic operant and respondent principles that underlie effective intervention (Linscheid, 1999). It is also critically important for clinicians to remember the overall goal of any intervention, which is to improve the overall quality of life for individuals with ASDs. Keeping this overall goal in mind will assist clinicians with the difficult decisions that arise when intervening to reduce problem behaviors in individuals with ASDs.

Although communication-based interventions can be highly effective, it is important to emphasize that FCT and the provision of choice-making opportunities are not always sufficient to reduce problem behavior. In addition, FCT and choice-making interventions might not be the only procedures necessary to produce clinically significant reductions in problem behavior. Clinicians will therefore require skills in combining FCT and choice-making interventions with other types of empirically supported interventions for addressing the communication deficits and problem behaviors of individuals with ASDs.

RESEARCH IMPLICATIONS AND FUTURE RESEARCH

Although a large number of applied intervention studies have consistently demonstrated the effectiveness of FCT and choice-making interventions, there remain several important research questions that have received rather limited attention in the literature. Specifically, there has been relatively little research into the prevention of problem behaviors, the integration of FCT and choice-making interventions, and the application of communication-based approaches for ameliorating other core symptoms associated with ASDs, such as resistance to change and insistence on sameness.

Preventing Problem Behaviors

Understandably, FCT and choice-making interventions have primarily been used to reduce existing behavior problems. However, the possibility of preventing the emergence of severe behavior problems through early introduction of FCT and choice-making interventions has not gone unrecognized (Sigafoos & O'Reilly, 2006). Although the potential preventative effects of FCT have been recognized, to our knowledge, no studies have evaluated its potential to prevent severe behavior problems in children with ASDs.

Early introduction of FCT may be resisted for several reasons. First, there may be a mistaken belief that the child is likely to out grow his or her problem behavior and hence there is no need for treatment. Emerging problem behaviors are also often easier for parents and preschool teachers to tolerate because the child is not yet strong enough to inflict serious injury or damage. There may also be a reluctance to introduce AAC as part of the FCT intervention because of fears that this will interfere with speech and language development.

All of the above reasons are ungrounded. If anything, problem behaviors are likely to become worse as the child ages (Einfeld & Tonge, 1996) and AAC is likely to facilitate rather than hinder language development (Mirenda, 1997). Strong evidence showed highly positive outcomes when parents used FCT to replace problem behaviors of young children with developmental disabilities (Wacker et al., 1998). Given the success of FCT when implemented by parents for treatment of problem behaviors in young children, early introduction of FCT might also be an effective preventative measure. Studies exploring this hypothesis would be a welcome addition to the literature.

Integrating FCT and Choice-Making Interventions

Because FCT and choice-making interventions are each effective, combining these two approaches may represent an even more powerful form of treatment. Studies are needed that can demonstrate effective ways of combining FCT and choice-making interventions. Along these lines, Peck Peterson et al. (2005) demonstrated the value of adding choice-making opportunities to an FCT intervention. These investiga-tors first used FCT with two boys diagnosed with developmental dis-abilities. A prior functional assessment showed that the boys' problem behaviors were maintained by escape from academic tasks. Instead of engaging in problem behavior to escape from task demands, these two children were taught to request a break using either manual signs or speech (e.g., *I want a break, please*).

Acquisition of these replacement requests was associated with decreased problem behavior. Unfortunately, task engagement also decreased because the two boys were constantly requesting breaks. To increase task engagement, the researchers then provided a choice between continuing the task a little bit longer versus taking an immediate break. If the boys chose to take an immediate break, they were given a 15-second break with no toys or attention. If they chose to work, however, they later got a 2-minute break that included access to toys and adult attention. Incorporating these choice opportunities with the FCT intervention not only kept problem behav-ior to low levels but also increased the boys' participation in important academic tasks.

These results show the benefit of integrating choice opportunities with FCT. Future research needs to evaluate the effects of other combinations of FCT and choice making. Successful integration of these two procedures may enable clinicians to design more effective interventions.

Extension to Other Core Features of Individuals with ASD

To date, FCT and choice-making interventions involving individuals with ASDs have been applied to self-injury, aggression, property destruction, tantrums, noncompliance, and stereotyped movements (Mancil, 2006). Future research should aim to extend the generality of communication-based interventions by evaluating their effectiveness for ameliorating some of the other behavioral problems associated with ASD.

Resistance to change and insistence on sameness are two such problems for which there are few empirically supported treatments. Resistance to change and insistence on sameness figured heavily in Kanner's (1943) description of 11 children with autism and remain dis-tinguishing features of ASD today. Individuals with ASDs often resist change and insist on sameness to a degree that is highly problematic. For example, the child may have an extreme tantrum if a piece of furni-ture is moved from its usual location or if the parent deviates from the usual route home. Despite their ubiquity in descriptions of individuals with ASDs, there has been almost no intervention research to address these two major problem areas for individuals with ASDs (cf., Marchant, Howlin, Yule, & Rutter, 1974).

It is possible that FCT and choice-making interventions could be modified to address these core features of ASD. For example, the child may be allowed to choose one of two routes that will be taken on the way home from school or taught to request changes in the environment that are more to his or her liking, rather than having a tantrum in response to any slight change. It remains to be determined if such approaches would be viable options for addressing these core features of ASD.

SUMMARY

FCT and choice-making interventions are sound and sensible approaches for addressing problem behaviors of individuals with ASDs. When implemented with care by skilled professionals, there is very good evidence to justify the use of these procedures. As with any intervention, however, the procedures will often need to be modified to suit the individual. Even when appropriately modified to suit the individual, intervention may fail to produce the desired effect.

FCT and choice making are good tools that can be very effective when used for the right job. However, these methods might not always be the best—or the only tools—because problem behavior may not always have a communicative basis. When problem behavior does have a communicative basis, then FCT and choice-making interventions are certainly good choices. FCT and choice-making interventions are consistent with the move toward evidence-based practice in AAC intervention (Schlosser, 2000).

There was a time when the presence of problem behavior often excluded an individual from receiving communication intervention. Today, the presence of problem behaviors should signal the need to consider FCT and choice-making interventions. We believe that FCT and choice-making interventions have a role in preventing the emergence of severe problem behaviors and therefore should be considered even when the individual does not have any major problem behavior. It would be unfortunate if clinicians began to exclude individuals from receiving these types of effective communication-based interventions because they did not have serious problem behavior.

REFERENCES

Bambara, L.M., Koger, F., Katzer, T., & Davenport, T.A. (1995). Embedding choice in the context of daily routines: An experimental case study. *Journal of The Association for Persons with Severe Handicaps, 20,* 185–195.

Beitchman, J.H., & Peterson, M. (1986). Disorders of language, communication, and the behavior in mentally retarded children: Some ideas on their co-occurrence. *Psychiatric Clinics of North America, 9*, 689–698.

Bopp, K.D., Brown, K.E., & Mirenda, P. (2004). Speech-language pathologists' roles in the delivery of positive behavior support for individuals with developmental disabilities. *American Journal of Speech-Language Pathology, 13*, 5–19.

Browder, D.M., Cooper, K.J., & Lim, L. (1998). Teaching adults with severe disabilities to express their choice of settings for leisure activities. *Education and Training in Mental Retardation & Developmental Disabilities, 33*, 228–238.

Cannella, H.I., O'Reilly, M.F., & Lancioni, G.E. (2005). Choice and preference assessment research with people with severe to profound developmental disabilities: A review of the literature. *Research in Developmental Disabilities, 26*, 1–15.

Carr, E.G., & Durand, V.M. (1985). Reducing behavior problems through functional communication training. *Journal of Applied Behavior Analysis, 18*, 111–126.

Carr, E.G., Levin, L., McConnachie, G., Carlson, J.I., Kemp, D.C., & Smith, C.E. (1994). *Communication-based intervention for problem behavior: A user's guide for producing positive change.* Baltimore: Paul H. Brookes Publishing Co.

Chamberlain, L., Chung, M.C., & Jenner, L. (1993). Preliminary findings on communication and challenging behaviour in learning difficulty. *British Journal of Developmental Disabilities, 39*, 118–125.

Didden, R., Duker, P., & Korzilius, H. (1997). Meta-analytic study of treatment effectiveness for problem behaviors for individuals who have mental retardation. *American Journal on Mental Retardation, 101*, 387–399.

Donnellan, A.M., Mirenda, P.L., Mesaros, R.A., & Fassbender, L.L. (1984). Analyzing the communicative functions of aberrant behavior. *Journal of The Association for Persons with Severe Handicaps, 9*, 201–212.

Duker, P., Didden, R., & Sigafoos, J. (2004). *One-to-one training: Instructional procedures for learners with developmental disabilities.* Austin, TX: PRO-ED.

Durand, V.M. (1986). Self-injurious behavior as intentional communication. *Advances in Learning & Behavioral Disabilities, 5*, 141–155.

Durand, V.M. (1990). *Severe behavior problems: A functional communication training approach.* Albany, NY: Guilford Press.

Durand, V.M. (1999). Functional communication training using assistive devices: Recruiting natural communities of reinforcement. *Journal of Applied Behavior Analysis, 32*, 247–267.

Einfeld, S., & Tonge, B.J. (1996). Population prevalence of psychopathology in children and adolescents with intellectual disability: II. Epidemiological findings. *Journal of Intellectual Disability Research, 40*, 99–109.

Goldstein, H. (2002). Communication intervention for children with autism: A review of treatment efficacy. *Journal of Autism and Developmental Disorders, 32*, 373–396.

Hagopian, L.P., Fisher, W.W., Sullivan, M,T., Acquisto, J., & LeBlanc, L.A. (1998). Effectiveness of functional communication training with and without extinction and punishment: A summary of 21 inpatient cases. *Journal of Applied Behavior Analysis, 31*, 211–235.

Horner, R.H., & Budd, C.M. (1985). Acquisition of manual signs use: Collateral reduction of maladaptive behavior, and factors limiting generalization. *Education & Training of the Mentally Retarded, 20,* 39–47.

Horner, R.H., & Day, M.D. (1991). The effects of response efficiency on functionally equivalent competing behaviors. *Journal of Applied Behavior Analysis, 24,* 719–732.

Iwata, B., Dorsey, M., Slifer, K., Bauman, K., & Richman, G. (1982). Toward a functional analysis of self-injury. *Analysis and Intervention in Developmental Disabilities, 2,* 3–20.

Iwata, B., Pace, G., Dorsey, M., Zarcone, J., Vollmer, T., Smith, R., et al. (1994). The functions of self-injurious behavior: An experimental-epidemiological analysis. *Journal of Applied Behavior Analysis, 27,* 215–240.

Kanner, L. (1943). Autistic disturbances of affective contact. *Nervous Child, 2,* 217–250.

Linscheid, T.R. (1999). Commentary: Response to empirically supported treatments for feeding problems. *Journal of Pediatric Psychology, 24,* 215–216.

Lovaas, O.I. (1982). Comments on self-destructive behaviors. *Analysis & Intervention in Developmental Disabilities, 21,* 115–124.

Mancil, G.R. (2006). Functional communication training: A review of the literature related to children with autism. *Education and Training in Developmental Disabilities, 41,* 213–224.

Marchant, R., Howlin, P., Yule, W., & Rutter, M. (1974). Graded change in the treatment of the behaviour of autistic children. *Journal of Child Psychology and Psychiatry, 15,* 221–227.

Martin, C.A., Drasgow, E., Halle, J.W., & Brucker, J.M. (2005). Teaching a child with autism and severe language delays to reject: Direct and indirect effects of functional communication training. *Educational Psychology, 25,* 287–304.

Matson, J.L., Dixon, D.R., & Matson, M.L. (2005). Assessing and treating aggression in children and adolescents with developmental disabilities: A 20-year overview. *Educational Psychology, 25,* 151–181.

Mirenda, P. (1997). Supporting individuals with challenging behavior through functional communication training and AAC. Research review. *Augmentative and Alternative Communication, 13,* 207–225.

O'Neill, R.E., Horner, R.H., Albin, R.W., Storey, K., & Sprague, J.R. (1997). *Functional analysis of problem behavior: A practical guide* (2nd ed.). Sycamore, IL: Sycamore Press.

O'Reilly, M.F., Cannella, H.I., Sigafoos, J., & Lancioni, G. (2006). Communication and social skills interventions. In J.K. Luiselli (Ed.), *Antecedent assessment and intervention: Supporting children and adults with developmental disabilities in community settings* (pp. 187–206). Baltimore: Paul H. Brookes Publishing Co.

Osterling, J., Dawson, G., & McPartland, J. (2001). Autism. In C.E. Walker & M.C. Roberts (Eds.), *Handbook of clinical child psychology* (3rd ed., pp. 432–452). New York: John Wiley & Sons.

Peck Peterson, S.M., Caniglia, C., Royster, A.J., Macfarlane, E., Plowman, K., Baird, S.J., & Wu, N. (2005). Blending functional communication training and choice making to improve task engagement and decrease problem behaviour. *Educational Psychology, 25,* 257–274.

Reichle, J., & Wacker, D.P. (Vol. Eds.). (1993). *Communicative alternatives to challenging behavior: Integrating functional assessment and intervention strategies.* In S.F. Warren & M.E. Fey (Series Eds.), *Communication and language intervention series: Vol. 3.* Baltimore: Paul H. Brookes Publishing Co.

Rotholz, D., Berkowitz, S., & Burberry, J. (1989). Functionality of two modes of communication in the community by students with developmental disabilities: A comparison of signing and communication books. *Journal of The Association for Persons with Severe Handicaps, 14,* 227–233.

Schlosser, R.W. (2000). *The efficacy of augmentative and alternative communication: Toward evidence-based practice.* Boston: Academic Press.

Sigafoos, J. (1998). Choice making and personal selection strategies. In J.K. Luiselli & M.J. Cameron (Eds.), *Antecedent control: Innovative approaches to behavioral support* (pp. 187–221). Baltimore: Paul H. Brookes Publishing Co.

Sigafoos, J. (2000). Communication development and aberrant behavior in children with developmental disabilities. *Education and Training in Mental Retardation and Developmental Disabilities, 35,* 168–176.

Sigafoos, J., Arthur-Kelly, M., & Butterfield, N. (Eds.). (2006). *Enhancing everyday communication for children with disabilities.* Baltimore: Paul H. Brookes Publishing Co.

Sigafoos, J., & Meikle, B. (1996). Functional communication training for the treatment of multiply determined challenging behavior in two boys with autism. *Behavior Modification, 20,* 60–84.

Sigafoos, J., & O'Reilly, M. (2006). Replacing problem behavior. In J. Sigafoos, M. Arthur-Kelly, & N. Butterfield (Eds.), *Enhancing everyday communication for children with disabilities* (pp. 87–106). Baltimore: Paul H. Brookes Publishing Co.

Skinner, B.F. (1988). The operant side of behavior therapy. *Journal of Behavior Therapy and Experimental Psychiatry, 18,* 171–179.

Snell, M.E., & Brown, F. (2006). *Instruction for students with severe disabilities* (6th ed.). Upper Saddle River, NJ: Pearson Education.

Vaughn, B., & Horner, R.H. (1995). Effects of concrete choice versus verbal choice systems on problem behavior. *Augmentative and Alternative Communication, 11,* 89–92.

Wacker, D.P., Berg, W.K., Harding, J.W., Derby, K.M., Asmus, J.M., & Healy, A. (1998). Evaluation and long-term treatment of aberrant behavior displayed by young children with disabilities. *Journal of Developmental and Behavioral Pediatrics, 19,* 260–266.

13

The Role of Aided AAC in Replacing Unconventional Communicative Acts with More Conventional Ones

KRISTA M. WILKINSON AND JOE REICHLE

This chapter will review the basic principles by which idiosyncratic or problem behaviors can be effectively replaced by more conventional communicative means, particularly aided forms of augmentative and alternative communication (AAC). First, the chapter will describe some well-established principles for responding to problem behaviors. These principles are based in longstanding research traditions and many have been incorporated into proven clinical intervention methodologies, such as functional communication training (see Chapter 12). Our goal is to relate these principles to their potential application with learners with autism spectrum disorders (ASDs) who could benefit from aided AAC intervention modalities. Thus, basic principles for replacing problem behavior will be outlined, paying special attention to the issues that arise when aided AAC modes are involved.

This chapter will examine potential ways in which aided AAC can function not only to replace existing problem behaviors (i.e., those that are already in a learner's repertoire) but also to promote new and desired behaviors. An old adage—"nature abhors a vacuum"—aptly describes many instances of the emergence of problem behaviors, in particular those that serve a communicative function. Learners who have few conventional means to communicate their intentions—either for instrumental purposes such as obtaining desired items or rejecting unwanted ones, or for social purposes such as attracting attention or maintaining social closeness—are likely to develop idiosyncratic means, some of which might be considered problematic by larger community groups. Planning proactively by offering systematic conventional means of communication may head off the development of problem behaviors, either before they start or before they become so well-established that they are difficult to replace.

Critical to the success of this effort is the selection of conventional acts that have equal or greater communicative power for the user. Because aided forms of communication present unique challenges as communication modes (in terms of their physical characteristics, the rate of message preparation, and so forth), specialized consideration is necessary when they are offered as alternatives to problem behavior. Accordingly, this chapter outlines some instructional approaches that are useful for replacing unwanted behaviors with aided symbols, as well as some evidence-based examples. These approaches offer a means for interventionists to maximize the likelihood that aided communication will successfully supplant unwanted problem behavior and are intended as complements to existing training technologies. Our intention is that these strategies will be integrated as appropriate with other communication goals that are relevant to each learner.

The final section focuses on an issue of specific relevance to individuals with ASDs. Here, our goal is to illustrate how the framework discussed in the two prior sections applies not only to communicative acts that regulate the behavior of others, which has been extensively researched in the area of AAC and ASD, but also to joint attention communicative acts, which have received little attention in AAC research despite their importance in ASD (Wetherby, 2006). Because there is little direct research concerning the ideas we discuss in this section, our comments are meant to be exploratory in nature. Nonetheless, we believe that it is useful to discuss some potential ways of integrating aided AAC for instruction on joint attention and to identify how current targeted approaches might benefit from including aided AAC modes. It is our hope that these ideas might help spur direct research on the topic.

REPLACING IDIOSYNCRATIC BEHAVIOR: AN OVERVIEW

Idiosyncratic and problem behaviors can either be social or nonsocial in their function (e.g., Johnston & Reichle, 1993). In this chapter, we focus on socially motivated problem behaviors in which the functional consequences of the behavior are mediated by a communication partner; such functions include obtaining or avoiding attention, objects, activities, or other desired or nondesired consequences. We have chosen this focus because socially motivated behaviors are potentially amenable to communication interventions such as those offered by aided AAC.

When establishing a conventional communicative repertoire, it is important that the new communicative form is an exact functional match for the idiosyncratic behavior that it is replacing. For example, if a learner is engaging in whining to escape a particular school activity, the communicative alternative must address escape. If the interventionist can not permit escape, some other intervention strategy will be required (Halle, Bambara, & Reichle, 2005). Additionally, it is important that the new communicative alternative is equally or more attractive to the learner than the existing communicative strategy—that is, that the new alternative is at least as efficient as the current one. A number of variables are helpful in operationalizing efficiency (Hernstein, 1961), including the immediacy of reinforcement, the rate of reinforcement, the physical/cognitive response effort required, and the quality of reinforcement.

Immediacy of Reinforcement

Consider the example of a learner who hits himself. Interventionists rush in to keep the learner from hurting himself; in so doing, they inadvertently reinforce his hitting behavior with attention. If one chooses to teach the learner to touch a symbol on a speech-generating device (SGD) that says "Please come here" as an alternative behavior to get attention, it is important that the interventionists' responses to his SGD use be as quick as (and preferably quicker than) their responses to the original hitting behavior. Otherwise, from the learner's perspective, the new communicative alternative will be a poor substitute. In addition, the desirability of the new alternative behavior can be enhanced by creating opportunities for the learner to use it for attention before he becomes anxious or even desperate to get a reaction from others.

Rate of Reinforcement

The rate of reinforcement refers to how many times or for how long the learner must engage in a behavior prior to obtaining the desired outcome. For example, when the teacher's back is turned, a learner may have to make silly or disruptive noises for a long time to get her to pay attention to him. If we structure the context such that selecting a message on an SGD results in the immediate delivery of her attention, we have created a situation in which the rate of reinforcement for attracting attention with aided communication is higher than that for undesired noises.

Physical and Cognitive Effort

Physical effort refers to the amount of physical exertion (i.e., the number of calories) required to complete an act. Behaviors that require less physical effort to achieve a goal will generally be preferred over those that take more effort (e.g., greater fine or gross motor coordination or strength). Any replacement behavior should require physical effort that is no greater and preferably less arduous than the behavior being replaced. This issue is particularly salient for AAC because aided modes of communication may require a learner to search and select symbols from an array. Many problem behaviors involve little physical effort; for example, hitting one's neighbor even once usually has immediate, predictable, and direct consequences. If a learner is accomplishing her goal with a single undesirable but relatively effortless act such as this, she is unlikely to exert more effort to accomplish the same goal by, for example, selecting a series of graphic symbols. Efforts to replace her problem behavior must accommodate this important consideration.

In addition to physical effort, cognitive effort may play a role in response efficiency. Some behaviors may occur so often in certain situations that they become automatic. Many of us have experienced the following: when driving to work each morning, we may not remember passing certain landmarks or turning at certain exits, yet we make it to work without an accident. In essence, we have become so mentally familiar with what to do that we no longer need to devote all of our thought to driving. A similar phenomenon appears to be at work with problem behaviors. Sometimes, learners engage in problem behavior because it has become well rehearsed and effortless to produce in a specific situation. If this is the case, the learner may view that behavior as more efficient than a newly introduced alternative. Johnston, Reichle, and Evans (2004) provided a tutorial on response efficiency that details numerous examples of this phenomenon.

Quality of Reinforcement

Quality of reinforcement is a bit more challenging to describe. Essentially, we must consider the relative value to the learner of what he or she obtains for engaging in the new alternative response as compared to the old, undesired response. This can be operationalized in terms of either 1) the quantity or duration of a reinforcer or 2) the availability of a reinforcer that has been identified as being especially powerful for the learner. The importance of identifying a learner's individual preference(s) among reinforcers becomes especially important as we seek to provide him or her with opportunities to engage in alternatives to problem behavior. Often, we offer feedback that we believe will be reinforcing to a learner such as social praise (e.g., "Nice job!"), treats, or activities (e.g., extra dessert, extra recess). If our belief is consistent with the learner's actual preferences, then the feedback will be an integral part of the intervention. If, however, the feedback is unmotivating (or perhaps even aversive) to the learner, it will not be successful and may even impede the targeted outcome. Thus, it is critical to evaluate, on a learner-by-learner basis, the feedback that truly reinforces target behaviors.

Taken together, these four parameters of response efficiency also address potential opportunities for collateral benefits. For instance, if a learner learns to raise his hand instead of making disruptive noises to get a teacher's attention, the teacher is likely to begin to offer him compliments (e.g., "Thanks for raising your hand!"). Another collateral benefit is the potential for improved peer interactions; peers who might have been afraid to approach a learner who engaged in problem behavior are more likely to initiate social exchanges once the problem behavior is no longer so prominent.

PROMOTING ACCEPTABLE ALTERNATIVE BEHAVIORS THROUGH AIDED AAC

Idiosyncratic behaviors, including problem behaviors, often emerge when learners have no conventional means of communicating. Learners produce actions that are part of their behavioral repertoires and, when others consistently react to these behaviors in accordance with the learners' desires, the behaviors are strengthened and become intentional. Intentional behavior, in turn, occurs along a continuum that ranges from socially acceptable to socially unacceptable. If learners are offered an equally efficient, effective, and effortless mode for self-expression, the problem behaviors that emerge in the absence of conventional ones may be replaced or even prevented. This section discusses methods for promoting viable aided alternatives that might be expected to compete with learner-initiated problem behaviors.

This section will focus on visual aided symbols, even though functional communication training for replacing idiosyncratic or problem behaviors can involve providing speech, manual signs, or visual symbols as alternatives. Of course, when unaided gestures or manual signs are understood by all partners, they can be equally efficient and effective as either unconventional acts or oral/spoken modes of communication. However, visual-graphic symbols such as pictures, words, icons, or other graphic modes offer some special challenges in this regard, as discussed in the sections that follow.

Focus and Disciplinary Philosophy

One longstanding debate within the disciplines of language intervention, ASD, and AAC concerns the appropriate context and form of intervention. Should we use naturalistic intervention that occurs in context by exploiting learning opportunities as they arise? Or, should we structure intervention to occur in pull-out therapy sessions, with highly planned targeted learning opportunities? Historically, this debate has been framed as an "either/or" proposition. However, there is growing acknowledgement across a number of disciplines that unique advantages may be offered by each approach, as well as by hybrid approaches that combine elements of both (e.g., Paul, 2007).

Fey (1986) discussed a *continuum of naturalness* with regard to language intervention approaches. He concluded that, while naturalistic approaches are to be preferred when everything else is equal, there is also a place for highly structured interventions that target specific goals. These circumstances are often related to specific communication goals and to individual learner temperaments or developmental characteristics. Kaiser, Yoder, and Keetz (1992) have demonstrated the effectiveness of adapting elements of both naturalistic and structured approaches to create hybrid interventions, while Warren and Yoder (1997) offered a review of the different uses of child-centered (i.e., naturalistic), clinician-directed (i.e., structured/contrived), and hybrid approaches.

An appreciation of the unique and complementary contributions of each approach has recently been echoed within the field of ASD (Mundy & Wetherby, 2006; Quill, 2006; Warren & Yoder, 1997). In this chapter, we extend the spirit of this philosophy to aided AAC interventions for learners with ASDs. The approaches reviewed here are largely (although not exclusively) situated toward the "less natural" end of the instructional continuum. Yet, although our discussion will focus on the utility of planned and clinician-structured learning opportunities for promoting AAC alternatives to problem behavior, we do not intend that these strategies be used instead of or as prerequisites to more naturalistic interventions. Rather, we offer evidence-based methods that can complement naturalistic interventions by providing additional opportunities for practicing specific skills or for working on goals that arise infrequently in natural conversations (Warren & Yoder,

1997). Our suggestions can also be used to supplement and/or enhance various naturalistic modeling and aided language input programs that have been demonstrated to be successful with children with disabilities, including ASDs (see Chapters 7–9).

Many of the techniques discussed in this chapter derive from learning principles in the discipline of behavioral psychology. In particular, the area of stimulus control analysis seeks to pinpoint the environmental supports that contribute to or impede functional behavior. Many of the strategies we offer rely on match-to-sample (MTS) tasks, in which a participant is expected to locate a target stimulus in an array on the basis of a target sample. Extensive research has demonstrated consistently that most individuals with intellectual and language limitations are readily able to perform MTS tasks, either independently or following simple instruction (e.g, Carter & Werner, 1978; Lattal & Perone, 1998; McIlvane, 1992; McIlvane, Dube, Green, & Serna, 1993; Wilkinson & Rosenquist, 2006).

From a practical standpoint, MTS tasks underlie many clinical assessment and intervention procedures, including the act of communicating itself. For instance, standardized tests of receptive vocabulary, such as the Peabody Picture Vocabulary Test (Dunn & Dunn, 2006) and the Receptive One Word Picture Vocabulary Test (Brownell, 2000), require that a learner match spoken words and pictures. Many research and clinical assessments of expressive or receptive symbol knowledge involve the presentation of either a symbol or its referent, with the expectation that the learner will select an appropriate match from an array of choices (e.g., Brady & Saunders, 1991; Franklin, Mirenda, & Phillips, 1996; Wilkinson & Rosenquist, 2006). Furthermore, initial AAC instruction almost always involves the use of modeling, prompting, or some combination thereof to teach the learner that a specific symbol (e.g., a photograph) refers to (i.e., matches) a specific referent (Bondy & Frost, 2001; Romski & Sevcik, 1996). Learners who use symbols to communicate are always engaging in the task of selecting an appropriate symbol to match to a desired referent.

Basic Principles of Replacing Behavior Through Aided AAC

One of the greatest challenges faced by individuals who use visual-aided AAC symbols to communicate is their relatively slow rate of message preparation. Beukelman and Mirenda (2005, p. 67) reviewed the "drastic" reduction in communication rate encountered by aided communicators relative to natural speakers. While spoken communication proceeds at a rate of approximately 150–250 words per minute, message construction with aided communication has been estimated to occur at less than 15 words per minute. The reduced rate of message preparation has direct implications for the efficiency of and effort required for aided communication, particularly when it comes to problem behavior. An act such as hitting one's neighbor to gain escape can be produced very rapidly and with very little effort. How do we replace such a behavior with a graphic symbol, given the visual and motoric effort and time that might be required to locate and select the symbol?

To accomplish this, the symbol being taught (e.g., *help, break*) should be very large in size, appear alone on a display, and/or be placed in a preferred location that is easy for the learner to access. This will allow the learner to find the target symbol with minimal search time, making the search highly efficient and relatively effortless. Second, it will be important for the learner to encounter an immediate response for using the new symbol, coupled with a less immediate response for engaging in the associated problem behavior. If the latter is not possible, the interventionist should consider making the quality of the response less effective for the problem behavior. For example, if a learner gets a 3-minute break from work after he uses his *break* symbol, he should get a much shorter break (e.g., 30–60 seconds) if and when he hits his neighbor to escape. Once we have considered such basic strategies related to response efficiency, we are well-positioned construct a program for individuals who are already engaging in intentional but unconventional communicative acts.

Advanced Strategies for Promoting Desired Communication Behaviors Using Aided Symbols

How can we promote a conventional aided communicative repertoire that is likely to compete with problem behavior? Among the many possible strategies, we have opted to review those that relate specifically to the unique challenges of aided communication. These include 1) assessing visual skills for aided AAC, 2) determining learners' sensitivity to antecedent cues and planned consequences, 3) implementing errorless instruction, 4) selecting appropriate functional targets for communication, 5) identifying and promoting the conditional use of communicative acts, and 6) expanding learners' existing symbolic repertoires.

Assessing Visual Skills for Aided AAC Interventions   Learners who produce problem behavior that serves one or more communicative functions often do so because they are unable to make use of the conventional communicative alternatives they have been offered. For example, the visual demands of a communication display may not be well matched to a learner's perceptual abilities. If a visual display is overly complex and/or the symbols are difficult for the user to see, the user will either develop or continue to use problem behaviors instead.

It is important to consider both basic and complex visual processes in the design of a communication display. At the basic level, we must consider both the relative placement and the size of symbols on the display. If the symbols are placed too close together (i.e., if the display is too crowded) or if the symbols are too small for accurate discrimination, the learner will not be able to use them in the intended fashion and may resort to problem behaviors instead. Thus, it is critical to evaluate the learner's ability to distinguish among symbols of varying sizes and proximities, not only individually but also as members of a display. Discussions of these issues and how to assess them using MTS strategies with many populations are available elsewhere (e.g., Utley, 2002; Wilkinson & McIlvane, 2002).

Some important issues to examine during such assessments include how well learners can discriminate among aided symbols that are similar in size and color (e.g., strawberry symbol versus apple symbol), how well they comprehend the relationship between a spoken word and an object or picture referent (e.g., selecting the apple symbol from an array of other symbols upon hearing the spoken word "apple"), and how well they are able to differentiate between spoken words that sound similar (selecting the correct symbol for *hat, cat,* and *bat* on the same array). Research has indicated that markers of comprehension such as these may be important predictors of learning rates and outcomes in individuals who use aided AAC, including those with ASD (Romski & Sevcik, 1996; Sevcik & Romski, 2005).

In addition to assessing basic perceptual processes related to visual acuity and existing symbol matching skills, clinicians need to be aware of a number of complex visual factors that might also be important in determining whether a learner will be able to process the symbols on a communication display efficiently and accurately. The literature suggests that learners with specific types of disabilities may have distinct patterns of visual processing. For instance, a phenomenon reported in individuals with intellectual disabilities or ASDs is overselective attention—attention that is narrowly focused on one minor feature of a stimulus (e.g., Gersten, 1980; Happe & Frith, 2006; Huguenin, 2004; Liss, Saulnier, Fein, & Kinsbourne, 2006; Litrownik, McInnis, Wetzel-Pritchard, & Filipelli, 1978; Wilhelm & Lovaas, 1976).

The presence of overselective attention has clear implications for aided display construction. If a learner focuses only on a small feature of a symbol (e.g., the presence of a stem on line drawings representing various fruits), she may have difficulty differentiating between the symbols for *cherry* and *apple*. Another feature of visual processing that appears to be characteristic of individuals with ASDs is a narrow focus within the visual field more generally (Wainwright & Bryson, 1996). This characteristic also has implications for aided display construction, as a learner's use of symbols that appear in certain locations on a display (e.g., the corners) might be affected. See Wilkinson, Carlin, and Thistle (2008) for further discussion of this and other visual-perceptual considerations.

Although the visual processing patterns of individuals with specific disabilities have not been documented beyond these initial observations, it stands to reason that visual processing abilities will vary across learners, such that a display that is visually appropriate for one learner might not be appropriate for another. This can occur not solely because of cognitive or communicative differences, but also because of mismatches between a learner's visual processing skills and the demands of a specific display. Such a problem can leave parents and professionals wondering why certain symbols are neglected while others are overused.

MTS tasks can be useful for assessing the visual processing skills of individuals with ASDs. Such tasks have been used to examine, for example, the breadth of observation within a stimulus or a field of view (McIlvane, Dube, & Callahan, 1996) and the extent to which a learner relies on visual cues such as location or color (Stephenson, 2007; Wilkinson, Carlin, & Jagaroo, 2006; Wilkinson et al., 2008). Such assessments can assist clinicians to make accommodations when designing communication displays so that they are appropriate to each learner's visual processing patterns.

Determining Sensitivity to Antecedent Cues and Planned Consequences Problem behavior that serves a communicative function results in an outcome that is sought by the learner. As noted previously, if the new behaviors that are selected to replace these idiosyncratic behaviors do not offer motivating consequences that are similar and/or more powerful, the problem behaviors will likely continue. Thus, it is important to determine the sensitivity of a learner to specific reinforcers and to design interventions that match the consequences the learner is seeking.

The first step in accomplishing this task is to determine the consequences that motivate a given learner. Often, interventionists seek to reinforce new communicative behaviors socially (i.e., verbally) by complimenting learners when they produce those behaviors. For many learners, such social/verbal consequences are reinforcing and result in increased use of new communicative behaviors over time. However, for others (particularly learners with ASDs), such social reinforcers may not be effective or may need to be modified to suit the learner's preferences and interests. Assessment techniques derived from MTS tasks and stimulus control analyses are available to evaluate the effectiveness of specific reinforcers and have been used successfully in this regard (e.g., Dube & McIlvane, 2002; McIlvane et al., 1996; Neef, Shade, & Miller, 1994).

Once the preferred reinforcers have been identified, the next step is to design interventions that incorporate them as consequences. Initially, such interventions may not be focused on spontaneous communication, but they can be critical building blocks for communication nonetheless. Once motivating consequences (i.e., reinforcers) are identified for a specific learner, it is necessary to offer as many opportunities as possible for the learner to engage in the behavior that will elicit those consequences. Doing so teaches the learner as rapidly as possible which behavior will result in which consequence. When the target communicative behavior is unlikely to occur spontaneously in conversation, it is often important to structure the environment to foster its occurrence (Warren & Yoder, 1997). Moreover, and just as importantly, doing so also allows the interventionist to participate in interactions with the learner that involve promoting positive behaviors rather than simply eliminating unwanted ones.

Finally, in some situations it may be important to increase the value of reinforcement to make the new communicative alternative more attractive. For example, consider the situation in which a learner is being taught to request a break instead of engaging in problem behavior related to escape. Rather than simply allowing the learner to push away from the table for a brief period when she uses the *break* symbol, we might allow her to play a computer game for a few minutes during the break as well. In this instance, the addition of tangible reinforcement is likely to make the use of the *break* symbol more attractive than the consequence that is intermittently available for problem. Identifying powerful reinforcers that can be delivered contingent on the production of a new communicative behavior also offers the interventionist the opportunity to become associated with positive consequences.

Using Errorless Learning Techniques MTS tasks can be exploited to teach communication behaviors that have been identified as replacements for problem behavior. MTS tasks can be useful either when the target communicative behavior does not arise frequently in natural conversations or when the interventionist wants to increase the number of opportunities the learner has to practice the behavior and experience the consequences. This approach can be conceptualized in part within the framework of "today" and "tomorrow" goals

(Beukelman & Mirenda, 2005). "Today" goals are those that maximize a learner's current functioning, given his or her existing communication repertoire and skill set. For example, we might provide an object schedule to help a beginning communicator understand what will happen next in his day (thus reducing tantrums at transition times). Or, we might arrange the environment to maximize this learner's ability to use his existing communication modes to express wants and needs, share information, and/or engage in social closeness interactions with friends and family members. "Tomorrow" goals are related to new skills and must be taught for the learner to communicate more effectively across settings and partners in the future. Tomorrow goals can include things such as teaching a learner who currently communicates through nonsymbolic modes (e.g., gestures, vocalizations) to use simple symbols such as objects or teaching a learner who communicates with object symbols to use a higher-order symbol set, such as photographs or line drawings. The advantage of doing so is that higher-order symbols are often more portable than objects and are also more suitable for expressing abstract concepts such as *stop* and *hot*.

In such situations, structured intervention strategies can serve as a bridge between the learner's current communication behaviors and the "tomorrow" mode that we envision. For example, for a learner who uses aggression to obtain escape, we would clearly want to 1) structure the environment to support appropriate, existing modes of communication and 2) model the use of symbols, such as objects, in as many natural interactions as possible to foster aided symbol use as an alternative to aggression. In addition, we might also want to design specific instructional sessions in which we teach the relationship between *break* symbol use and getting a break, thus providing optimal practice and experience under both natural and structured conditions.

MTS Tasks as Alternatives to Trial-and-Error Instruction

Some instructional methods use trial-and-error techniques, in which the learner is encouraged to guess the correct response and learn from the consequences (i.e., reinforcement when correct and no response when incorrect). Because it is fairly simple, this is a tempting place to start an instructional program. However, many professionals have probably encountered learners who, once they make an error, have difficulty shifting away from the error pattern. For such learners, trial-and-error techniques can be counterproductive because they set up error patterns that then must be eliminated. Thus, trial-and-error learning is often rejected by individuals with ASDs because of their vulnerability to failure (Richmond & Bell, 1986; Sidman & Stoddard, 1967). Recent research that compared directly the efficacy of error-correction techniques and an MTS-based errorless instructional technique (exclusion learning, described later in the chapter) reported superior outcomes for the errorless technique in establishing relations between photographs and objects, with children with autism diagnoses (Carr & Felce, 2008).

Aided symbol instruction for beginning communicators can be accomplished using simple MTS tasks in which the learner is initially taught to match identical symbols within an array (e.g., finding an identical line drawing within an array of line drawings). As the learner progresses, instruction can include matching on the basis of either shared features (e.g., finding a line drawing in an array that matches a photograph) or arbitrary features (e.g., finding a line drawing in an array that matches a written word; Wilkinson & McIlvane, 2002). Such alternative instructional approaches can also be used to reduce errors and promote positive feedback opportunities.

Consider a learner for whom we seek to establish identity-matching behavior. At the outset, this learner cannot reliably select a specific shape from an array of shapes. For example, when presented with a triangle, he cannot select a matching triangle from array containing a triangle and several other shapes. To enhance the learner's likelihood of locating the identical stimulus in an array, we can exploit some basic visual-perceptual characteristics of the array in an MTS task. One way to focus his attention is through presentation of a single "odd-man-out" stimulus (i.e., an oddity task). To do so, we present a triangle within an array made up of repeated instances of a single other shape (e.g., one triangle among three identical squares). Presenting the triangle as the odd-man-out among an otherwise uniform display serves to make it appear to "pop out" to the viewer. Gradually, the number of distracters (in this case, the squares) is systematically diminished until only one target symbol and one distracter remain as choices to match to the sample. Research has supported the effectiveness of such methods at teaching identity matching skills to individuals with developmental and intellectual disabilities, not only with regard to shapes but also with regard to colors or other stimulus features (e.g., Carlin, Soraci, Dennis, Strawbridge, & Chechile, 2002; Mackay, Soraci, Carlin, Dennis, & Strawbridge, 2002).

Additional errorless learning techniques can be used to teach feature-based or arbitrary matching. Sample stimulus shaping procedures allow interventionists to gradually "morph" a stimulus (e.g., a line drawing) into another (e.g., associated written word) during the course of instruction. Using this technique, we can move a learner through increasingly difficult tasks that begin with identity matching (e.g., line drawing to line drawing), proceed to matching on the basis of shared features (e.g., line drawing to photograph or line drawing to object), and terminate in arbitrary matching (e.g., line drawing to written word). Such systematic instruction may be important for a learner whose goals include moving from more to less iconic symbols (e.g., from photographs to line drawings, or from line drawings to written words). Although time and effort consuming, such techniques have been used successfully to teach matching relations to individuals with severe intellectual disabilities (see Carr, Wilkinson, Blackman, & McIlvane, 2000; Serna, Wilkinson, & McIlvane, 1998).

All of these examples illustrate instructional methods that exploit the antecedent cues and reinforcing consequences that are inherent in aided communication displays, while also maximizing the likelihood that the new communicative act will compete successfully with existing problem behavior as the preferred method of communication. These simple methods can be effective for a number of reasons. First, they allow a learner to experience desired consequences for performing conventional (albeit simple) communicative behaviors. If we have properly assessed and chosen reinforcers, then performing the new behaviors will be a positive experience for the learner, making it more likely that he or she will perform them more often (and will also perform undesired behaviors less). Moreover, if we have properly chosen the target behavior, then the learner will be taught at least two important components of the communication task simultaneously—how to visually locate a specific target symbol from an array and how to select a target symbol that is identical to an intended referent. Together, these two components are the underpinnings of conventional aided communication.

In addition, these methods may be effective because they allow numerous opportunities for the interventionist to interact with the learner in positive ways and to become associated with the presentation of desired reinforcers. By promoting positive interactions and conventional communicative alternatives, these methods are a means to compete with problem behaviors that serve to obtain desired reinforcers.

Requesting or Rejecting as the Target Function During Initial Instruction
Initial instruction aimed at building a communicative repertoire usually involves teaching learners to request or reject objects or events in their environments (i.e., behavior regulation). Requesting and rejecting are developmentally among the very earliest communicative functions to emerge, making them appropriate initial targets for intervention (e.g., Reichle, Drager, & Davis, 2002; Sigafoos et al., 2004). Furthermore, requesting and rejecting are the communicative functions that are the most robust in many individuals in ASDs (Wetherby, 2006) and thus offer a reliable and motivating context for instruction.

It is essential to select communicative behaviors that directly match the social functions served by existing idiosyncratic behaviors (e.g., problem behaviors such as aggression). For example, if an interventionist determines that a learner is engaging in a communicative act to escape an event, a variety of communicative behaviors can be taught. One option is to teach the learner to use a symbol to request a break, as in the example provided previously. Another option that is especially appropriate for learners who attempt to escape because the work required is very difficult (rather than because of its duration) is to teach use of a *help* symbol that will result in additional assistance rather than a break. In the short run, this option will significantly lessen task difficulty for the learner; in the long run, it will also provide the interventionist with opportunities to teach the learner to be more independent as the level of assistance is gradually faded. A third option is to teach an *I don't want to do this* symbol to learners who attempt to escape because they dislike the activity, even though it is brief and they can accomplish it independently.

To determine which communicative alternative to teach, we have found it useful to manipulate specific features of the situation associated with problem behavior systematically. For example, in a task that requires problems to be solved, we may choose to alternate between tasks that the learner can complete successfully less than 25% of the time with tasks that he can complete more than 75% of the time. If problem behavior occurs substantially more often in the 25% condition than in the latter, teaching the learner to request assistance may be an appropriate communicative alternative.

In another example, suppose that a preschooler engages in problem behavior to escape participation in a morning "circle time." Manipulating features of this activity might involve comparing the proportion of 30-second intervals in which problem behavior occurs when the activity lasts 5 minutes compared to when it lasts 15 minutes. If problem behavior is more prevalent in the 15-minute condition, then teaching the learner to request a break might be a reasonable communicative alternative.

In both of these examples, we have taken care to identify the specific conditions of a task that might provoke the desired outcome of escape.

Using New Communicative Functions Conditionally   One of the main challenges for a significant number of beginning communicators is using communicative acts conditionally—that is, using such acts in only specific circumstances (i.e., conditions) rather than all of the time. For interventionists, an equal challenge is differentiating between situations in which a learner's failure to produce newly taught communicative behaviors stems from problems with conditional use and those in which it stems from a lack of generalization. For example, Dragsow, Halle, and Ostrosky (1998) taught three young children with significant developmental disabilities to use conventional requests rather than idiosyncratic communicative means (i.e., problem behaviors) to obtain desired activities. The learners' classrooms served as the acquisition settings, but the activities that were the focus of the requesting intervention were also available in the children's homes. The children learned to request desired activities in their classrooms, but they did not use their newly acquired requesting behaviors at home; rather, they continued to engage in problem behavior to get what they wanted. Their parents were then taught to refrain from reinforcing the idiosyncratic behaviors at home. Once these behaviors were rendered inefficient, two of the three children began to produce the new communicative acts instead.

It may seem that the learners' failure to produce the new communicative behaviors at home stemmed from a failure to generalize the learned behavior to a new setting (i.e., from school to home). However, when the consequences for problem behavior at home were changed to make the alternative behaviors more efficient, two of the three learners immediately showed corresponding changes in their behavior in that setting. If the issue had been solely a failure to generalize, the interventionist would have had to teach the new communicative form directly in the children's homes. However, the results suggested that at least two of the learners began to use their new conventional communicative acts at home when it was simply made clearer to them that it was more efficient to do so.

Conditional use comes into play extensively when teaching any new communicative function. Reichle and his colleagues conducted a series of studies to examine the conditional use of requests for assistance, in which they taught children when to ask for help and when to refrain from doing so (Reichle & Johnston, 1999; Reichle & McComas, 2004; Reichle et al., 2005). In Reichle and McComas (2004), the intervention involved first teaching the learner to request assistance upon encountering work (in this case, math) that was beyond his current skill level. Following this, the interventionist began to gradually fade the physical assistance provided in response to his requests for help; thus, across teaching sessions, the learner became increasingly more competent and independent. Finally, the learner was offered a more attractive reinforcer when he completed the assigned work successfully and independently then when he asked for assistance. Results indicated that, once this conditional-use phase was implemented, he asked for assistance only when he really needed it (i.e., for subtraction problems) and refrained from doing so when he did not (i.e., for addition problems).

Expanding the Size of the Symbol Repertoire   Thus far, we have considered very simple aspects related to visual processing and the reinforcement-based foundations for problem behaviors, as well as the more complex challenges of placing these basic foundations within communication contexts. This section concludes by illustrating one final MTS-based "errorless" method for expanding a symbol repertoire for an individual who has well-established communicative skills.

It would be frustrating to anyone who understands the power of communication and is motivated to express herself to be unable to do so because of a lack of available vocabulary. In such situations, a learner may develop idiosyncratic or problem behaviors to express the messages that are missing from her communication display. Individuals who have not yet learned to read and who use aided symbols to communicate are especially at risk for experiencing frustration related to this issue; this is because the vocabulary available to them is limited to the symbols included on their communication aids or displays. The potential for creating this frustration arises whenever supporters who are responsible for programming or constructing communication displays fail to anticipate the numerous topics a communicator might want to express. Thus, it is important to examine some strategies for expanding the content of an existing aided symbol repertoire.

Other chapters in this volume offer detailed descriptions of various programmatic approaches to this issue, which include aided language modeling and other naturalistic methods. Thus, we have opted to review a specific set of studies that incorporate MTS procedures to examine vocabulary expansion for aided symbols, which have direct application to individuals with ASDs and intellectual disabilities.

Wilkinson and her colleagues initiated a series of studies in children both with and without communication and intellectual disabilities, using a process referred to as "disambiguation and fast mapping" or "learning by exclusion" (Wilkinson, 2005, 2007; Wilkinson & Albert, 2001; Wilkinson & Green, 1998). *Fast mapping* refers to a learner's ability to acquire a partial map of word meanings rapidly and after very little exposure. Most often, fast mapping procedures take the form of simple matching tasks. A learner is first shown an array containing a number of visual stimuli (e.g., objects, photographs, line drawings, or written words). On baseline trials, the learner is presented with an array of known items and asked to point to one of them; for example, a learner might be presented with photographs of a tree, an apple, and a cat and asked to point to *apple*.

In fast mapping trials (also called "disambiguation trials" by Wilkinson and colleagues; see Wilkinson, 2007 for discussion of the terminology used in the literature), the array contains one novel or unnamed stimulus that is presented alongside an array of well-known items. For example, the array might contain photographs of a tree, an apple, and an unusual object (e.g., a garlic press). In these trials, the learner is provided with nonsense word and is asked to point to the object that matches it (e.g., *Show me the pafe*) to determine if the learner understands that the novel word refers to the unnamed photograph (e.g., the garlic press) rather than to the photographs of well-known and previously labeled items. Selection of the novel photograph under these circumstances is initial evidence for fast mapping ability, which is then confirmed by some type of later demonstration that the learner has made an initial map between the nonsense word and the novel referent.

Typically developing children begin to demonstrate fast mapping (i.e., the reliable selection of a novel item when presented with a novel label) by 15–18 months of age (Markman, 1989). Individuals with intellectual and developmental disabilities, including ASDs, also show evidence of fast mapping when presented with a single novel word (Chapman, Kay-Raining Bird, & Schwartz, 1990; Mervis & Bertrand, 1995; Romski, Sevcik, Robinson, Mervis, & Bertrand, 1996; Stevens & Karmiloff-Smith, 1997).

In her studies, Wilkinson and colleagues (Wilkinson, 2005, 2007; Wilkinson & Albert, 2001; Wilkinson & Green, 1998) adapted the usual fast mapping procedures to examine the acquisition of multiple words by learners with severe intellectual disabilities, including those with ASDs. Although, as expected, the participants in these studies reliably selected a novel referent upon hearing a novel word, the map learned during this initial exposure was more vulnerable to interference in individuals with intellectual disabilities than in vocabulary-matched children (Wilkinson, 2005, 2007). For instance, in a direct examination of instructional procedures for teaching two new words, Wilkinson (2005) found that the protocols for introducing new words to individuals with intellectual disabilities had to be structured more carefully; these individuals also required more systematic practice of each novel word prior to the introduction of additional words. However, in two case studies in which these protocols were individualized to specific learners, they were highly successful in teaching aided sight word vocabulary (Wilkinson & Albert, 2001). These studies provided initial evidence that indirect natural learning processes such as fast mapping can be exploited for vocabulary instruction of aided communicators. Carr and Felce (2008) recently demonstrated that for children with ASDs, instruction adapted from exclusion resulted in more reliable acquisition of photograph-object relations than instruction using an error-correction technique.

Summary

Aided AAC can used to replace problem behaviors that have social functions in a number of ways. Systematic application of the basic principles for replacing unconventional behaviors can be effective in this regard, especially if instruction takes into account the specific challenges involved in teaching an aided mode of communication (e.g., accommodations related to the rate of communication, visual processing capabilities, instructional concerns, and symbol teaching issues). This chapter will now examine the application of these basic principles in the use of aided AAC to address joint attention, one of the special considerations in the communicative profiles of individuals with ASDs.

AIDED AAC IN TARGETED INTERVENTIONS THAT SUPPORT BIDS FOR JOINT ATTENTION

An important contributor to early language and social development is the ability to share coordinated attention to an object with a partner, which is generally known as *joint attention* (see Bakeman & Adamson, 1984). As Yoder and McDuffie (2006) noted, a number of definitions of joint attention have been proposed in the literature. Some of these are based on the presence of specific behaviors (e.g., eye gaze, pointing), whereas others emphasize the learner's engagement in an episode of shared reference, regardless of specific behaviors. When considering the very earliest (i.e., prelinguistic) emergence of joint attention, Yoder and McDuffie observed that most definitions stipulate that "the infant demonstrates simultaneous or sequential coordinated attention between object and person" (p. 118). They distinguished two subtypes of prelinguistic joint attention that appear to be important for predicting both a learner's response to treatment and later language outcomes—responding to joint attention and initiating joint attention. When responding to joint attention, the learner responds to (i.e., follows) an adult's behavior or focus of attention, whereas when initiating joint attention, the learner initiates a behavior for the purpose of sharing content or commenting.

Both responding to and initiating joint attention are clear predictors of later receptive and expressive language outcomes in typically developing learners (e.g., Watt, Wetherby, & Shumway, 2006; Yoder & McDuffie, 2006). Research has confirmed that individuals with ASDs are characterized by a specific and selective deficit in the ability to coordinate attention between a communication partner and an object or event in the environment (Mundy, Sigman, & Kasari, 1994; see Wetherby, 2006, for a review and analysis). Unusual patterns of both responding to and initiating joint attention have been reported in pre-school learners with ASDs; the extent to which these behaviors are evident very early in life predict later diagnosis and/or language development (Charman et al., 2003; Sullivan et al., 2007; Toth, Munson, Meltzoff, & Dawson, 2006; Warreyn, Roeyers, Van Wetswinkel, & De Groote, 2007; Wetherby, 2006). The presence of at least some prelin-guistic joint attention is also associated with other cognitive and adap-tive outcomes in young children with ASDs (Toth, Munson, Meltzoff, & Dawson, 2006).

Given the importance of joint attention, recent research has exam-ined whether it is possible to enhance its development through direct intervention in children with ASDs (Kasari, Freeman, & Paparella, 2006; Dube, MacDonald, Mansfield, Holcomb, & Ahearn, 2004; Jones, Carr, & Feeley, 2006; Martins & Harris, 2006; Whalen & Schriebman, 2003). Kasari et al. (2006) conducted a controlled intervention study with preschoolers with ASDs who were assigned randomly to one of three groups: joint attention intervention, symbolic play intervention, or a control group. Behavioral prompting techniques were used to elicit the behaviors that were targeted in each condition. The children who received the joint attention intervention showed significantly greater gains in both responding to and initiating joint attention behaviors compared to the control group, both in experimental assessments and in generalization assessments during interactions with parents.

Although there are many other important aspects of this elegant study, the key point for our purposes is that, when joint attention is operationalized in terms of measurable behaviors, it is indeed amenable to change through intervention. Additional studies of joint attention instruction within an applied behavior analytic paradigm have reported similarly positive outcomes (Dube, Klein, MacDonald, O'Sullivan, & Wheeler, 2006; Jones et al., 2006; Martins & Harris, 2006; Whalen & Schriebman, 2003).

Aided AAC as a Potentially Useful Accessory in Joint Attention Interventions

One potential role of aided AAC is to enhance a learner's ability to share reference with a partner—that is, to engage in joint attention (Light, 1989, 2006; Wilkinson & Hennig, 2007). In fact, some of the fea-tures of aided symbols make them particularly well suited to enhance interventions aimed at increasing joint attention in learners with ASDs.

First, aided AAC that makes use of visual symbols is well matched to the visual learning strengths of many learners with ASDs. Furthermore, aided AAC can be readily integrated into many of the activities that elicit joint attention behaviors.

Despite this potential, virtually no AAC research has directly examined interventions that specifically target joint attention. A keyword search for the terms *joint attention* and both *augmentative and alternative communication* and *aided or visual symbols* resulted in no hits within four major databases (Academic Search Premier, PsycInfo, PsychArticles, and ComDisDome). Thus, we must extrapolate from research whose main purpose was not to examine joint attention but whose results are nonetheless relevant to a discussion of the potential contributions of aided AAC to joint attention outcomes.

One such study (Yoder & Stone, 2006) examined the general rates of communication during aided AAC interventions. It is important to note that the study was designed to compare the overall efficacy of two communication interventions and was not designed to target joint attention specifically. Yoder and Stone compared the types of communicative acts that emerged under two intervention conditions— responsive prelinguistic milieu teaching and the Picture Exchange Communication System (PECS). Increases in joint attention behaviors were observed during and after PECS intervention, especially in learners with very low levels of joint attention at the outset (i.e., during the baseline phase). This finding suggests that—even without direct targeting of the joint attention function—increases in related behaviors can emerge during aided symbol intervention in the form of PECS.

Another avenue to explore with regard to aided symbol use and joint attention concerns storybook reading. The relationship between book reading and joint attention is somewhat obvious, given the fact that book reading requires a shared focus of attention between an adult and child. Indeed, a book-reading activity is one of the communication temptations used to elicit joint attention behaviors in the Communication and Symbolic Behavior Scales™ assessment tool (Wetherby & Prizant, 1993). Shared book reading has long been used as a content for spoken language intervention and recent AAC research has promoted it use for teaching aided symbol use as well (Liboiron & Soto, 2006; Trudeau, Cleave, & Woelk, 2003). Thus far, none of the participants in these studies have been diagnosed with ASDs. Nonetheless, there is considerable potential for integrating aided symbols into the rich instructional context provided by storybook reading to elicit and reinforce joint attention. This remains an important area for both clinical and research attention.

Another potential application for which aided communication may be well suited pertains to the restricted interests of learners with

ASDs. Many learners with ASDs become so captivated by specific interests that they are reluctant to share them with others (e.g., they focus on playing with trains but do not welcome others playing with them). Interventionists might incorporate aided symbols into such activities to foster or facilitate sharing of the interest. With the symbols available (e.g., attached with Velcro to the relevant parts of a train setup), other individuals could comment on the learner's interest (thus seeking to enhance the response to joint attention) or elicit commenting by the learner him or herself (thus seeking to enhance initiation of joint attention). Again, clinical and research application of this idea remains to be examined.

CONCLUSION

In this chapter, we have developed a beginning communicative repertoire for individuals with ASDs. We suggested that most learners with ASDs already have functional communicative strategies (often in the form of problem behaviors) that they are able to produce prior to the time that formal communication interventions are introduced. Thus, interventionists must attend to the literature that describes how to replace existing communicative means with socially appropriate alternatives via functional communication training. In this discussion, we focused on the challenges related to acquiring the discriminative use of symbols, learning to use the new communicative behaviors conditionally, and being able to use the new communicative behaviors in relevant situations that may not have been addressed during acquisition.

We also focused on joint attention, a communicative function that has received limited attention in the AAC literature to date. Of course, as in any chapter, there are important topics that we did not address as well, such as how to establish extended communicative interactions for conversational repair. Although this competence often begins to emerge in beginning communicators, we chose instead to focus on the types of brief episodic exchanges for requesting and rejecting that are more often targeted in interventions related to problem behavior reduction.

Effective instructional strategies that are available to persons who support beginning communicators with ASDs have proliferated over the past decade or more. Increasingly, interventionists are able to choose and implement strategies that have a high likelihood of producing useful communicative repertoires, which can enable beginning communicators with ASDs to lead the most inclusive life possible.

REFERENCES

Bakeman, R., & Adamson, L.B. (1984). Coordinating attention to people and objects in mother-infant and peer-infant interaction. *Child Development, 55,* 1278–1289.

Beukelman, D.R., & Mirenda, P. (2005). *Augmentative and alternative communication: Supporting children and adults with complex communication needs* (3rd ed.). Baltimore: Paul H. Brookes Publishing Co.

Bondy, A., & Frost, L. (2001). The picture exchange communication system. *Behavior Modification, 25,* 725–745.

Brady, N.C., & Saunders, K.J. (1991). Considerations in the effective teaching of object to symbol matching. *Augmentative and Alternative Communication, 7,* 112–116.

Brownell, R. (2000). *Receptive One Word Picture Vocabulary Test, 2000 Edition.* Novato, CA: Academic Therapy Products.

Carlin, M.T., Soraci, S.A., Dennis, N.A., Strawbridge, C.P., & Chechile, N.A. (2002). Guided visual search in individuals with mental retardation. *American Journal on Mental Retardation, 107,* 237–251.

Carr, D., & Felce, J. (2008). Teaching picture-to-object relations in picture-based requesting by children with autism: A comparison between error prevention and error correction teaching procedures. *Journal of Intellectual Disability Research, 52,* 309-317.

Carr, D., Wilkinson, K.M., Blackman, D., & McIlvane, W.J. (2000). Equivalence classes in individuals with minimal verbal repertoires. *Journal of the Experimental Analysis of Behavior, 74,* 101–114.

Carter, D.E., & Werner, T.J. (1978). Complex learning and information processing by pigeons: A critical analysis. *Journal of the Experimental Analysis of Behavior, 29,* 565–601.

Chapman, R.S., Kay-Raining Bird, E., & Schwartz, S.E. (1990). Fast mapping of words in event contexts by children with Down syndrome. *Journal of Speech and Hearing Disorders, 55,* 761–770.

Charman, T., Baron-Cohen, S., Swettenham, J., Baird, G., Drew, A., & Cox, A. (2003). Predicting outcomes in infants with autism and pervasive developmental disorder. *International Journal of Language and Communication Disorders, 38,* 265–285.

Drasgow, E., Halle, J.W., & Ostrosky, M.M. (1998). Effects of differential reinforcement on the generalization of a replacement mand in three children with severe language delays. *Journal of Applied Behavior Analysis, 31,* 357–374.

Dube, W.V., Klein, J.L., MacDonald, R.P.F., O'Sullivan, G.A., & Wheeler, E.E. (2006). Joint attention deficits in preschool children and discrimination of adult gaze direction: Assessment and training. *Proceedings of the 39th Annual Gatlinburg Conference on Research and Theory in Intellectual and Developmental Disabilities,* 86.

Dube, W.V., MacDonald, R.P.F., Mansfield, R.C., Holcomb, W.L., & Ahearn, W.H. (2004). Toward a behavioral analysis of joint attention. *The Behavior Analyst, 27,* 197–207.

Dube, W.V., & McIlvane, W.J. (2002). Quantitative assessments of sensitivity to reinforcement contingencies in mental retardation. *American Journal on Mental Retardation, 107,* 136–145.

Dunn, L.M., & Dunn, L.M. (2006). *Peabody Picture Vocabulary Test—4th Edition.* Circle Pines, MN: American Guidance Service.

Fey, M.E. (1986). *Language intervention with young children.* San Diego: College Hill Press.

Franklin, K., Mirenda, P., & Phillips, G. (1996). Comparison of five symbol assessment protocols with nondisabled preschoolers and learners with severe intellectual disabilities. *Augmentative and Alternative Communication, 12,* 63–77.

Gersten, R.M. (1980). In search of the cognitive deficit in autism: Beyond the stimulus overselectivity model. *Journal of Special Education, 14,* 47–65.

Halle, J., Bambara, L., & Reichle, J. (2005). Teaching alternative skills. In L. Bambara & L. Kern (Eds.), *Individualized supports for students with problem behaviors: Designing positive behavioral support plans* (pp. 237–274). New York: Guilford Press.

Happe, F., & Frith, U. (2006). The weak coherence account: Detail-focused cognitive style in autism spectrum disorders. *Journal of Autism & Developmental Disorders, 36,* 5–25.

Hernstein, R. (1961). Rate and absolute strength of responses as a function of frequency of reinforcement. *Journal of the Experimental Analysis of Behavior, 4,* 267–272.

Huguenin, N.H. (2004). Assessing visual attention in young children and adolescents with severe mental retardation utilizing conditional-discrimination tasks and multiple testing procedures. *Research in Developmental Disabilities, 25,* 155–182.

Johnston, S.S., & Reichle, J. (1993). Designing and implementing interventions to decrease problem behaviors. *Language, Speech, and Hearing Services in Schools, 24,* 225–235.

Johnston, S.S., Reichle, J., & Evans, J. (2004). Supporting AAC use by beginning communicators with severe disabilities. *American Journal of Speech-Language Pathology, 13,* 20–30.

Jones, E.A., Carr, E.G., & Feeley, K.M. (2006). Multiple effects of joint attention intervention for children with autism. *Behavior Modification, 30,* 782–834.

Kaiser, A., Yoder, P., & Keetz, A. (1992). Evaluating milieu teaching. In S.F. Warren & J. Reichle (Series & Vol. Eds.), *Communication and language intervention series: Vol. 1. Causes and effects in communication and language intervention* (pp. 9–47). Baltimore: Paul H. Brookes Publishing Co.

Kasari, C., Freeman, S., & Paparella, T. (2006). Joint attention and symbolic play in young children with autism: a randomized controlled intervention study. *Journal of Child Psychology & Psychiatry, 47,* 611–620.

Lattal, K.A., & Perone, M. (Eds.). (1998). *Handbook of research methods in human operant behavior.* New York: Plenum Press.

Liboiron, N., & Soto, G. (2006). Shared storybook reading with a student who uses alternative and augmentative communication: A description of scaffolding practices. *Child Language Teaching and Therapy, 21,* 69–95.

Light, J.C. (1989). Toward a definition of communicative competence for individuals using augmentative and alternative communication systems. *Augmentative and Alternative Communication, 5,* 137–144.

Light, J.C. (2006). Designing dynamic display AAC systems for young children with complex communication needs. *Perspectives on Augmentative and Alternative Communication, 15,* 2–7.

Liss, M., Saulnier, C., Fein, D., & Kinsbourne, M. (2006). Sensory and attention abnormalities in autistic spectrum disorders. *Autism: The International Journal of Research & Practice, 10,* 155–172.

Litrownik, A.J., McInnis, E.T., Wetzel-Pritchard, A.M., & Filipelli, D.L. (1978). Restricted stimulus control and inferred attentional deficits in autistic and retarded children. *Journal of Abnormal Psychology, 87,* 554–562.

Mackay, H.A., Soraci, S., Carlin, M., Dennis, N.A., & Strawbridge, C.P. (2002). Guiding visual attention during acquisition of matching-to-sample. *American Journal on Mental Retardation, 107,* 445–454.

Markman, E.M. (1989). *Categorization and naming in children.* Cambridge, MA: MIT Press.

Martins, M.P., & Harris, S.L. (2006). Teaching children with autism to respond to joint attention initiations. *Child & Family Behavior Therapy, 28,* 51–68.

McIlvane, W.J. (1992). Stimulus control analysis and nonverbal instructional methods for people with intellectual disabilities. In N.W. Bray (Ed.), *International review of research in mental retardation. Vol. 1* (pp. 55–109). San Diego: Academic Press.

McIlvane, W.J., Dube, W.V., & Callahan, T.D. (1996). Attention: A behavior analytic perspective. In G.R. Lyon & N.A. Krasnegor (Eds.), *Attention, memory, and executive function* (pp. 97–117). Baltimore: Paul H. Brookes Publishing Co.

McIlvane, W.J., Dube, W.V., Green, G., & Serna, R.W. (1993). Programming conceptual and communication skill development. In S.F. Warren & J. Reichle (Series Eds.) & A.P. Kaiser & D. Gray (Vol. Eds.), *Communication and language intervention series: Vol. 2. Enhancing children's communication: Research foundations for early language intervention* (pp. 242–285). Baltimore: Paul H. Brookes Publishing Co.

Mervis, C.B., & Bertrand, J. (1995). Acquisition of the novel-name-nameless-category (N3C) principle by young children who have Down syndrome. *American Journal on Mental Retardation, 100,* 231–243.

Mundy, P., Sigman, M., & Kasari, C. (1994). Joint attention, developmental level, and symptom presentation in autism. *Development and Psychopathology, 6,* 389–401.

Mundy, P., & Wetherby, A. (2006, November). *Autism spectrum disorders: Challenges in early differential diagnosis.* Symposium presented at the Annual Meeting of the American Speech-Language-Hearing Association, Boston.

Neef, N.A., Shade, D., & Miller, M.S. (1994). Assessing influential dimensions of reinforcers on choice in students with serious emotional disturbance. *Journal of Applied Behavior Analysis, 27,* 575–583.

Paul, R. (2007). *Language disorders from infancy through adolescence* (3rd ed.). St. Louis: Mosby.

Quill, K. (2006, November). *Translating complex treatment for autism into an organized conceptual framework.* Symposium presented at the Annual Meeting of the American Speech-Language-Hearing Association, Boston.

Reichle, J., Drager, K., & Davis, C. (2002). Using requests for assistance to obtain desired items and to gain release from nonpreferred activities: Implications for assessment and intervention. *Education and Treatment of Children, 25,* 47–66.

Reichle, J., & Johnston, S.S. (1999). Teaching the conditional use of communicative requests to two school-age children with severe developmental disabilities. *Language, Speech, and Hearing Services in Schools, 10,* 324–334.

Reichle, J., & McComas, J. (2004). Conditional use of a request for assistance. *Disability and Rehabilitation, 226,* 1255–1262.

Reichle, J., McComas, J., Dahl, N., Solberg, G., Pierce, S., & Smith, D. (2005). Teaching an individual with severe intellectual delay to request assistance conditionally. *Educational Psychology, 34,* 275–286

Richmond, G., & Bell, J. (1986). Comparison of trial-and-error and graduated stimulus change procedures across tasks. *Analysis and Intervention in Developmental Disabilities, 6,* 127–136.

Romski, M.A., & Sevcik, R.A. (1996). *Breaking the speech barrier: Language development through augmented means.* Baltimore: Paul H. Brookes Publishing Co.

Romski, M.A., Sevcik, R.A., Robinson, B.F., Mervis, C.B., & Bertrand, J. (1996). Mapping the meanings of novel visual symbols by youth with moderate or severe mental retardation. *American Journal on Mental Retardation, 100,* 391–402.

Serna, R.W., Wilkinson, K.M., & McIlvane, W.J. (1998). Blank-comparison assessment of stimulus-stimulus relations in individuals with mental retardation. *American Journal on Mental Retardation, 103,* 60–74.

Sevcik, R., & Romski, M.A. (2005). Early visual-graphic symbol acquisition by children with developmental disabilities. In L. Namy (Ed.), *Symbol use and symbolic representation: Developmental and comparative perspectives* (pp. 155–170). Mahwah, NJ: Lawrence Erlbaum Associates.

Sidman, M., & Stoddard, L.T. (1967). The effectiveness of fading in programming a simultaneous form discrimination for retarded children. *Journal of the Experimental Analysis of Behavior, 10,* 3–15.

Sigafoos, J., Drasgow, E., Reichle, J., O'Reilly, M., Green, V., & Tait, K. (2004). Teaching communicative rejecting to children with severe disabilities. *American Journal of Speech-Language Pathology, 13,* 31–42.

Stephenson, J. (2007). The effect of color on the recognition and use of line drawings by children with severe intellectual disabilities. *Augmentative and Alternative Communication, 23,* 44–55.

Stevens, T., & Karmiloff-Smith, A. (1997). Word learning in a special population: Do individuals with Williams syndrome obey lexical constraints? *Journal of Child Language, 24,* 737–765.

Sullivan, M., Finelli, J., Marvin, A., Garrett-Mayer, E., Bauman, M., & Landa, R. (2007). Response to joint attention in toddlers at risk for autism spectrum disorders: a prospective study. *Journal of Autism and Developmental Disorders, 37,* 37–48.

Toth, K., Munson, J., Meltzoff, A.N., & Dawson, G. (2006). Early predictors of communication development in young children with autism spectrum disorder: Joint attention, imitation, and toy play. *Journal of Autism & Development Disorders, 36,* 993–1005.

Trudeau, N., Cleave, P., & Woelk, E.J. (2003). Using augmentative and alternative communication approaches to promote participation of preschoolers during book reading: A pilot study. *Child Language Teaching and Therapy, 19,* 181–210.

Utley, B.L. (2002). Visual assessment considerations for the design of AAC systems. In D.R. Beukelman & J. Reichle (Series Eds.) & J. Reichle, D.R. Beukelman, & J.C. Light (Vol. Eds.), *Augmentative and alternative communication series. Exemplary practices for beginning communicators: Implications for AAC* (pp. 353–394). Baltimore: Paul H. Brookes Publishing Co.

Wainwright, J.A., & Bryson, S.E. (1996). Visual-spatial orienting in autism. *Journal of Autism and Developmental Disorders, 26,* 423–438.

Warren, S.F., & Yoder, P. (1997). Emerging model of communication and language intervention. *Mental Retardation and Developmental Disabilities Research Reviews, 3,* 358–362.

Warreyn, P., Roeyers, H., Van Wetswinkel, U., & De Groote, I. (2007). Temporal coordination of joint attention behavior in preschoolers with autism spectrum disorder. *Journal of Autism and Developmental Disorders, 37,* 501–512.

Watt, N., Wetherby, A., & Shumway, S. (2006). Prelinguistic predictors of language outcome at 3 years of age. *Journal of Speech, Language, and Hearing Research, 49,* 1224–1237.

Wetherby, A.M. (2006). Understanding and measuring social communication in children with autism spectrum disorders. In T. Charman & W. Stone (Eds.), *Social and communication development in autism spectrum disorders: Early identification, diagnosis, and intervention* (pp. 3–34). New York: Guilford Press.

Wetherby, A.M., & Prizant, B.M. (1993). *Communication and Symbolic Behavior Scales™ (CSBS).* Baltimore: Paul H. Brookes Publishing Co.

Whalen, C., & Schreibman, L. (2003). Joint attention training for children with autism using behavior modification procedures. *Journal of Child Psychology and Psychiatry, 44,* 456–468.

Wilhelm, H., & Lovaas, O. (1976). Stimulus overselectivity: a common feature in autism and mental retardation. *American Journal of Mental Deficiency, 81,* 26–31.

Wilkinson, K.M. (2005). Disambiguation and mapping of new word meanings by individuals with intellectual/developmental disabilities. *American Journal on Mental Retardation, 110,* 71–86.

Wilkinson, K.M. (2007). The effect of "missing" information on retention of fast mapped labels by individuals with receptive vocabulary limitations associated with intellectual disability. *American Journal on Mental Retardation, 112,* 40–53.

Wilkinson, K.M., & Albert, A. (2001). Adaptations of fast mapping for vocabulary intervention with augmented language users. *Augmentative and Alternative Communication, 17,* 120–132.

Wilkinson, K.M., Carlin, M., & Jagaroo, V. (2006). Preschoolers' speed of locating a target symbol under different color conditions. *Augmentative and Alternative Communication, 22,* 123–133.

Wilkinson, K.M., Carlin, M., & Thistle, J. (2008). Sensitivity of children with and without Down syndrome to color cuing in aided symbol displays. *American Journal of Speech-Language Pathology, 17,* 179–193.

Wilkinson, K.M., & Green, G. (1998). Implications of "fast mapping" for vocabulary expansion in individuals with mental retardation. *Augmentative and Alternative Communication, 14,* 162–170.

Wilkinson, K.M., & Hennig, S. (2007). The state of research and practice in augmentative and alternative communication for children with developmental/intellectual disabilities. *Mental Retardation and Developmental Disabilities Research Reviews, 13,* 58–69.

Wilkinson, K.M., & McIlvane, W.J. (2002). Considerations in teaching graphic symbols. In D.R. Beukelman & J. Reichle (Series Eds.) & J. Reichle, D.R. Beukelman, & J.C. Light (Vol. Eds.), *Augmentative and alternative communication series. Exemplary practices for beginning communicators: Implications for AAC* (pp. 273–322). Baltimore: Paul H. Brookes Publishing Co.

Wilkinson, K.M., & Rosenquist, C. (2006). Demonstration of a method for assessing semantic organization and category membership in individuals with autism spectrum disorders and receptive vocabulary limitations. *Augmentative and Alternative Communication, 22,* 242–257.

Yoder, P., & McDuffie, A.S. (2006). Treatment of responding to and initiating joint attention. In T. Charman & W. Stone (Eds.), *Social and communication development in autism spectrum disorders* (pp. 117–142). New York: Guilford Press.

Yoder, P., & Stone, W.L. (2006). Randomized comparison of two communication interventions for preschoolers with autism spectrum disorders. *Journal of Consulting and Clinical Psychology, 74,* 426–435.

IV

AAC-Related Issues

14

Literacy in Individuals with Autism Spectrum Disorders Who Use AAC

DAVID A. KOPPENHAVER AND KAREN A. ERICKSON

- - - - - But surpassing all stupendous inventions, what sublimity of mind was his who dreamed of finding means to communicate his deepest thoughts to any other person, though distant by mighty intervals of place and time! Of talking with those who are in India; of speaking to those who are not yet born and will not he born for a thousand or ten thousand years; and with what facility, by the different arrangements of twenty characters upon a page!

Galileo Galilei, 1632

Galileo long ago recognized the value of written language in communicating across time and place. Even today, nearly 400 years later, his written language facility beautifully elucidates his argument. However, only recently have scholars recognized the power of written language, not just for distance communications but also for meeting the more immediate and face-to-face communication needs of individuals who use augmentative and alternative communication (AAC; Blackstone, 1989). In relation to individuals with autism spectrum disorders (ASDs) who use AAC, only recently have scholars begun to discuss written language as anything more than aberrant, as in the case of hyperlexia (e.g., Cobrinik, 1974); questionable, as in the case of facilitated communication (e.g., Green & Shane, 1994); or unattainable, as in a readiness view of literacy learning (e.g., Koppenhaver, Coleman, Kalman, & Yoder, 1991).

The first major review of literacy as it relates to individuals with ASDs who use AAC was published in 2000 (Mirenda & Erickson, 2000) and was followed soon after by a themed journal issue focused on the same topic (Bedrosian & Koppenhaver, 2003). The goals of this chapter are to extend and broaden some of the issues initiated in those two previous reviews, focusing especially on literacy intervention issues. In this chapter, literacy in its various iterations first will be defined and described. Next, parallel models of separate aspects of literacy (i.e., both reading and writing) will be overviewed. Finally, the research literature on persons with ASDs, particularly those who use AAC, will be explored before implications for clinical practice and research are discussed.

DEFINITION AND DESCRIPTION OF LITERACY

Literacy has become an increasingly nebulous construct in recent years, with the creation of terms like *cultural literacy, media literacy, computer literacy,* and arguments that digital technologies have brought about *new literacies* (e.g., Leu, Leu, & Coiro, 2004). It is clear that culture, media, technology, and a host of other factors affect literacy learning. They are not viewed in this chapter, however, as forms of literacy but rather as separate competencies in and of themselves that may— but do not inherently—affect written language learning.

Literacy is defined in this chapter quite simply as reading and writing (i.e., the cognitive processes of comprehending and composing meaning in written texts). Reading or spelling words in isolation are subskills that are necessary but not solely sufficient to meet the criteria of these definitions of reading and writing. Literacy is a powerful tool for achieving a wide range of communication and learning activities both in real time (e.g., face-to-face interactions involving initial letter cuing or abbreviation/expansion techniques) and across time and distance (e.g., grocery lists compiled during the morning at home and used in the afternoon at the store).

Theoretical Foundations

The discussion of literacy in this chapter references a pair of cognitive models of reading with comprehension and writing to compose a message. The models provide the theoretical foundations for examining and interpreting the literacy research involving individuals with ASDs who require AAC. Use of the models in this chapter is based on the premise that the cognitive processes of children with ASDs who require AAC are similar to those of typically developing children in that relative learning success is a result of both individual skill and learning opportunities. More than a philosophical perspective, such a view is supported by Nation and colleagues' review of the literature (Nation, 1999) and examination of the learning characteristics of individuals with ASDs (Nation, Clark, Wright, & Williams, 2006).

A Reading Model   Cunningham's whole-to-part model (1993) is based on the premise that the ultimate goal of reading instruction or intervention is to teach students to read silently with comprehension. The term *whole-to-part* is used to indicate that the whole construct, reading silently with comprehension, is made up of parts, each of which is a whole construct itself. The parts, or components, can each be assessed and taught in isolation or in integration with the other components to help students read silently with comprehension. The components include word identification, language comprehension, and print processing of text.

Word identification is defined as the cognitive process of making print-to-sound links to translate both familiar and unfamiliar printed words into their pronunciations. The translation need not be vocal; in fact, it is typically subvocal or neurological in skilled readers (e.g., Cunningham & Cunningham, 1978). Familiar words are translated automatically without conscious attention of the reader. Unfamiliar words are mediated, or decoded, by the reader using a variety of phonic or morphemic strategies. *Language comprehension* refers specifically in this model to written language comprehension or the intersection of language skills required to understand text whether it is read orally, silently, or presented in another mode (e.g., signed or read aloud). Language comprehension comprises both knowledge of the world and knowledge of text structures. *Print processing* of text involves cognitive control of eye movements across and down pages of text, making links directly from printed words to their meanings, using inner speech to monitor relative reading success, projecting prosody, and integrating the use of these four skills. All of these cognitive skills are carried on beyond the single-word level in print processing. An elaborated discussion of this model with respect to students who use AAC was presented in Erickson, Koppenhaver, and Cunningham (2006).

A Writing Model   The model of written composition described here draws on the work of Flower and Hayes (1981), with modest adaptations to include Singer and Bashir's (2004) view of the role of production in composition. It is also described as a whole-to-part model because the individual constructs are wholes themselves but contribute as parts to the overall ability to convey meaning through writing. The components of written composition include planning, translating, reviewing, text production, and monitoring.

Planning is composed of the processes of setting goals, generating ideas, and organizing thoughts relative to a written text. *Translating* requires the writer to convey ideas such as images, sensory impressions, and spoken language into written language that follows print conventions. *Reviewing* is composed of both revision (i.e., reorganizing existing text) and evaluation (i.e., appraising the degree to which a text fulfills the writer's plan). *Text production* refers to the speed and mode of recording printed words on or in various media and is influenced by the writer's graphomotor skills (Singer & Bashir, 2004) and the availability of individually appropriate writing tools (e.g., pencils, keyboards, spelling prediction software, and other technologies). Text production is particularly relevant to understanding the composition process of people who use AAC tools as their writing instruments. Such tools typically require conscious attention to the tool itself, which, verbal efficiency theory (Perfetti, 1985) suggests would limit cognitive resources available to other composition processes. Finally, *monitoring* refers to the writer's ability to attend to and adjust the application of these component processes while composing a given text.

Emergent Literacy   A final definition and description is required before addressing the literature on literacy skills of individuals with ASDs who use AAC. Each of the models described above refers to conventional literacy (i.e., reading and writing that follows the conventions of spelling, grammar, and use that facilitate communication between literate individuals). However, literacy also may take emergent forms.

Emergent literacy refers to the nonconventional and often idiosyncratic behaviors and understandings that developing learners exhibit prior to achieving conventional literacy. Emergent literacy is evident when a preschooler with developmental disabilities uses the language of a favorite book, *Millions of Cats* (Gág, 2002), to describe her drawing, saying "I made hundreds of dots, thousands of dots, millions and billions and trillions of dots" (Butler, 1980). It is no less evident in the adult with ASD who spells *vacuum* as *vacm, sponge* as *spoj,* or *broom* as *brum* when writing opportunities are introduced into his supported employment setting (Foley & Staples, 2003).

Emergent literacy is more a function of experience than of development. Emergent literacy, because of its reliance on nonconventional print forms, depends on either an individual's oral interpretation of what he or she has written or on a reader's knowledge of the individual's background. *Conventional literacy,* on the other hand, is more independent in nature because it follows conventions of form. Individuals who are conventionally literate can write and read texts created by other conventionally literate individuals; the same cannot be said of individuals who are emergent readers and writers.

Conventional literacy is not a unitary construct that is achieved at a particular point in time. Rather, conventional literacy exists along a continuum from beginning literacy, demonstrated by many young readers and writers in their first few years of formal schooling, to the highly sophisticated forms of literacy exhibited by authors, poets, philosophers, or scholars in any field of human endeavor. Conventional literacy, thus, is a normative concept; children in school are said to be conventionally literate if they read and write at levels of competence comparable to other typically developing children of the same age (Perfetti, 1985).

LITERACY IN ASD AS REFERENCED TO MODELS OF LITERACY

Prior to 1990 and the introduction of facilitated communication (Biklen, 1990), research on literacy for individuals with ASDs focused largely on two areas of study: hyperlexia and sight word instruction. These lines of research demonstrated that some individuals with autism could learn to identify words through a variety of different teaching approaches but that their comprehension of those words, particularly in text, often lagged far behind (e.g., Cobrinik, 1974).

With the publication of Biklen's 1990 paper on facilitated communication, the research focus shifted to investigations of literacy as a means to support communication, largely in the form of experimental studies attempting to (in)validate authorship. On the basis of these experimental studies, it was concluded that facilitated communication, with rare exceptions (e.g., Cardinal, Hanson, & Wakeham, 1996), led to messages constructed more by facilitators than the individuals with ASDs they had been intending to assist (e.g., Green & Shane, 1994). Neither of these areas of study resulted in information that could be translated easily to inform practice, nor were they completed with reference to models of literacy development and use that could be employed to frame the results in a broader context. The focus of the remainder of this literature review will be on contextualizing the literacy research in this regard and examining other types of studies with reference to the whole-to-part models of reading and writing described above. Not all of the research studies provide specific information regarding the communication skills of individual participants; however, this information is provided whenever available.

Reading

In the largest existing study of reading profiles in this area, Nation et al. (2006) reported on 41 children with ASDs, ages 6–15 years, who had language skills that were sufficient for their participation in traditional, unadapted assessments of various aspects of reading. When examined with reference to the whole-to-part model of reading, the findings of this study revealed common profiles of strengths and weaknesses that have clinical and research implications. The specific components of the whole-to-part model that were assessed by Nation et al. included mediated word identification, which was assessed using a nonsense word task and an untimed word identification task. Although no measures of automatic word recognition were employed, print processing was assessed with a proxy task requiring the participants to read connected text aloud. Language comprehension for text (e.g., understanding text read aloud by another person) was not assessed, but the subskill of knowledge of the world was assessed with a single-word receptive vocabulary test and a sentence-level comprehension test.

Nine of the children in the study were unable to complete any of the assessment tasks and were excluded from further analyses. The mean performance of the 32 remaining children in mediated word identification tasks and print processing was within the normal range, but reading comprehension was approximately 1 standard deviation below population norms. The researchers noted that there was extreme variability within the sample, with performance on nearly every assessment ranging from floor to ceiling levels. Children who struggled with reading comprehension in general performed more poorly on the language comprehension measures than children with average and above-average reading comprehension scores. Nonsense word decoding tasks proved particularly difficult, with 42% of the sample performing at least 1 standard deviation below population norms.

Five children with average word identification performance scored at floor level on the nonsense-word reading test, perhaps supporting contentions that nonsense word reading tasks may introduce a level of complexity to decoding that does not accurately tap phonics knowledge (Cunningham et al., 1999). Nonsense words represent an attempt to insure that students must use decoding skills to complete the assessment task. However, they differ markedly from real-word decoding, because they do not involve manipulating the print-to-sound match to identify a known word. Instead, nonsense word tasks require the reader to make a print-to-speech match and judge its accuracy by comparing that speech match to known real words that might share the spelling pattern. Consequently, nonsense word tasks require a level of metalinguistic awareness that is not required when decoding real words. Such tasks may present substantial confusion for children with ASDs because they are reported to have widespread and significant language comprehension deficits (e.g., Kjelgaard & Tager-Flusberg, 2001; Lord & Paul, 1997).

Nation et al. (2006) suggested that their data demonstrated that "reading is not a unitary construct and that component skills may dissociate in cases of developmental disorder" (p. 918). However, the differential performance achieved across measures of word identification, print processing, and language comprehension may also furnish evidence that the whole-to-part model is applicable to individuals with ASDs. Component skills may dissociate for all sorts of causes, both intrinsic and extrinsic to the child. For example, children who receive an instructional emphasis on sight word recognition with little attention to other reading components would be likely to test well on word-level measures and less well on text-level or language comprehension tasks. It is also common for typically developing readers to demonstrate relative strengths and needs across the components of the whole-to-part model. Typical readers who perform poorly on general measures of language comprehension tend to perform poorly on measures of reading comprehension, as did the children in the Nation et al. study. These strengths and needs typically change from year to year in response to experience and instruction. The underlying causes of the observed performance of children with ASDs in this study and whether they might respond to focused interventions remain to be studied.

Myles et al. (2002) assessed the reading skills of 16 students with Asperger syndrome, age 6–16 years, using an informal reading inventory. Reported assessment results suggested that students' word identification, print processing, language comprehension, and overall reading performance were all approximately at grade level. Given the foundational role of language in reading (e.g., Catts & Kamhi, 2005), such a profile for developing readers suggests that language comprehension was the greatest area of need; a reader's ability to listen with comprehension typically exceeds the ability to read with comprehension until overall reading skills reach high school level (Erickson et al., 2006). This interpretation is further supported by the fact that participants demonstrated significantly greater difficulties responding accurately to inferential questions than to literal questions. One additional finding of note was that little difference was found between the children's instructional level (i.e., the text difficulty level at which children would achieve optimal learning with a teacher's guidance) and frustration level (i.e., the text difficulty level at which children would find it difficult to learn even with a teacher's assistance). The critical insight for clinical practice is that practitioners would need to devote considerable attention to assessing and monitoring relative text difficulty to achieve positive learning outcomes for children with ASDs.

Word Identification   As confirmed by the findings of Nation et al. (2006) and Myles et al. (2002), individuals with ASDs typically have demonstrated a relative strength in accurate word identification. Despite this evidence to suggest that intervention efforts should focus on building the language comprehension skills that are a relative weakness for this population, instead a good deal of research has focused on a wide variety of methods to teach accurate word identification with little attention to language comprehension.

Hyperlexia   Perhaps the most widely researched aspect of literacy in individuals with ASDs, hyperlexia refers to a significant discrepancy between well-developed word identification skills and difficulties in reading comprehension. While hyperlexia is not specific to ASD, most individuals with hyperlexia are on the autism spectrum (Grigorenko et al., 2002). Researchers have proposed that the prevalence of hyperlexia in individuals with ASDs is attributable to their relative strengths in perceptual processing along with relative deficits in associative and reasoning skills (Happé, 1994), obsessive and repetitive behaviors (Tirosh & Canby, 1993), and a specific deficit in using context to construct meaning (Frith, 2003). Nation (1999)—in reviewing the range of research pertaining to literacy development, ASDs, and hyperlexia—concluded that hyperlexia in people with ASDs is best understood as "a consequence of individual differences in a number of reading-related skills, and as such, their reading development can be well accommodated within a theoretical framework of normal reading development" (p. 352).

Influence of AAC   Most beginning communicators who require AAC depend on graphic symbols to communicate, at least until they develop sufficient literacy skills to allow them to use print to interact with others (Beukelman, Mirenda, & Sturm, 2005). The influence of graphic symbol use in AAC on the development of word identification skills remains unclear. When words are paired with graphic symbols as part of a comprehensive communication intervention, the symbols and words may be learned, even without direct instruction (Romski & Sevcik, 1996). However, research also has indicated that pairing graphic symbols and words is less effective than words used alone in the context of reading instruction (Rose & Furr, 1984; Singer, Samuels, & Spiroff, 1973; Singh & Solman, 1990).

Language Comprehension Severe oral language impairments have been widely documented in children with ASDs (e.g., Tager-Flusberg & Joseph, 2003). A consistent finding in studies of children with ASDs has been that they tend to demonstrate difficulties not just in reading comprehension tasks but also when listening to texts read aloud by others, suggesting underlying language comprehension deficits (Nation, 1999). Importantly, these deficits have been linked to overall cognitive and linguistic abilities. For example, while children with ASDs and cognitive impairments in a study by Snowling and Frith (1986) performed poorly on experimental sentence and text-level comprehension tasks, children with ASDs and no cognitive impairments performed comparably to typically developing children who were matched for reading age. Therefore, like typically developing children, the children with ASDs in this study tended to read with comprehension at levels comparable to their overall language comprehension levels.

Of relevance to language comprehension is *theory of mind*, a theoretical construct widely researched and reported to be delayed or impaired in as many as 80% of individuals with ASDs (Baron-Cohen, Leslie, and Frith, 1985). In fact, Baron-Cohen (1995) and others have asserted that the significant social impairments evident in children with ASDs are caused by impaired theory of mind. Theory of mind refers to the ability to perceive "oneself and others in terms of mental states—the desires, emotions, beliefs, intentions, and other inner experiences that result in and are manifested in human action" (Wellman, Cross, & Watson, 2001, p. 655).

In the whole-to-part model, theory of mind is an aspect of background knowledge (e.g., understanding of character motivation) that would assist in explaining some of the difficulties observed in language comprehension for individuals with ASDs. In fact, stories have been used to aid students with ASDs in developing a greater understanding of theory of mind (e.g., Nelson, 1996). However, research has yet to thoroughly explore the relationship of language development and theory of mind (Astington, 2001).

Teaching Vocabulary Meaning Word identification has long been recognized as a relative strength in students with ASDs. Consequently, investigators have addressed a good deal of attention to strategies for teaching students with ASDs word meanings and the use of those words for receptive and expressive communication. Several early studies demonstrated that individuals with ASDs and intellectual disabilities can learn to use printed words to enhance their communication by requesting or labeling a preferred object (Hewitt, 1964; LaVigna,

1977; McGee, Krantz, & McClannahan, 1986) and communicating their wants and needs (Hewitt, 1964). Recent studies have provided a closer examination of the types of behavioral approaches that are most effective in teaching word reading skills to individuals with ASDs.

Eikeseth and Jahr (2001) compared rates of acquisition of receptive and expressive word reading and sign language use to support communication. The four participants with ASDs used a combination of printed words, pictures, and signs across four conditions. The first condition was reading (receptive) in which the child was shown three pictures and asked to match a printed word with the correct picture. In the writing (expressive) condition, the child was presented with three printed words and asked to match a picture to the correct word. In the receptive signing condition, the child was provided with three pictures and was asked to find the picture that matched a sign produced by the researcher. In the expressive signing condition, the child was provided with three pictures and asked to produce the correct sign in response to the question "What is it?" The instruction in each condition was the same: Correct responses were met with praise, smiles, and individualized reinforcements, whereas incorrect responses resulted in a verbal response of "no" and the removal of the training stimuli. The results suggested that the receptive reading condition was acquired more easily than any other. Two of the participants never acquired receptive signing and one never acquired either of the expressive skills (writing or signing). Furthermore, all four participants demonstrated maintenance of the reading skills they acquired. The results of this study suggested that children with ASDs can learn to match printed words to pictures given sufficient trials.

Fossett and Mirenda (2006) compared picture-to-text matching with a paired associate learning task. Two of the participants in this study learned to read five individual words by matching those words with pictures during the intervention. However, they were relatively unsuccessful in acquiring five words presented through paired association with a picture. Furthermore, they retained the five words learned through text-to-picture matching when assessed 4 months after the intervention was terminated. The authors suggested that the active role the participants played in physically matching the word to a picture allowed the instructional strategy to overcome the well-known blocking effect that appears to occur when words are simply paired with pictures (Didden, Prinsen, & Sigafoos, 2000; Singh & Solman, 1990).

One final study of note by McGee, Krantz, and McClannahan (1986) involved an investigation of incidental teaching procedures to promote word reading in children with ASDs. Two participants in the study quickly learned to read words to request desired toys and locate toys stored in boxes. The instructional approach differed markedly from the picture-to-text matching procedures mentioned previously in that the use of the text was supported incidentally when the researcher interacted with the child participant in a play session. Much like the development of emergent literacy skills noted by Koppenhaver and Erickson (2003) in the context of child-led interactions, these children learned to read the words because they could use them in personally meaningful ways to gain desired toys. Furthermore, the children maintained their understanding and use of the words and transferred their knowledge of the words to novel stimuli 15 and 25 days following the completion of the intervention.

Interestingly, this final study is one of the few that bears any resemblance to best practice in vocabulary instruction for typically developing children. Best practice recommendations include immersing students in language-rich environments, helping students make connections between their existing vocabulary and words to be learned, providing students with multiple examples of appropriate use of the target vocabulary in meaningful contexts, and providing students with opportunities to use and reuse target vocabulary (Beck, McKeown, & Kucan, 2002). Although studies of word reading skills have provided evidence that individuals with ASDs can learn to read words and use those words to communicate with others, it is far from clear if the strategies studied are the most efficient or effective, or the extent to which learned skills generalize. These issues are particularly important for individuals with ASDs who require AAC because written words provide an important means of communication. Furthermore, these individuals need to acquire these words in large numbers while maintaining and transferring that knowledge to maximize communicative competence.

Teaching Comprehension of Text   Few intervention studies of text-based language comprehension have been found in the literature. One of note is the study by O'Connor and Klein (2004) on "procedural facilitation" (p. 117)—that is, text structure modifications intended to prompt various executive processes the researchers believed might improve comprehension. Participants included 25 students with ASDs, age 14–17 years, who were perceived as high functioning. Texts at the sixth-grade level were modified in one of three ways: 1) prereading questions were added to facilitate reader consideration of personal knowledge and experiences related to the text's main ideas; 2) a cloze version of each passage was made in which blanks could be completed with words other than pronouns by attending to information within the three preceding sentences; and 3) an anaphoric cueing version of the passage was made in which 12 pronouns were underscored and three possible referents provided for each.

All three adaptations were essentially different forms of assessment from a reading education perspective. Anaphoric cueing resulted in significantly better performance on postreading comprehension questions, perhaps because it alone was a modification that provided rather than requested information, albeit accompanied by two distractors. On postreading questions, participants tended to provide list-like recall of main events rather than story grammar elements in retellings, partial information rather than complete responses in main idea items, and titles referring to main characters or objects but not main ideas. The results suggested language-related difficulties and pointed to the importance of distinguishing between assessment and teaching procedures when designing interventions for people with ASDs.

Individuals Who Use AAC   Reports in the literature have indicated considerable variation across individuals who use AAC in their semantic and specific vocabulary knowledge (Udwin & Yule, 1990). Some children have demonstrated the ability to acquire vocabulary through the same fast-mapping channels as their peers without disabilities, but the process has been slow at best (Romski, Sevcik, & Robinson, 1996). Children with the most developed language skills and internal lexicon appear to have made up for limitations in the external lexicons in their AAC systems by employing a variety of metalinguistic compensation strategies, such as the use of synonyms, homonyms, and modification markers (e.g., "It's in the same category as…."; Soto, 1999).

Unfortunately, the severe oral language impairments that have been widely documented in children with ASDs (e.g., Tager-Flusberg & Joseph, 2003) and the limited research with young children with ASDs who use speech to communicate (e.g., McDuffie, Yoder & Stone, 2006) both suggest that children with ASDs who use AAC typically encounter great difficulty with fast mapping and the use of metalinguistic compensation strategies. As a consequence, they have been at risk for restricted vocabulary development over time and consequent difficulties with both oral and written language comprehension.

The positive relationship between vocabulary knowledge and comprehension of both oral and written language has been well documented (e.g., Muter, Hulme, Snowling, & Stevenson, 2004; National Institute of Child Health and Human Development, 2000). Children without disabilities have been reported to possess oral language vocabularies approaching 14,000 words by the age of 6 years (Clark, 1993). Given the difficulty young children with ASDs who require AAC are likely to encounter in acquiring new vocabulary and the complexity of organizing large vocabulary sets of use in AAC (Yorkston, Dowden, Honsinger, Marriner, & Smith, 1988), acquiring even 10% of this vocabulary for use in communication and literacy learning is often a daunting task.

Print Processing   There has been a lack of research into print processing in the ASD literature. Nonetheless, case study reports and studies of the facilitative effects of written language on language learning have indicated that print processing also may be a relative strength of students with ASDs. Broderick and Kasa-Hendrickson (2001), for example, reported the case an adolescent with autism who initially used facilitated communication for approximately 8 years, then learned to type independently, and finally began to speak at the age of 12–13 years. The researchers noted a variety of supportive experiences that led to the child's use of speech, including instances in which he 1) typed and read aloud what he typed and 2) listened to what he typed read aloud on his speech-generating device, a Lightwriter, as he followed the scrolling text with his eyes.

Similarly, Craig and Telfer (2005) reported the case of a child diagnosed with pervasive developmental disorder-not otherwise specified. The boy was described as hyperlexic, scoring at the 95th percentile in decoding, the 84th percentile in oral reading accuracy (i.e., a proxy measure of print processing), and the 16th percentile in comprehension on standardized tests of reading as a second grader. The researchers not only observed his greater attention and success with written rather than oral language, but also used it to improve his receptive language and reading comprehension skills. For example, he was observed to respond much more successfully to *wh–* questions in the context of storybook reading than in conversation. Written words were used to cue his response to questions, build his oral language vocabulary, and introduce new language concepts; these were gradually faded. In upper elementary school, the boy often wrote elaborated responses to questions that he was not capable of generating orally. Written schedules, notes, outlines, and other visual materials were used to prepare and support his learning in various classes.

Relative strengths in word identification and print processing may have contributed to the successful use of written language to modify the behavior of individuals with ASDs. Two commonly reported intervention techniques have been written schedules (e.g., McClannahan & Krantz, 1999) and Social Stories (e.g., Delano & Snell, 2006). Written schedules have been used within tasks to support greater independence in completing specific tasks and between tasks to assist participants in predicting what will happen next (see Chapter 11; also,

Mirenda & Erickson, 2000). Written schedules have been found to reduce aggression, self-injury, and the need for other supports such as adult direction or discrete trial training (Flannery & Horner, 1994; Stromer, Kimball, Kinney, & Taylor, 2006).

Social Stories initially were introduced by Gray and Garand (1993) as an intervention aimed at helping children with ASDs negotiate social situations. In addition to detailing the most important aspects of social situations, Social Stories provide information about the likely reactions of others in the situation and describe appropriate interactions. Reading and discussing Social Stories have been found to lead to decreases in incidences of inappropriate behavior, increases in appropriate behaviors, and greater social engagement, although results across studies have not been consistent (Delano & Snell, 2006).

In keeping with the whole-to-part reading model, the relative strengths of students with ASDs in word identification and print processing may be strategic rather than aberrant or in some way an intrinsic aspect of ASD. That is, individuals with ASDs who demonstrate an orientation to written language—and find it facilitative of language learning, scheduling, or behavior improvement—may be relying on their relative strengths in word identification and print processing to compensate for their relative difficulties with language comprehension. The profile of the boy in the Craig and Telfer (2005) study, discussed earlier, begs such an interpretation. Whether such a profile would be found in other individuals with ASDs, who experience benefits from written language interventions to address behavioral goals, has yet to be explored.

Writing

Mayes and Calhoun (2006) investigated the overall written language capabilities of 124 children with ASDs, age 6–16 years, who had been evaluated in their outpatient diagnostic clinic or child psychiatry unit. Using a battery of standardized tests, the researchers found that 60% of the children with intelligence within the normal range had learning disabilities in written expression; their criterion for this judgment was a Wechsler Individual Achievement Test (Wechsler, 1992) written expression subtest score that was significantly lower than predicted, based on the child's Wechsler Intelligence Scale for Children–Third Edition (Wechsler, 1991) full-scale IQ. At the same time, learning disabilities in reading and spelling were identified in just 6%–9% of this same group of children. That written expression broadly, but not spelling specifically, would be such a widespread and significant difficulty for this sample of children with ASDs parallels the findings in reading reported by Nation et al. (2006), who found relative strengths in word identification and significant challenges with language comprehension.

Other studies of writing, although not numerous, also provide insight into various aspects of the writing process in individuals with ASDs. The whole-to-part model of writing (Flower & Hayes, 1981) is used below as a framework for discussing this work.

Translation and Writing Quality   Rousseau, Krantz, Poulson, Kitson, and McClannahan (1994) studied sentence-combining as a strategy for increasing adjective use and writing quality in three adolescents with autism, moderate cognitive impairments, and language delays. In doing so, they borrowed from the best practice literature in writing instruction for typically developing children (Hillocks, 1984). The authors used a multiple-baseline design to compare the relative effects of reinforcement for adjective use to those of sentence combining. During two baseline phases, the students first wrote in response to a picture prompt, receiving no reinforcement for adjective use and then receiving a penny to be used in a token economy during the baseline with reinforcement phase.

During intervention, students were taught to combine shorter sentences into longer single sentences (e.g., *The ^ horse is brown. The horse is fast.* = *The fast horse is brown.*) by inserting an underlined adjective from the second sentence into the space marked with a caret in the first sentence. After 13 sessions, the carets were removed. Immediately following the sentence-combining activities, the students wrote responses to picture prompts and received reinforcement for the use of adjectives in their writing. Overall results showed improved writing quality, a significant increase in adjective use when writing, and continued increases in the use of new adjectives during the maintenance period after sentence-combining activities were discontinued. On the basis of the whole-to-part writing model, it can be argued that the practice of combining simple sentences into more complex structures provided practice in the skill of translating ideas into language more efficiently, thereby enabling greater attention to other components of the writing process and enhancing overall writing quality.

Planning, Translation, and Writing Quality   Colasent and Griffith (1998) explored the effects of reading aloud thematically related stories on writing quality and quantity in three young adolescents with ASDs, ages 12–15 years. Student abilities, based on a variety of standardized measures, were in the range of second to third grade in spelling and word recognition, 51–64 in verbal IQ, and either untestable or unreported in reading comprehension. Students were asked to retell three thematically related stories, first orally and then using writing and drawing. Writing and drawing were found to result in more complete retellings. All three students wrote longer texts with more elaborated vocabulary and sentences following the third story.

In keeping with the whole-to-part model of writing, it is likely that improved writing was due to at least two factors. First, the oral retelling and use of pictures may have assisted planning by enabling students to capture larger ideas efficiently, visualize story details, rehearse those ideas, and organize the ideas before and during writing. Second, repeated readings in thematically-related stories may have increased knowledge of core concepts and vocabulary, thereby facilitating the process of translating the story retelling into written text.

Planning, Translation, Production, Reviewing, and Writing Quality

In the most complete intervention study of writing process in ASD to date, Bedrosian, Lasker, Speidel, and Politsch (2003) reported on the decision-making process and outcomes of an intervention for an adolescent with ASD who used AAC. The intervention involved use of technological supports, including multimedia writing software and task-specific vocabulary programmed into an AAC device. Explicit instruction was provided in both the use of the technologies and the collaborative writing process. Both a clinician and peer-modeled turn taking, negotiating story content, writing process, and completion of story maps. Finally, the clinician provided prompting as needed in the collaboration and the peer provided scaffolding for the writing of the adolescent with ASD.

Across four stories, the adolescent demonstrated an increase in the percentage of ideas contributed during the story map planning, hand-written and typed entries, and the percentage and range of edits and revisions. Both the adolescent with ASD and his peer partner indicated on a questionnaire that they believed their communication and writing skills had also improved as a result of the intervention. The study provides a model for decision making, design, and reporting of intervention studies as a means of developing the evidence base to support literacy practices for individuals with ASDs who use AAC.

Relative to the whole-to-part model, it is understandable why the intervention was effective. Planning was supported by story boards and peer interaction. Translation was supported by peer modeling and interaction, story-specific vocabulary, and repeated experience in the process across four stories. Production was supported by the use of multimedia writing software and turn taking in authorship with peers. Reviewing was facilitated by peer interactions, teacher feedback, and the story boards. Thus, nearly every aspect of the writing process was supported by peers, the clinician, and technologies.

Emergent Literacy

There is little emergent literacy research involving children with ASDs who use AAC. However, two existing lines of research have seemed particularly promising: studies of storybook reading and integration of print experiences into environments serving individuals with ASDs to provide increased learning opportunities. Both may provide opportunities for children with ASDs who use AAC to employ relative strengths in word identification and print processing to promote early language learning.

Storybook Reading   Skotko, Koppenhaver, and Erickson (2004) reported on the use of parent–child storybook reading as a context for teaching early communication using AAC to young girls with Rett syndrome. Research participants were mothers and their four daughters, age 3½–7 years. The girls all had severe communication impairments and the hand-wringing and/or hand-mouthing behaviors that are characteristic of Rett syndrome. All had normal hearing and vision; age equivalent scores were 5–19 months on the Bayley Scales of Infant Development (Bayley, 1993) and 9–17 months on the Vineland Adaptive Behavior Scales (Sparrow, Balla, & Cicchetti, 1984). The four-phase study included baseline during which 1) mothers read with their daughters, then 2) hand splints were introduced to increase functional hand use, 3) AAC devices and symbols were provided, and 4) training and guidance were provided in use of the AAC devices and symbols to support communication.

Although none of the girls communicated symbolically prior to the study, over the course of the intervention, all showed increased use of a single-message speech generating device (SGD) with a Picture Communication Symbol, using it appropriately for labels and comments 58%–72% of the time. Mothers modified their behaviors across the study in several specific ways that led to increased child participation and success. First, they increased wait time after making a comment or asking a question. Next, they modeled the use of Picture Communication Symbols by pointing until their daughters saw where they were pointing. Finally, they encouraged the natural use of the SGD to label or make predictions by asking questions or making comments to which the child's available symbols were a logical communication turn.

Correlation and multiple regression analyses suggested that, for each of the girls, a different combination of the mothers' behaviors led to increasingly successful communication attempts. For example, one mother's confirmations, requests for clarification, use of directives, and prediction questions were significantly associated with increased eye-pointing and activation of a single-message SGD for her daughter. Another mother's labeling and requests for clarification were associated with her child's increased labeling, page turning, and use of the single-message SGD. Although girls with Rett syndrome have not presented the same profile associated with individuals who have other forms of ASDs, the success of the intervention for these children with multiple disabilities points to the importance of early intervention and the value of predictable language routines such as storybook reading.

Bellon, Ogletree, and Harn (2000) examined the efficacy of repeated storybook reading supported by adult scaffolding to increase spontaneous language use by a speaking preschooler with ASD, age 3 years 10 months. Five adult–child storybook reading interactions were conducted across eight 45-minute intervention sessions. Scaffolding strategies included cloze statements (e.g., *She said, "Get me some _____."*), binary choices (e.g., *Do you want to swim or splash?*), expansions (e.g., after a child says, "cow," the adult might say, "The cow jumped"), and constituent questions (e.g., *What happened?*). Repeated storybook reading with scaffolding proved successful in decreasing echolalic responses and increasing spontaneous language.

Together, these studies suggest that storybook reading is an activity that is relatively easily modified and supportive of early print awareness and AAC. Storybook interactions can be constructed so as to promote language expression in young children with ASDs. Early interventions such as these have the potential to begin to address the language deficits reported in so many school-age children with ASDs.

Increased Learning Opportunities   Two studies involving individuals with ASDs have indicated that learning opportunities may be at least as important as individual capability in promoting literacy and communication development. As described below, the participants in these two studies had cognitive and linguistic impairments that led to limited literacy learning opportunities. However, when the environments and interactions were modified to provide greater learning opportunities, significant improvements in emergent literacy understandings and skills resulted.

Koppenhaver and Erickson (2003) reported on a study of three preschoolers with ASDs who required AAC. The children, age 3 years 3 months to 3 years 7 months, had delays in cognitive performance (0–12 months), cognitive verbal ability (4–17 months), and communication development (6–12 months). The intervention focused first on increasing natural opportunities for emergent literacy learning in the children's self-contained preschool classroom. Researchers provided a print-rich environment, a wide variety of reading and writing tools, and time for children to explore the print and the tools. During free play, the three children chose to explore reading materials 23%–85% of the time and writing tools 9%–12% of the time. The three children progressed from refusals to explore and random markings for their names to letter-like shapes and, in one case, conventional spelling.

The children's names became a cornerstone of several important literacy activities. A sign-in routine was employed each time the children interacted with the research team. Wanting the children to learn the form of their name after being motivated by its function, the researchers always encouraged the children to write their names first. Then, using hand-over-hand modeling, the researchers helped the children write their names conventionally, completing the activity with, "That's how you wrote your name. This is how I write your name. Let's go play." Additionally, after the students' names were added to morning circle activities, two of the children learned to identify all six of their classmates' names in print.

Other demonstrations of learning emerged from the variety of print experiences. One child was able to identify most of the letters of the alphabet and picked up sight words quickly from language experience texts, such as a repeated-line story about a field trip to the zoo. Another spelled out *bingo* independently during playtime after the song title had been available for several months as a morning circle activity choice. In this study, the children with ASDs who required AAC were easily engaged in emergent literacy activities that were playful and exploratory, and were able to demonstrate their growing understanding of print through choices, behaviors, writing, and use of picture communication symbols.

Foley and Staples (2003) described how they integrated AAC and literacy interventions into a supported employment setting serving five adults with ASD. The intervention involved four integrated strategies: 1) modification of the supported employment setting to increase communication and literacy learning opportunities; 2) theme-based, age-appropriate literacy content; 3) comprehensive literacy intervention involving reading skills and comprehension, writing, and reading motivation; and 4) intentional attempts to support transfer of learned skills to other community settings. Following intervention, all of the participants demonstrated gains in communicative competence and generalization to other settings. Four participants produced longer utterances through multiple communication modes and expressed a wider array of communicative intents. All five improved their ability to retell stories and use story vocabulary spontaneously, and all five were highly engaged in and motivated by the intervention.

Like the research on typically developing children, these two emergent literacy interventions suggest that opportunity to learn is at least as important as individual capability. Participants in both studies had performed poorly on cognitive and linguistic measures, leading professionals serving them to 1) assume reduced learning capability, 2) place them in print-deprived environments, 3) provide them few opportunities to use print materials, and 4) interact with them only rarely about print use. All participants demonstrated significant improvements in emergent literacy understandings and skills when the environments were made more print-rich and interactions increased around the integrated use of that print.

CLINICAL IMPLICATIONS

Dr. James Cunningham of the University of North Carolina–Chapel Hill frequently told students in his graduate courses on reading diagnosis and intervention that, in the absence of truth, it is important to diversify. That is, when the best solution is unknown, it is wise to try a variety of approaches. This axiom holds also when considering the clinical implications of the work discussed above.

Conventional Literacy

The whole-to-part models used to organize this chapter represent ways of diversifying intervention programs systematically. Each is an attempt to represent reading and writing as cognitive skills composed of whole parts, which can be assessed and taught in isolation or integration. Adapted informal assessments exist to examine the relative strengths and needs of students with ASDs who use AAC across these whole parts of reading (Erickson et al., 2006) and writing (Foley, Koppenhaver, & Williams, in press).

An important application of these assessments has been to determine individual needs given the prevalence of hyperlexia in the general population of individuals with ASDs. Schools in the United States are required by federal law to provide scientifically based instruction, derived largely from the National Reading Panel's review of reading in typically developing children (National Institute of Child Health and Human Development, 2000). The conclusion from that research is that beginning readers—including struggling learners—benefit from instruction focused on word-level skills and subskills (e.g., phoneme awareness). Most beginning and special reading programs currently employed in public schools focus largely or even exclusively on teaching skilled decoding and/or sight word reading. For children with strengths in word identification but significant needs in written language comprehension, such interventions do little to address their primary learning needs, language comprehension and language expression. Assessments based on the whole-to-part models can be used to identify student needs and to monitor student response to the proffered interventions.

Emergent Literacy

The prevalent profile of school-age children with ASDs presented in the literature is that of a significant strength in word identification and significant need in language comprehension. Furthermore, the AAC and language development literature demonstrate that access to expressive communication is severely limited for most individuals who use AAC. Integrating expressive and receptive communication development with emergent reading and writing opportunities may enable young children to make greater sense of language through their strengths in identifying and spelling words.

Likewise, interactions structured around storybook reading would seem to offer greater support to early language learning than play-based activities lacking print integration. Storybook interactions can offer the repetition with variety that will enable children with ASDs to learn not just the word reading and spelling that seem to come relatively easily, but also the meaning and use of the language represented by that print. The written language of books—supported by pictures, modeling, play, and interaction—offer these students opportunities to examine and reexamine the use and meaning of language more intensively than the less observable oral language they seem to find relatively difficult to comprehend.

Finally, although best practice in emergent literacy suggests that integrating reading and writing opportunities into the environment is effective, it would seem especially critical in the case of children with ASDs who use AAC. Adding menus and a waitress notepad to a preschool restaurant play center, for example, provides the support of print to the learning of language, social routines, and AAC use. Every opportunity to communicate with and around print may provide the experience that enables these students to make greater sense of language content and use through their relative ease in learning its written forms.

RESEARCH IMPLICATIONS

With respect to the whole-to-part models of reading and writing and emergent literacy, three factors were considered in determining that the following areas of study might be the most fruitful in advancing knowledge of written language awareness and development in children with ASDs, particularly those who use AAC. First, the vast body of emergent and conventional literacy research involving typically developing children was examined in relation to those aspects that have led to the greatest advances in understanding. Second, the research on ASDs was reviewed with regard to what it suggested are significant areas of delay or difficulty across the models of emergent and conventional literacy. Finally, practitioners' experiences were examined as they attempted to support written language learning in children with ASDs who do and do not use AAC.

Aspects of the Whole-to-Part Model of Reading

Efforts to understand conventional literacy learning for children with ASDs who use AAC will be enhanced by improving understanding of the underlying causes of advanced word reading relative to comprehension skill demonstrated by many children with ASDs. Furthermore, research directed toward understanding the ways children with these profiles respond to interventions focused in areas of weakness, such as language comprehension, is needed.

Related to investigations of language comprehension, research that examines the environmental factors that best support broad and deep vocabulary learning in children with ASDs who use AAC are required. One currently untapped and potentially rich direction for such research would be an examination of how children with ASDs who use AAC respond to a wide variety of rich vocabulary instructional strategies that have been identified in the literature for typically developing children (e.g., Beck, McKeown, & Kucan, 2002).

Specific investigations of the oral language outcomes that result when children with ASDs who use AAC participate in reading comprehension lessons might address the impact of different forms of aided AAC, vocabulary selection techniques, reading materials, or lesson formats. Specific attention should be directed to comprehension instruction methods that increase student understanding of social stories or character motivation and whether such interventions influence theory of mind development for children with ASDs who use AAC.

Aspects of the Whole-to-Part Model of Writing

Although the research base in reading for children with ASDs is limited, the base in writing is even more so. Expanding on the use of sentence combining as an intervention to address syntactic complexity in writing with an additional focus on oral language or improved AAC device use is one obvious starting place. Other future directions for research in conventional writing might explore interventions that focus on revising texts for different audiences and the impact such interventions have on written language outcomes and the development of theory of mind.

Emergent Literacy

Storybook interactions have been the focus of investigations regarding early language and literacy development for typically developing young children and other populations (e.g., Teale & Sulzby, 1986; Van Kleeck, Vander Woude, & Hammett, 2006). Given that many children with ASDs have an orientation toward print materials, it is reasonable to expect that manipulating social interactions, vocabulary selection and representation in AAC, materials, and the learning environment during storybook reading could positively influence written and oral language outcomes.

The development of writing—from earliest reflections of alphabetic knowledge through the development of phonemic awareness, concept of word, and the accurate representation of letter sound relationships in words—presents another important area in need of future research. Koppenhaver and Erickson (2003) provided some initial evidence to suggest that young children with ASDs who use AAC can develop as writers given opportunities to engage in self-directed writing. Investigations of the effects of manipulating adult–child interactions around writing, the use of assistive technologies or AAC in early writing development, materials, or the learning environment would inform current understandings and future practice.

CONCLUSION

Individuals with ASDs, including those who use AAC, appear to find exploring in print interesting and relatively easy. It is long overdue for research and clinical practice to systematically investigate how this strength in understanding and use of the forms of print might be more effectively employed to address the greater challenges that these students find in understanding and using language in meaningful and communicative ways. There will no doubt be surprises to be discovered once scholars and practitioners move beyond the current constraints of an underresearched understanding of literacy in children with ASDs who use AAC.

REFERENCES

Astington, J.W. (2001). The future of theory-of-mind research: Understanding motivational states, the role of language, and real-world consequences. *Child Development, 72,* 685–687.

Baron-Cohen, S. (1995). *Mindblindness: An essay on autism and theory of mind.* Cambridge, MA: The MIT Press.

Baron-Cohen, S., Leslie, A.M., & Frith, U. (1985). Does the autistic child have a 'theory of mind'? *Cognition, 21,* 37–46.

Bayley, N. (1993). *Bayley Scales of Infant Development* (2nd ed.). San Antonio, TX: Harcourt Assessment.

Beck, I.L., McKeown, M.G., & Kucan, L. (2002). *Bringing words to life: Robust vocabulary instruction.* New York: Guilford Press.

Bedrosian, J.L., & Koppenhaver, D.A. (2003). Foreword. *Topics in Language Disorders, 23*(4), 269–270.

Bedrosian, J.L., Lasker, J., Speidel, K., & Politsch, A. (2003). Enhancing the written narrative skills of an AAC student with autism: Evidence-based research issues. *Topics in Language Disorders, 23*(4), 305–324.

Bellon, M.L., Ogletree, B.T., & Harn, W.E. (2000). Repeated storybook reading as a language intervention for children with autism: A case study on the application of scaffolding. *Focus on Autism and Other Developmental Disabilities, 15,* 52–58.

Beukelman, D.R., Mirenda, P., & Sturm, J. (2005). Literacy development of children who use AAC. In D.R. Beukelman & P. Mirenda (Eds.). *Augmentative and alternative communication: Supporting children and adults with complex communication needs* (3rd ed.). Baltimore: Paul H. Brookes Publishing Co.

Biklen, D. (1990). Communication unbound: Autism and praxis. *Harvard Educational Review, 60,* 291–314.

Blackstone, S.W. (1989). The 3 R's of reading, writing, and reasoning. *Augmentative Communication News, 2,* 1–3.

Broderick, A.A., & Kasa-Hendrickson, C. (2001). "Say just one word at first": The emergence of reliable speech in a student labeled with autism. *Journal of The Association for Persons with Severe Handicaps, 26,* 13–24.

Butler, D. (1980). *Cushla and her books.* Boston: Horn Book.

Cardinal, D., Hanson, D., & Wakeham, J. (1996). Investigation of authorship in facilitated communication. *Mental Retardation, 34,* 231–342.

Catts, H.W., & Kamhi, A.G. (Eds.). (2005). *The connections between language and reading disabilities.* Mahwah, NJ: Lawrence Erlbaum Associates.

Clark, E. (1993). *The lexicon in acquisition.* Cambridge, England: Cambridge University Press.

Cobrinik, L. (1974). Unusual reading ability in severely disturbed children. *Journal of Autism and Childhood Schizophrenia, 4,* 163–175.

Colasent, R., & Griffith, P.L. (1998). Autism and literacy: Looking into the classroom with rabbit stories. *Reading Teacher, 51,* 414–420.

Craig, H.K., & Telfer, A.S. (2005). Hyperlexia and autism spectrum disorder: A case study of scaffolding language growth over time. *Topics in Language Disorders, 25*(4), 364–374.

Cunningham, J.W. (1993). Whole-to-part reading diagnosis. *Reading and Writing Quarterly: Overcoming Learning Difficulties, 9,* 31–49.

Cunningham, J.W., Erickson, K.A., Spadorcia, S.A., Koppenhaver, D.A., Cunningham, P.M., & Yoder, D.E. (1999). Assessing word attack from an onset-rime perspective. *Journal of Literacy Research, 31,* 391–414.

Cunningham, P.M., & Cunningham, J.W. (1978). Investigating the "print-to-meaning" hypothesis. In P.D. Pearson & J. Hansen (Eds.), *Reading: Disciplined inquiry in process and practice. 27th Yearbook of the National Reading Conference* (pp. 116–120). Clemson, SC: National Reading Conference.

Delano, M., & Snell, M.E. (2006). The effects of social stories on the social engagement of children with autism. *Journal of Positive Behavior Interventions, 8,* 29–42.

Didden, R., Prinsen, H., & Sigafoos, J. (2000). The blocking effect of pictorial prompts on sight-word reading. *Journal of Applied Behavior Analysis, 33,* 317–320.

Eikeseth, S., & Jahr, E. (2001). The UCLA reading and writing program: An evaluation of the beginning stages. *Research in Developmental Disabilities, 22,* 289–307.

Erickson, K.A., Koppenhaver, D.A., & Cunningham, J.W. (2006). Balanced reading intervention and assessment in augmentative communication. In M.E. Fey & R.J. McCauley (Eds.), *Treatment of language disorders in children* (pp. 309–345). Baltimore: Paul H. Brookes Publishing Co.

Flannery, B., & Horner, R. (1994). The relationship between predictability and problem behavior for students with severe disabilities. *Journal of Behavioral Education, 4,* 157–176.

Flower, L., & Hayes, J. (1981). A cognitive process theory of writing. *College Composition and Communication, 32,* 365–387.

Foley, B.E., & Staples, A.H. (2003). Developing augmentative and alternative communication (AAC) and literacy interventions in a supported employment setting. *Topics in Language Disorders, 23*(4), 325–343.

Foley, B.E., Koppenhaver, D.A. & Williams, A. (in press). Writing assessment for students with AAC needs. In D.R. Beukelman & J. Reichle (Series Eds.) & G. Soto & C. Zangari (Vol. Eds.), *Augmentative and alternative communication series. Practically speaking: Language, literacy, and academic development for students with AAC needs.* Baltimore: Paul H. Brookes Publishing Co.

Fossett, B., & Mirenda, P. (2006). Sight word reading in children with developmental disabilities: A comparison of paired associate and picture-to-text matching instruction. *Research in Developmental Disabilities, 27,* 411–429.

Frith, U. (2003). *Autism* (2nd ed.). Oxford, England: Blackwell Publishing.

Gág, W. (2002). *Millions of cats.* Toronto: Penguin Books.

Galilei, G. (1632). *Dialogue concerning the two chief world systems.* Retrieved April 2, 2007, from http://webexhibits.org/calendars/year-text-Galileo.html

Gray, C., & Garand, J. (1993). Social stories: Improving responses of students with autism with accurate social information. *Focus on Autistic Behavior, 8,* 1–10.

Green, G., & Shane, H. (1994). Science, reason, and facilitated communication. *Journal of The Association for Persons with Severe Handicaps, 19,* 151–172.

Grigorenko, E.L., Klin, A., Pauls, D.L., Senft, R., Hooper, C., & Volkmar, F. (2002). A descriptive study of hyperlexia in a clinically referred sample of children with developmental delays. *Journal of Autism and Developmental Disorders, 32,* 3–12.

Happé, F.G.E. (1994). Wechsler IQ Profile and theory of mind in autism: A research note. *Journal of Child Psychology and Psychiatry, 35,* 1461–1471.

Hewitt, F.M. (1964). Teaching reading to an autistic child through operant conditioning. *Reading Teacher, 17,* 613–618.

Hillocks, G., Jr. (1984). What works in teaching composition: A meta-analysis of experimental treatment studies. *American Journal of Education, 93,* 133–170.

Kjelgaard, M.M., & Tager-Flusberg, H. (2001). An investigation of language impairment in autism: Implications for genetic sub-groups. *Language and Cognitive Processes, 16,* 287–308.

Koppenhaver, D.A., Coleman, P., Kalman, S.L., & Yoder, D.E. (1991). The implications of emergent literacy research for children with developmental disabilities. *American Journal of Speech-Language Pathology, 1,* 38–44.

Koppenhaver, D.A., & Erickson, K.A. (2003). Natural emergent literacy supports for preschoolers with autism and severe communication impairments. *Topics in Language Disorders, 23*(4), 283–292.

LaVigna, G.W. (1977). Communication training in mute, autistic adolescents using written word. *Journal of Autism and Childhood Schizophrenia, 7,* 135–149.

Leu, D.J., Jr., Leu, D.D., & Coiro, J. (2004). *Teaching with the internet: New literacies for new times* (4th ed.). Norwood, MA: Christopher-Gordon.

Lord, C., & Paul, R. (1997). Language and communication in autism. In D.J. Dohen & F. Volkmar (Eds.), *Handbook of autism and pervasive developmental disorders* (pp. 195–225). New York: John Wiley & Sons.

Mayes, S.D., & Calhoun, S.L. (2006). Frequency of reading, math, and writing disabilities in children with clinical disorders. *Learning and Individual Differences, 16,* 145–157.

McClannahan, L.E., & Krantz, P.J. (1999). *Activity schedules for children with autism: Teaching independent behavior.* Bethesda, MD: Woodbine House.

McDuffie, A., Yoder, P., & Stone, W. (2006). Fast-mapping in young children with autism spectrum disorders. *First Language, 26,* 421–438.

McGee, G.G., Krantz, P.J., & McClannahan, L.E. (1986). An extension of incidental teaching procedures to reading instruction for autistic children. *Journal of Applied Behavior Analysis, 19,* 147–157.

Mirenda, P., & Erickson, K.A. (2000). Augmentative communication and literacy. In S.F. Warren & J. Reichle (Series Eds.) & A.M. Wetherby & B.M. Prizant (Vol. Eds.), *Communication and language intervention series: Vol. 9. Autism spectrum disorders: A transactional developmental perspective* (pp. 333–367). Baltimore: Paul H. Brookes Publishing Co.

Muter, V., Hulme, C., Snowling, M.J., & Stevenson, J. (2004). Phonemes, rimes, vocabulary, and grammatical skills as foundations of early reading development: Evidence from a longitudinal study. *Developmental Psychology, 40,* 665–681.

Myles, B.S., Hilgenfeld, T.D., Barnhill, G.P., Griswold, D.E., Hagiwara, T., & Simpson, R. (2002). Analysis of reading skills in individuals with

Asperger syndrome. *Focus on Autism and Other Developmental Disabilities,* *17,* 44–47.

Nation, K. (1999). Reading skills in hyperlexia: A developmental perspective. *Psychological Bulletin, 125,* 338–355.

Nation, K., Clarke, P., Wright, B., & Williams, C. (2006). Patterns of reading ability in children with autism spectrum disorder. *Journal of Autism and Developmental Disorders, 36,* 911–919.

National Institute of Child Health and Human Development. (2000). *Report of the National Reading Panel. Teaching children to read: An evidence-based assessment of the scientific research literature on reading and its implications for reading instruction* (NIH Publication No. 00-4769). Washington, DC: U.S. Government Printing Office.

Nelson, K. (1996). *Language in cognitive development.* New York: Cambridge University Press.

O'Connor, I.M., & Klein, P.D. (2004). Exploration of strategies for facilitating the reading comprehension of high-functioning students with autism spectrum disorders. *Journal of Autism and Developmental Disorders, 34,* 115–127.

Perfetti, C.A. (1985). *Reading ability.* New York: Oxford University Press.

Romski, M.A., & Sevcik, R.A. (1996). *Breaking the speech barrier: Language development through augmented means.* Baltimore: Paul H. Brookes Publishing Co.

Romski, M.A., Sevcik, R.A., & Robinson, B.F. (1996). Mapping the meaning of novel visual symbols by youth with moderate or severe mental retardation. *American Journal on Mental Retardation, 100,* 391–402.

Rose, T.L., & Furr, P.M. (1984). Negative effects of illustrations as word cues. *Journal of Learning Disabilities, 17,* 334–337.

Rousseau, M., Krantz, P., Poulson, C., Kitson, M., & McClannahan, L. (1994). Sentence-combining as a technique for increasing adjective use by students with autism. *Research in Developmental Disabilities, 15,* 19–39.

Singer, B.D., & Bashir, A.S. (2004). Developmental variations in writing composition. In C.A. Stone, E.R. Silliman, B.J. Ehren, & K. Apel (Eds.), *Handbook of language and literacy: Development and disorders* (pp. 559–582). New York: Guilford Press.

Singer, H., Samuels, S.J., & Spiroff, J. (1973). The effect of pictures and contextual conditions on learning responses to printed words. *Reading Research Quarterly, 9,* 555–567.

Singh, N.N., & Solman, R.T. (1990). A stimulus control analysis of the picture-word problem in children who are mentally retarded: The blocking effect. *Journal of Applied Behavioral Analysis, 23,* 525–532.

Skotko, B.G., Koppenhaver, D.A., & Erickson, K.A. (2004). Parent reading behaviors and communication outcomes in girls with Rett syndrome. *Exceptional Children, 70,* 145–166.

Snowling, M., & Frith, U. (1986). Comprehension in "hyperlexic" children. *Journal of Experimental Child Psychology, 42,* 392–415.

Soto, G. (1999). Understanding the impact of graphic sign use on the message structure. In F.T. Loncke, J. Clibbens, H.H. Arvidson, & L.L. Lloyd (Eds.), *Augmentative and alternative communication: New directions in research and practice* (pp. 40–48). London: Whurr.

Sparrow, S.S., Balla, D.A., & Cicchetti, D.V. (1984). *Vineland Adaptive Behavior Scale*. Circle Pines, MN: American Guidance Service.

Stromer, R., Kimball, J.W., Kinney, E.M., & Taylor, B.A. (2006). Activity schedules, computer technology, and teaching children with autism spectrum disorders. *Focus on Autism and Other Developmental Disabilities, 21*, 14–24.

Tager-Flusberg, H., & Joseph, R.M. (2003). Identifying neurocognitive phenotypes in autism. *Philosophical Transactions of the Royal Society of London Series B-Biological Sciences, 358*, 303–314.

Teale, W.H., & Sulzby, E. (Eds.). (1986). *Emergent literacy: Writing and reading*. Norwood, NJ: Ablex.

Tirosh, E., & Canby, J. (1993). Autism with hyperlexia: A distinct syndrome? *American Journal on Mental Retardation, 98*, 84–92.

Udwin, O., & Yule, W. (1990). Augmentative communication systems taught to cerebral palsied children: A longitudinal study. I. The acquisition of signs and symbols, and syntactic aspects of their use over time. *British Journal of Disorders of Communication, 25*, 295–309.

Van Kleeck, A., Vander Woude, J., & Hammett, L.A. (2006). Fostering literal and inferential language skills in Head Start preschoolers with language impairment using scripted book sharing discussions. *American Journal of Speech-Language Pathology, 15*, 85–95.

Wechsler, D. (1991). *Wechsler Intelligence Scale for Children* (3rd ed.). San Antonio, TX: Harcourt Assessment.

Wechsler, D. (1992). *Wechsler Individual Achievement Test*. San Antonio, TX: Harcourt Assessment.

Wellman, H.M., Cross, D., & Watson, J. (2001). Meta-analysis of theory-of-mind development: The truth about false belief. *Child Development, 72*, 655–684.

Yorkston, K.M., Dowden, P.A., Honsinger, M.J., Marriner, N., & Smith, K. (1988). A comparison of standard and user vocabulary lists. *Augmentative and Alternative Communication, 4*, 189–210.

15

Membership, Participation, and Learning in General Education Classrooms for Students with Autism Spectrum Disorders Who Use AAC

MICHAEL MCSHEEHAN,
RAE M. SONNENMEIER, AND CHERYL M. JORGENSEN

- - - - - What would happen if the place in which students with [ASD] had access to the general curriculum was in the general education classroom; if students with [ASD] pursued the same learner outcomes as students without disabilities; and if augmentative communication supports were developed, monitored and expanded until students with ASD could communicate the same messages—and to the same extent socially and academically—as students without disabilities?

(McSheehan, Sonnenmeier, Jorgensen, & Turner, 2006, p. 267)

This research was supported in part by the U.S. Department of Education, Office of Special Education Programs (Grant No. H324M020067) to the University of New Hampshire, Institute on Disability/UCED. The opinions expressed by the project do not necessarily represent those of the U.S. Department of Education or the University of New Hampshire.

In the past, students with intellectual and developmental disabilities, including those with autism spectrum disorders (ASDs), were typically educated in special schools or self-contained classrooms for students with disabilities. Initial changes in practices toward inclusive education focused on the social inclusion of students with disabilities; the early inclusion research addressed the social value of welcoming students with disabilities into general education classrooms (Stainback & Stainback, 1996). The emphasis on social inclusion was (and is) critical for enabling students with ASDs to learn appropriate communication, behavior, and social skills. However, even in the context of social inclusion, students with ASDs often continue to receive specialized curricular content that is implemented within general education classrooms but that focuses primarily on separate learning goals and instruction.

A growing body of evidence has demonstrated that students with intellectual and developmental disabilities, including ASDs, can be academically engaged, develop communication and social skills, demonstrate literacy skills, and show improvements on standardized measures of reading and math skills when they are included in general education curricular content (Baker, Wang, & Wahlberg, 1994/1995; Blackorby, Chorost, Garza, & Guzman, 2003; Downing, Morrison, & Berecin-Rascon, 1996; Erickson, Koppenhaver, Yoder, & Nance, 1997; McGregor & Vogelsberg, 1998; Ryndak, Morrison & Sommerstein, 1999; Wehmeyer, Lattin, Lapp-Rincker, & Agran, 2003). For example, in the United States, data from two longitudinal studies of students with disabilities found that—after controlling for differences in disability, functioning level, demographics, and household factors—students who spent more time in general education classrooms were more engaged, made greater academic gains, and were more socially adjusted at school (Blackorby et al., 2007; Wagner, Newman, Cameto, & Levine, 2006). However, it is clear that simply placing students with ASD in the same classrooms with typically developing peers is not enough; students with ASDs need individualized supports to learn within general education classrooms. Unfortunately, these same two longitudinal studies, with nationally representative samples, indicated that the educational programs of students with ASDs and related disabilities often fall short with respect to evidence-based practices and subsequent educational outcomes. Specifically, the reports noted that:

- Students with ASDs are more likely to take courses in special rather than general education settings.
- Of the students with ASDs in special education classes, 10% are exposed to the general education curriculum with some

modifications, 15% have substantially modified curricula, 64% receive a specialized or individualized curriculum, and 10% have no curriculum at all.

- Among all students with disabilities, students with ASDs are the least likely to take science and social studies courses.

- As they progress through the elementary grades, students with ASDs, traumatic brain injuries, or multiple disabilities are the most likely to lose ground with respect to achieving grade-level performance in reading and mathematics.

- Students with ASDs participate less actively than other students in general education classes.

- Less than 20% of students with ASDs use computers in their classes on a regular basis; computers are used most frequently for academic drills.

- Students with ASDs are less likely to graduate with standard diplomas, in comparison with students who both do and do not experience disabilities (U.S. Department of Education, 2007).

Some researchers examining the inclusion of students with ASDs in general education classrooms have focused on specific strategies for supporting inclusion (such as priming, self-management strategies, and peer-mediated interventions) and their impact on social and academic outcomes (see Harrower & Dunlap, 2001, for a review). Other researchers have focused on examining integrated models that address the needs of educators and students with ASDs alike. For example, Simpson, de Boer-Ott, and Smith-Myles (2003) described the Autism Spectrum Disorder Inclusion Collaboration Model, which addresses specific instructional methods (such as task analysis, transition methods, and generalization of skills) as well as educators' attitudinal and social supports, collaboration needs for implementing curricular adaptations and instructional methods (such as appropriate training, planning time, availability of paraeducators, and reduced class size), and recurrent evaluation of inclusive practices.

The goal of this chapter is to provide theoretical perspectives, research findings, and practical applications that pertain to academic learning and the use of AAC supports in general education classrooms. In the first section of the chapter, we discuss elements of inclusive education that are relevant to all students. In the second section, we discuss a model for continuous improvement that educators may use in their efforts to develop and enhance these elements of inclusive education in their classrooms.

ELEMENTS OF INCLUSIVE EDUCATION

To be successful in supporting student learning of the general education curriculum, educators need to provide the appropriate instruction,
supports, and accommodations to students with ASDs and must have
a vision for inclusive education that goes far beyond just "being there."
This requires educators to 1) reframe their expectations regarding students' learning to hold high expectations and presume competence, 2)
promote classroom membership, 3) plan for participation in instructional routines, 4) prioritize academic learning, and 5) engage in effective collaborative teaming practices.

Hold High Expectations and Presume Competence

Presuming that students with ASDs are competent to communicate and
to learn general curriculum challenges a number of long-held beliefs
about the nature of this disability itself. Although the criteria for autism
in the *Diagnostic and Statistical Manual of Mental Disorders, Fourth Edition, Text Revision* do not include a judgment regarding cognitive ability,
the authors of the current manual note that "in most cases, there is an
associated diagnosis of mental retardation, which can range from mild
to profound" (American Psychiatric Association, 2000, p. 71). Edelson
(2006) examined the evidence used as the basis for such claims, reviewing 215 articles published between 1937 and 2003. Results indicated that
74% of the claims came from nonempirical sources, 53% of which never
traced back to empirical data. Nonetheless, Edelson noted that "the
practice of claiming that a majority of children with autism are mentally
retarded continues largely unabated" (p. 74). Based on these mostly
unsubstantiated claims, many students with ASDs are presumed to be
less able than their peers to learn to read, write, do mathematics, think
critically, solve problems, perform functional life skills, and demonstrate age-appropriate receptive and expressive language skills.

A growing number of parents, educators, and researchers are
challenging this assumption. In their view, presuming students' competence to learn is not only justified, but it is an essential practice
that is related to positive educational outcomes (Jorgensen, 2005a;
Kasa-Hendrickson, 2005). This competence view is supported by
several rationales, including the potential for causing harm as a result
of inaccurate and inappropriately low expectations (e.g., Biklen, 1999;
Jorgensen, 2005a). In particular, Donnellan's (1984) principle of the
"least dangerous assumption" provides a foundation for this competence view. The application of the least dangerous assumption in educational programming requires educators to provide opportunities
consistent with high expectations because *to assume incompetence and*

not to provide such opportunities could be harmful if proved to be wrong. Thus, educational programming based on the assumption that a student has limited capacity to learn to read, write, or do math, for example, could result in limited instruction in these areas. If the student does have the capacity to learn such skills, such an educational program would result in great harm, with the student missing out on valuable learning opportunities. Educational decisions ought to be based on the best information available at the time and on the values that schools and communities hold about diversity and disability, while at all costs avoiding the possibility of harming the student. When educators make the least dangerous assumption to presume a student's competence, they are more likely to make decisions that promote a student's full membership within general education classrooms, provide supports for participation and engagement in classroom activities, and plan for learning the general education curriculum content (Jorgensen, McSheehan, & Sonnenmeier, 2007).

Promote Classroom Membership

Educators have reported that a student's presence in the classroom as a member of the learning community and the social and academic activities thereof is an essential component for raising team expectations for student learning (McSheehan et al., 2006). Kent-Walsh and Light (2003) reported on general education teachers' experiences with inclusion of students who use AAC. The teachers in their study noted several benefits, such as increased interactions between AAC users and their classmates without disabilities, classmates' increased acceptance of individuals with disabilities, and teachers' personal growth and learning. Clearly, membership has its benefits.

Membership in the general education classroom is characterized by students having access to valued social roles and to related "symbols of belonging," such as having a desk, being given class jobs, going on field trips, and having their names called during attendance (e.g., Jorgensen, McSheehan, & Sonnenmeier, 2002; McSheehan et. al., 2006). The first and most obvious sign of membership is attendance in the general education classroom; thus, a first step toward promoting a student's membership in the general education classroom is to monitor the percentage of the day that a student is physically present. Additionally, there are aspects of membership that are more affective, having to do with a sense of belonging (Kluth, 2003). Robertson, Chamberlain, and Kasari (2003) reported generally positive relationships between the general education teachers in their study and second- and third-grade students with ASDs who were included in their classrooms on a full-time basis. These researchers found that, as teachers perceived their relationships with included students with ASDs to be more positive, the students' levels of behavior problems were lower and they were more socially included in the class. Williams and Downing (1998), through a series of focus groups and interviews, found that middle school students' perceptions of membership incorporated components such as feeling comfortable, welcomed, wanted, and respected by classmates and teachers; feeling as if they belong to a group and/or to the class as a whole; and having fun. These studies suggest that general education teachers' relationships with included students and the students' perceptions of membership are both components of inclusive education that educational teams can influence positively.

Figure 15.1 presents a checklist format for monitoring indicators of class membership and the degree to which each indicator is present for an individual student. Based on these indicators, the educational team

Sample indicators	Present	Partial	Absent	Action steps
Attends the general education classroom, daily (Percent time spent in the classroom: approx __%)				
Follows the same schedule as classmates 　　Attends academics (reading, math, science) 　　Attends recess, lunch 　　Attends specials/unified arts 　　Attends assemblies, field trips				
Has own desk				
Desk is grouped with classmates' desks				
Has a textbook for each academic/subject area				
Has the same materials/handouts as classmates				
Homework is assigned				
Has a homework folder for turning in assignments				
Is on the attendance list; class list				
Has a mailbox, cubby, locker				
Gets a class job (as opposed to being a class job)				
Is acknowledged by teacher in the same way as are classmates				
Other indicators:				

Figure 15.1. Sample checklist to document indicators of class membership.

may recognize the need to make changes in their practices to promote a student's membership within the classroom. This might involve changes in daily routines that were established previously, changes in educators' expectations for student involvement, and/or changes to the types of supports provided to the student. The vignettes in Table 15.1 provide some examples.

Plan for Participation in Instructional Routines

Participation is defined as students actively accessing the social, communication, and instructional life of the classroom (McSheehan et al., 2006). There is well-documented concern that students who rely on AAC may be primarily passive participants in communicative interactions (Light, 1989). Students with ASDs who use AAC are participating members of general education classrooms when they take part in the same conversations, activities, and instructional routines as their classmates without disabilities. Examples of participation include being called on in class to give an answer and having a defined role during cooperative learning groups.

Given the scope of this chapter, we will emphasize participation in academic instruction which, of course, requires access to AAC supports for communication in many cases. Classroom instruction includes a variety of routines such as seatwork, one-on-one instruction, partnering

Table 15.1.   Examples of practices that promote class membership

- Jamie always arrived 5 minutes late for homeroom, missing opportunities to socialize with classmates and missing the morning announcements, because of issues with transportation. An administrator talked with those in charge of transportation schedules and arranged with Jamie's parents for him to arrive at school 5 minutes earlier.

- Previously, Sally's name was listed as a "class job" for another student ("Sally's peer buddy/assistant"). Now, Sally's name is not listed as a "job"; rather, choices for class jobs have been programmed into her speech-generating device (SGD). Each week, she indicates her preference for the class job she would like to do when asked (e.g., "Which class job would you like to try: line leader, attendance taker, or fish feeder?")

- In the past, Adam's desk was placed at the back of class and was not aligned with the rows of the rest of his class. This year, his desk was moved up to be in a row, alongside his classmates.

- Often, Thomas was pulled out of group read-aloud activities because it was difficult to support him to sit on the floor during reading. To address this, the occupational therapist (OT) and speech-language pathologist (SLP) conducted observations of the reading group. The OT generated a list of accommodations to support Thomas's seating and attending (e.g., bean bag chair, fidget tools). The SLP developed a communication board with the characters and scenes from the activity so that Thomas could read along with the rest of the class. The OT and SLP then provided services in class to model for the teacher how to provide these accommodations so that Thomas was able to remain in class during reading group activities.

with a classmate, small-group instruction, cooperative learning activities, large-group lectures, and large-group interactive sessions. Similar to tracking the percentage of time a student spends in the class as a membership indicator, educators can also track the occurrence and distribution of a student's engagement in instructional routines. Figure 15.2 presents a format for documenting a student's degree of participation in different instructional routines. The ultimate goal is to increase involvement in the same routines as the student's classmates, in the same proportion and at the same times of day, while allowing for variability to accommodate needs for individualized instruction.

Through the lens of participation (contrasted with the lens of learning), the goal is for the target student to be engaged in the instruction with his or her classmates. Even though the student may not yet be demonstrating learning of the same curriculum content as his or her classmates, the student is engaged in the learning process as a full participant, similarly to his or her classmates. Educators can support a student's participation in instructional routines by emphasizing both process and content. For example, during partner or small-group reading activities, a target student might demonstrate participation in the reading process by making comments and/or requests with his or her speech-generating device (SGD) (e.g., *What page are you on? It's your turn, I like this part of the story, Let's read some more*). During another part of the lesson, the teacher might lead a prereading activity to activate background knowledge or to recall what has been read thus far. In response to a teacher probe, classmates might brainstorm ideas or call out events from the book. Participation in a brainstorming activity does not require that a student has read, decoded, and comprehended the text via silent reading. Rather, a student's participation in this activity

Instructional routine	Number of occurrences for class	Number of occurrences for target student	Action steps (including fostering use of AAC)
Seat work— independent			
One-to-one instruction			
Small group— teacher directed			
Large group— teacher directed			

Figure 15.2. Sample worksheet to document and plan for a student's participation in instructional routines.

could involve sharing information the student heard a classmate mention or could simply be a guess at an answer. A student might have access to a communication display (e.g., a board, a series of index cards with symbols ands text) of possible correct answers related to events read from the book. Any of the messages selected from the display would communicate a viable answer. Thus, the student would be able to participate and stay engaged with the content of the lesson, without necessarily demonstrating learning of specific content. For beginning AAC users, the focus could be on developing their skills to activate a display or become familiar with the use of their SGD during a classroom activity. For a more advanced AAC users, this situation allows for repeated interactions with relevant academic vocabulary to foster learning of the general curriculum content.

An instructional planning process that presumes that a student is competent to learn and promotes a student's participation and engagement in instructional routines will look somewhat different than other planning models and processes that are not based on presuming competence. In other models, a framing question for instructional planning might be "What can this child do during this class lesson?" When presuming competence, educators instead might ask, "What would it take for this student to actively participate in the same lesson, in the same or a similar way as his/her classmates?" A framework for such instructional planning includes the following four steps.

1. Identify the content area (e.g., reading, math) and what all students are expected to do within the instructional activity.

2. Identify how students will demonstrate that they are engaged in the instructional activity (e.g., during reading students hold and look at age/grade-level books; track text with their eyes and/or index fingers; turn pages; and make comments, ask questions, and share information regarding the reading).

3. Identify how the target student can demonstrate those same or similar behaviors, possibly with an alternative way of demonstrating participation (such as AAC) as needed (e.g., Joe can hold, look at, and turn pages in a book; he can track text with his index finger with assistance; and can use his communication display to make comments, ask questions, and share information).

4. Identify what supports are needed for the target student to participate in the instructional routine (e.g., adapted book with text at student's reading level, possibly enhanced with pictures or symbols; hand-over-hand assistance for tracking text; communication displays with likely comments, questions, and information to be shared; an experienced communication partner to model or encourage use of the AAC display).

Activity content area	Typically, all students show they are engaged by:	This student shows the same types of engagement as his/her peers by (include use of AAC as means of communication):	This student may require the following supports in order to show that engagement (i.e., to participate and learn):	Preparation by team (what/who/by when)

Figure 15.3.   Sample worksheet to document planning for participation and learning within instructional routines.

Figure 15.3 presents a format that can be used to plan for students' participation (and learning) in instructional activities. Examples of participation in instructional routines are presented in Table 15.2.

Prioritize Academic Learning

Historically, students with ASDs have been "seen as 'too cognitively impaired' or 'not ready for' instruction" (Mirenda, 2003, p. 271) in general education academics. This concern has been discussed by a number of authors in relation to literacy learning (Kliewer & Biklen, 2001; Mirenda, 2003; Mirenda & Erickson, 2000). In the areas of math and science, these issues have also been raised in the literature on students with significant cognitive disabilities (Browder, Spooner, Ahlgrim-Delzell, Wakeman, & Harris, 2008; Courtade, Spooner, & Browder, 2007).

Researchers have called for instruction in academics to be an educational priority if students are to achieve desired outcomes and make progress (Browder, Wakeman, Spooner, Ahlgrim-Delzell, & Algozzine, 2006; Erickson & Koppenhaver, 1995). As discussed in the introduction to this chapter, there is some research supporting the idea that students with significant cognitive disabilities, including those with ASDs, can learn academic content. Comprehensive reviews of the literature related to reading (Browder et al., 2006), mathematics (Browder et al., 2008), and science (Courtade et al., 2007) provide additional examples of these students acquiring academic skills.

Table 15.2.   Examples of participation in instructional routines

Example 1: Supporting Jay's participation in reviewing homework assignments

- Activity: At the beginning of the math lesson, the classroom teacher checks home-work by calling on individual students to give answers.
- What all students are doing: Students look at their homework sheets and follow along as each item is reviewed. Students provide an answer when called upon by the teacher.
- Plan for Jay's participation: Previously, the classroom teacher did not call on Jay to provide answers when checking class homework because he was not given homework. To remedy this, the classroom teacher began to assign a few home-work problems to Jay. He completes the homework with his parents and practices giving the answer when requested, using his speech-generating device (SGD). In class, the teacher calls on him to share an answer for one of the problems he was assigned.

Example 2: Supporting Jeff's participation as the master of ceremonies of a fourth-grade play

- Activity: The entire fourth-grade social studies class is preparing a play to be presented to the school community based on content they have been studying in class. Students are to be organized into teams of 4–5 to prepare a section of the play. Jeff's group is in charge of the script for a master of ceremonies, who will introduce and manage transitions for the play.
- What all students are doing: Students will show participation in the preparation phase by discussing the emcee role, possible script ideas, and a process for assigning the emcee role. The group needs to generate ideas, agree and disagree with each others' ideas, and take notes. The emcee needs to speak out loud.
- Plan for Jeff's participation: Jeff uses his SGD to participate in discussions during the preparation work. Jeff can show agreement/disagreement with ideas by select-ing *yes* or *no* from his SGD. Classmates need to be coached on how to support Jeff in the small group work and supported to ask yes/no questions for group discussion. Jeff's teaching assistant and classroom teacher are available to assist Jeff's group as needed and then fade away to support other groups.

These syntheses, along with other qualitative studies and anec-dotal reports, suggest that learning of general academics is not only relevant but a priority for this population (see, for example, Erickson et al., 1997). Additionally, many researchers are beginning to rethink the notion that students with ASDs may progress through the curricu-lum in a way that is quite different from students without disabilities. Mirenda (2003) noted that:

- - - - - Research supports that learners with and without disabilities may be more similar than previously thought... most—if not all—students with autism can benefit from literacy instruction that incorporates the use of multiple instructional strategies that are carefully matched to the stages or phases of development through which all readers pass on their way from emergent reading to skilled reading. (p. 275)

Bedrosian, Lasker, Speidel, and Politsch (2003) reported on an intervention study designed to enhance the skills needed in the planning and writing of stories by an adolescent with ASD who used AAC. While working with a typically speaking peer as a partner, the student with ASD used a story grammar map, a joint story writing and revision process, story boards, and story writing software to support generation of the story. The researchers described positive outcomes for both the student's participation with the peer in the writing process and his achievement of learning goals that were aligned with the general education writing curriculum. This example highlights the type of preparation that is often needed to facilitate learning in instructional routines for students with ASDs who rely on AAC (e.g., selecting AAC vocabulary that is derived from a typical academic activity and that will be useful not only to the target student but also to classmates and teachers).

Pursuing the four-step instructional planning process described previously sets the stage for a student's demonstration of both anticipated and unanticipated learning. By using this process, educators have reported evidence of student learning that was not previously expected (McSheehan et al., 2006). For example, a student with ASD and little functional speech had never been exposed to grade-level novels. Beginning in fifth grade, books were rewritten for him from a fifth-grade reading level to a second-grade reading level, while preserving the essential content. The text was enhanced with Picture Communication Symbols that were consistent with those on his SGD. Initially, these supports were put into place to foster his participation with age-appropriate materials, on the same topics as his classmates. However, toward the end of the school year after repeated engagement with the adapted novels, the student began vocalizing as he independently turned pages in his books and tracked text with his index finger. He varied his intonation and began to pause on words and at the ends of sentences—similar to his classmates reading aloud. Additionally, he participated in quizzes, tests, and an end-of-year review of all of the novels by selecting from multiple-choice formats programmed into his SGD. By selecting some of the right answers, he demonstrated that he had not only participated in the various instructional routines, but also had learned some of the academic content expected of his classmates—which previously had not been expected of him.

Engage in Effective Collaborative Teaming Practices

The relationship between effective collaborative teaming and student learning is well documented in the literature (Blackstone, 1989; Edelman & Giangreco, 1995; Giangreco, 2000; Giangreco, Cloninger,

Dennis, & Edelman, 1994; Giangreco, Cloninger, & Iverson, 1998; Hunt, Soto, Maier, Muller, & Goetz, 2002; McCarthy et al., 1998; Snell & Janney, 2005; Villa, Thousand, Stainback, & Stainback, 1992). Collaborative teaming occurs when a group of individual team members with diverse but complementary expertise work together to achieve agreed-upon and mutually defined goals (e.g., Snell & Janney, 2005; Thousand & Villa, 1992). Effective collaborative teaming is particularly important when team members need to incorporate AAC displays and technologies to support the participation and learning of students in the general education classroom (Erickson et al., 1997; Koppenhaver, Spadorcia, & Erickson, 1998).

Hunt and her colleagues (Hunt et al., 2002; Soto, Muller, Hunt, & Goetz, 2001a, 2001b) identified several themes related to the ability of team members to work together collaboratively to support the successful inclusion of students with AAC needs. They described a set of professional skills for effective collaboration that is consistent with generally accepted inclusive practices, including 1) holding regular team meetings with contributions from all team members; 2) treating all team members with respect; 3) establishing good interpersonal and communication skills; 4) identifying team members' roles and responsibilities while being flexible about role boundaries; 5) identifying a team leader; 6) establishing common, action-oriented goals; and 7) establishing processes to maintain accountability among team members.

Teams frequently face numerous systemic and organizational barriers that inhibit effective and efficient team collaboration (Garmston & Wellman, 1999). These barriers can be amplified when students have ASDs and/or AAC needs (Hunt et al., 2002; Simpson et al., 2003; Soto et al., 2001a, 2001b). Barriers to effective collaborative teaming include lack of 1) administrative support for inclusion; 2) clarity about team members' roles and responsibilities; 3) time for regular team meetings, planning, and preparation of materials; 4) access to professional development and training in the use of technology and instructional strategies for students with ASDs and AAC needs; and 5) access to effective related service delivery models (Jorgensen, Fisher, Sax, & Skoglund, 1998; Jorgensen, Schuh, & Nisbet, 2005, McCarthy et al., 1998; Rainforth, York, & Macdonald, 1992; Soto et al., 2001a; Villa & Thousand, 1995). Additionally, some researchers have acknowledged the importance of access to a mentor—a "critical friend"—who can guide and support teams to learn new skills and collaborative processes and can help to institute organizational changes that are sustainable (Fullan, 2001; Fullan & Miles, 1992; Jorgensen et al., 2005, Olson, 1994).

Summary

The five elements of inclusive education described in this section provide a focus for designing effective instruction, interventions, and supports, including AAC for students with ASDs who are included in general education classrooms. Each element in and of itself is necessary but not sufficient for successful inclusive education. Presuming a student is competent to learn the general curriculum and "dumping" him into a general education classroom without appropriate instructional planning will no doubt fail. Providing only individualized instruction on the curriculum with no connection to the rich and meaningful social context of the classroom is also inadequate. Although making progress in all areas requires well-coordinated, systematic efforts, "few models and procedures have been advanced to facilitate the successful placement and maintenance of learners with ASD in general education classrooms" (Simpson et al., 2003, p. 117). The Beyond Access model integrates the key elements of inclusive education that support educational teams to promote the learning of general education curriculum content by students with significant disabilities.

THE BEYOND ACCESS MODEL

From 2002 through 2006, the Beyond Access model was designed and evaluated as part of a federally funded grant from the Office of Special Education Programs, U.S. Department of Education. Students who participated in the development and evaluation of the Beyond Access model used a variety of unaided communication modes (including facial expressions, natural gestures, sign language, and speech) and aided communication strategies (including Picture Communication Symbols, switches, and electronic SGDs). Students were included in general education classrooms for at least 50% of the day in at least two core academic areas (e.g., language, arts, math, social studies).

The Beyond Access model (see Figure 15.4) was developed to address the research-to-practice gaps that exist in schools that are attempting to include students with significant disabilities (including those with ASDs) who use assistive technology and AAC in general education classrooms. As a professional development and student support planning model, it assists teams with translating emerging research and promising instructional strategies into a daily practice. It structures collaborative teaming through a set of processes to identify, try out, and systematically evaluate the instructional and communication strategies that students need to be successful academic learners. Expectations for student membership, participation, and learning—along with supports

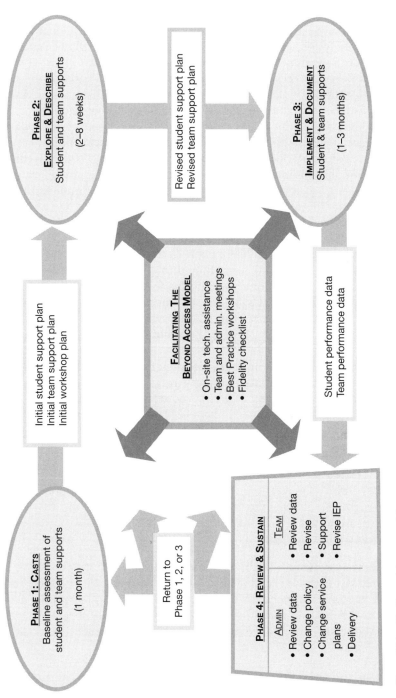

PHASE 2:
EXPLORE & DESCRIBE
Student and team supports

(2–8 weeks)

Revised student support plan
Revised team support plan

PHASE 3:
IMPLEMENT & DOCUMENT
Student & team supports

(1–3 months)

Initial student support plan
Initial team support plan
Initial workshop plan

FACILITATING THE
BEYOND ACCESS MODEL

• On-site tech. assistance
• Team and admin. meetings
• Best Practice workshops
• Fidelity checklist

Student performance data
Team performance data

PHASE 1: CASTS
Baseline assessment of
student and team supports

(1 month)

Return to
Phase 1, 2, or 3

PHASE 4: REVIEW & SUSTAIN

ADMIN	TEAM
• Review data	• Review data
• Change policy	• Revise
• Change service	• Support
plans	• Revise IEP
• Delivery	

Figure 15.4. The Beyond Access model.

for collaborative teaming and the use of AAC and other forms of assistive technology—are essential elements of this model (e.g., Jorgensen, McSheehan, & Sonnenmeier, in press; Jorgensen et al., 2007; McSheehan et al., 2006; Sonnenmeier, McSheehan, & Jorgensen, 2005).

The Beyond Access model engages teams in an iterative process of 1) assessment; 2) exploration of various instructional strategies, AAC and assistive technology strategies, supports, and accommodations; 3) implementation of the most promising practices based on the exploration; and 4) evaluation of the efficacy of those practices to support an individual student's learning. All members of a student's team participate in model activities, including parents/guardians, general educators, special educators, related service providers, and administrators.

Preliminary research on use of the Beyond Access model with elementary-age students with significant disabilities, including ASDs, shows promising outcomes (Jorgensen et al., 2007; McSheehan et al., 2006; Sonnenmeier et al., 2005). Schools that use the Beyond Access model have demonstrated commitment to engage collaborative teaming practices including administrative leadership and support for staff to attend monthly professional development workshops and weekly team meetings; an in-district staff person to assume leadership in using the model; and an administrative team that monitors implementation of the model and works on systems for sustainability. By engaging in collaborative practices, teams enhance their capacity to plan for, implement, and evaluate students' membership, participation, and academic learning within the context of general education classrooms.

Components of the Beyond Access Model

In this section, we describe the key components of the Beyond Access model, which include an emphasis on best practices, the participation of a Beyond Access consultant, the use of an in-district Beyond Access mentor, the establishment of an administrative review team, the provision of an initial team orientation, and the provision of ongoing professional development workshops.

Best Practices   The foundation of the Beyond Access model is a set of values-based, promising, and evidence-based best practices (see Chapter 15 appendix). Each of the Beyond Access model best practices includes a list of indicators that are used to document each team member's knowledge and skill level of each practice over time (Jorgensen et al., 2002).

Consultant   A core component of the Beyond Access model is the active participation of a "critical friend" who is knowledgeable in the best practices and implementation of the model. This person might be a private consultant, a university faculty member, or any person with extensive experience supporting the inclusive education of students with significant disabilities. It is important for teams to have support from a critical friend because the model challenges them to change their practices related to how they work together as a team *and* how they promote the learning of the general education curriculum by students with ASDs. Team members also need support in changing their perspectives on student's presumed levels of competence. The Beyond Access consultant guides the team through the initial implementation of the phases of the model while simultaneously mentoring the in-house Beyond Access Facilitator.

In-District Facilitator   Essential to long-term sustainability is the identification and mentoring of an in-district staff person (e.g., inclusion facilitator, school special education coordinator) who is positioned within the school to assume a leadership role in the implementation of the Beyond Access model. This person takes the lead in supporting teams in the day-to-day implementation of the model. Over time, this person assumes more responsibility for facilitating the phases of the model, supporting review and problem solving regarding the team's practices, and oversight regarding the implementation fidelity.

Administrative Review Team   The establishment of an administrative review team is critical to the model's success and sustainability. The Beyond Access consultant meets regularly with key administrators to discuss both the progress being made and the challenges that may prevent full model implementation. The administrative review team includes at least the school principal, special education coordinator, and the special education teacher who supports Beyond Access students. Once a month, the Beyond Access consultant meets with these individuals and the district special education administrator to monitor implementation of the model. In addition, we encourage the superintendent to join the monthly administrative review meetings two to three times each year.

Initial Team Orientation   Members of each student's educational team participate in a 2-day orientation to learn about the underlying assumptions and practices of the Beyond Access model. The orientation provides informed consent for team members to more fully understand the potential successes and struggles of using this approach. In an era of accountability and an emphasis on evidence-based practice, this is an important step in the process and encourages team members develop a mindset for designing defensible educational programs that include practices that may be values based or promising but that do not yet have a strong research base. Topics addressed in the orientation session include

- Historical perspectives on practices for educating students with ASDs and those who use AAC
- Beyond Access model overview, with an emphasis on the iterative phases of the model and on collaborative teaming practices
- Understanding what constitutes access to, participation in, and learning of the general education curriculum, with an emphasis on the Beyond Access Best Practices (Jorgensen et al., 2002)
- The least dangerous assumption of presumed competence (Jorgensen, 2005a)

Professional Development Workshops Team members participate in monthly professional development workshops on topics related to their implementation of the Beyond Access model. Workshops may include topics such as presuming students' competence (Jorgensen, 2005a); effective teaming practices such as collaborative teaming, problem solving, conflict resolution, and evaluating student and team progress (e.g., Jorgensen et al., 2002); instructional planning, accommodations, and curriculum modifications (Jorgensen, 2005b); AAC and assistive technology; positive behavior supports; literacy instruction; and writing standards-based individualized education program.

Beyond Access Model Phases

There are four main phases involved in Beyond Access model implementation related to assessment, exploration, implementation, and review.

Phase 1: Comprehensive Assessment of Student and Team Support The Comprehensive Assessment of Student and Team Supports (CASTS) is an assessment of a student's learning and supports in the context of current school and team practices, and how those practices align with the model's best practices (see Chapter 15 appendix). The findings from the CASTS provide a baseline from which the team establishes priorities and documents progress.

Two focus questions guide the CASTS:

1. What supports are needed for the student's membership in the general education classroom and his or her full engagement in and learning of the general education curriculum content?

2. How does the team need to work together to support the student's full engagement and learning?

Data are typically collected by a consultant or team point person over a 2- to 3-week period (see Table 15.3) and include a thorough review of the student's educational records (e.g., individualized education program, evaluations, behavior charts, academic performance data, and work samples); completion of questionnaires by each team member; interviews with each team member; observations of the student at school and home; and observations of team collaboration or team meetings.

The Beyond Access consultant synthesizes the information, summarizes themes, notes areas of agreement and discrepancies, and identifies representative examples of student and team performance. The consultant also compares and contrasts the team's current practices

Table 15.3. Data sources for comprehensive assessment of student and team supports (CASTS)

Activity
1. Conduct an initial assessment of current use of evidence-based and promising practices (e.g., Beyond Access Best Practices Rating Scale; McSheehan et al., 2006).
2. Review the student's educational records, including individualized education programs (current and past) and evaluation reports (e.g., achievement, communication, occupational and physical therapy, psychology, medical).
3. Administer a questionnaire addressing the student's interests, learning style, and communication profile; overall strengths/weaknesses in the student's educational program including indicators of membership and participation; and the team's collaborative practices.
4. Review team and school artifacts (e.g., team meeting minutes, school's professional development model, building-wide behavior procedures, school newsletter, mission statement).
5. Conduct observations at school and record description of a day in the life of the student from the student's perspective (Jorgensen, Schuh, & Nisbet, 2005).
6. Review student work samples, current augmentative communication devices and strategies, and instructional supports such as adapted materials.
7. Conduct observations at student's home and interview parent(s)/guardian(s) and sibling(s).
8. Conduct interviews with each team member to expand on information gathered from questionnaires and observations.
9. Observe a team meeting.
10. Identify the alignment between the student's educational program (including team practices) and best practices that promote the learning of the general education curriculum in the general education classroom by students with significant disabilities (McSheehan et al., 2006; Sonnenmeier et al., 2005).
11. Meet with team to review CASTS findings and obtain agreement with findings.
12. Meet with team to review, obtain agreement, and prioritize recommendations.

Note: "Team members" includes parents/guardians. Typically, the CASTS process is completed over the course of 2–3 weeks.

with Beyond Access Best Practices (see Chapter 15 appendix), then reports the findings to the team members. As each summary finding from the CASTS is reported, team members engage in a consensus-building process in which they add any missing and highly relevant information, seek clarification or propose revisions to any inaccurate information, and finally state their level of agreement with the accuracy of each category of information using six levels of agreement (adapted from Kaner, 1996). Any findings that do not achieve full team agreement are discussed, clarified, and edited until agreement is obtained.

Once the summary findings are approved, the team reviews four categories of recommendations: student supports, team supports, professional development needs, and team member responsibilities. The consultant engages the team in a process similar to the one related to the Beyond Access Best Practices to reach agreement on the recommendations. These recommendations are intended to build team capacity aligned with the Beyond Access model and to promote team collaboration and student membership, participation, and learning.

Phase 2: Explore and Describe   The team then begins initial implementation of the CASTS results to address the two guiding questions. The BA consultant guides the team to explore and describe instructional, AAC, and assistive technology strategies and supports to promote the student's membership in the classroom (e.g., having a desk, being assigned a classroom job, being called on for attendance); participation in social activities and routines (e.g., playing with classmates during recess, chatting during snack, talking about current events); participation in academic activities and routines (e.g., cooperative learning groups, brainstorming sessions, teacher directed lectures, laboratory activities); and ability to demonstrate learning (e.g., giving answers, completing worksheets, writing essays). Supports to promote team collaboration are also determined (e.g., effective meeting structures, decision-making processes, and team communication skills). Throughout the remainder of the school year, team members attend professional development workshops that are needed to enhance their knowledge and skills to achieve the desired student and team outcomes.

During Phase 2, team members are encouraged to embrace a try-and-see approach. This approach encourages the team to be creative and open-minded, particularly if specific team members are unsure about how a given strategy might work. The consultant models instructional approaches; facilitates team meetings; coaches team members on the effective use of interventions; assists in the creation of instructional, AAC, and assistive technology materials; and arranges monthly professional development workshops.

By the end of Phase 2, the team selects one of four actions based on dialogue and discussion of their experiences with trying out the recommendation for the prescribed time period: 1) continue exploration of the recommendation; 2) abandon the recommendation; 3) adapt/alter the recommendation and extend exploration; or 4) adopt the recommendation for Phase 3. The efficacy of a support in this phase is based on the team's overall impressions and the team members' professional judgments regarding questions such as

1. Does this recommendation seem to be moving us toward our vision for the student and for ourselves?

2. Does the recommendation seem to positively address the framing questions regarding membership, participation, learning, and/or collaborative teaming?

Student and team supports that are endorsed at the end of Phase 2 are prioritized for implementation and more formal evaluation in Phase 3.

Phase 3: *Implement and Document*   During Phase 3, the team focuses on improving the consistency and quality of the instructional, AAC, and assistive technology strategies and supports provided to the student, as well as documenting the efficacy of those strategies and supports. By reviewing student work samples, communication displays, observations, and videotapes of lessons, the team is able to describe the fidelity of implementation of the supports, as well as the student's performance using AAC and other techniques to engage in classroom activities over time. Concurrently, by reviewing evaluations of team meetings, the team is able to describe the fidelity of implementation of their collaborative teaming practices. These data are essential for establishing a defensible, sustainable educational program.

Throughout Phase 3, the team continues to attend professional development workshops related to the desired student and team outcomes. Additional mentoring from the school-based mentor and from the consultant is provided to ensure team members are providing the necessary supports accurately and consistently.

Phase 4: *Review and Sustain*   During team meetings, reflective practice methods are used to evaluate the delivery of student and team supports systematically and to reflect on the patterns of student and team performance. The aim of Phase 4 is to determine if the supports result in increases in student membership, student participation in social and academic activities and instruction, student demonstration of learning, and team collaboration. Student and team supports that have demonstrated efficacy are maintained. Those supports that do not demonstrate efficacy may be referred for further training, implementation, data collection, and analysis of student and team performance (revisit Phase 3) or may be discontinued. Additional student or team supports may be recommended for exploration as well (revisit Phase 2). This iterative process leads to increased team confidence in designing the educational program. Equally important is analysis of the student's work for evidence of learning that may be seen to represent performance with consistent, quality supports. This lessens the chance that judgments will be made about student performance or capacity in isolation from a consideration of the quality of instruction and individualized supports.

CONCLUSION

The Beyond Access model illustrates that educating students with ASDs who use AAC not only requires effective service delivery through collaboration by a group of skilled professionals, but also requires a deep commitment to the inherent dignity, value, and competence of students with ASD. With the growing number of students who are diagnosed with ASDs, the field of education is at a critical decision-making juncture about these students' educational programs. Do we continue to focus on student deficits and remediation? Do we require students to demonstrate specific sets of skills before they can be included with their classmates without disabilities? Or, do we develop approaches that foster both skill development and engagement with typical peers in natural settings?

The students, families, and professionals with whom we have worked tell us that they have come to believe that students with ASDs using AAC are "fine, just as they are" and that our job is to support their full membership, participation, and learning within the mainstream of general education. Our research suggests that the Beyond Access model provides teams with both the grounding principles and the practical strategies to help achieve those goals. We acknowledge that other educational models may accomplish the same outcomes equally well. However, in the final analysis, the efficacy of the Beyond Access model or any other set of values- and evidence-based practices will be measured by the degree to which our students are happy, learned, and responsible citizens who are able to fully participate in their schools and communities.

REFERENCES

American Psychiatric Association. (2000). *Diagnostic and statistical manual of mental disorders* (4th ed., text. rev.). Washington, DC: Author.

Baker, E., Wang, M., & Wahlberg, H. (1994/1995). The effects of inclusion on learning. *Educational Leadership, 52,* 33–35.

Bedrosian, J., Lasker, J., Speidel, K., & Politsch, A. (2003). Enhancing the written narrative skills of an AAC student with autism: Evidence-based research issues. *Topics in Language Disorders, 23*, 305–324.

Beukelman, D.R., & Mirenda, P. (2005). *Augmentative and alternative communication: Supporting children and adults with complex communication needs* (3rd ed.). Baltimore: Paul H. Brookes Publishing Co.

Biklen, D. (1999). The metaphor of mental retardation: Rethinking ability and disability. In H. Bersani, Jr. (Ed.), *Responding to the challenge: Current trends and international issues in developmental disabilities: Essays in honor of Gunnar Dybwad* (pp. 35–52). Cambridge, England: Brookline.

Blackorby, J., Chorost, M., Garza, N., & Guzman, A. (2003). The academic performance of secondary students with disabilities. In M. Wagner, C. Marder, J. Blackorby, R. Cameto, L. Newman, P. Levine, et al. (2003). *The achievements of youth with disabilities during secondary school. A report from the National Longitudinal Transition Study-2 (NLTS2)*. Menlo Park, CA: SRI International.

Blackorby, J., Knokey, A.-M., Wagner, M., Levine, P., Schiller, E., & Sumi, C. (2007). *Special Education Elementary Longitudinal Study (SEELS): What makes a difference? Influences on outcomes for students with disabilities*. Menlo Park, CA: SRI International.

Blackstone, S. (1989). The 3 R's: Reading, writing, and reasoning. *Augmentative Communication News, 2*, 1–8.

Browder, D.M., Spooner, F., Ahlgrim-Delzell, L., Wakeman, S.Y., & Harris, A. (2008). A meta-analysis on teaching mathematics to students with significant cognitive disabilities. *Exceptional Children, 74*(4), 407–432.

Browder, D.M., Wakeman, S., Spooner, F., Ahlgrim-Delzell, L., & Algozzine, B. (2006). Research on reading instruction for individuals with significant cognitive disabilities. *Exceptional Children, 72*, 392–408.

Courtade, G., Spooner, F., & Browder, D. (2007). Review of studies with students with significant cognitive disabilities which link to science standards. *Research and Practice for Persons with Severe Disabilities, 32*, 43–49.

Danielson, C. (1996). *Enhancing professional practice: A framework for teaching*. Alexandria, VA: The Association for Supervision and Curriculum Development.

Donnellan, A. (1984). The criterion of the least dangerous assumption. *Behavioral Disorders, 9*, 141–150.

Downing, J.E., Morrison, A.P., & Berecin-Rascon, M.A. (1996). Including elementary school students with autism and intellectual impairments in their typical classrooms: Process and outcomes. *Developmental Disabilities Bulletin, 24*, 20–45.

Edelman, S., & Giangreco, M. (1995). VISTA: A process for planning educationally necessary support services. *Language Learning and Education (Special Interest Division Newsletter of the American Speech-Language-Hearing Association), 2*, 17–18.

Edelson, M.G. (2006). Are the majority of children with autism mentally retarded? A systematic evaluation of the data. *Focus on Autism and Other Developmental Disabilities, 21*, 66–83.

Erickson, K.A., & Koppenhaver, D.A. (1995). Developing a literacy program for children with severe disabilities. *The Reading Teacher, 48*, 676–684.

Erickson, K., Koppenhaver, D., Yoder, D., & Nance, J. (1997). Integrated communication and literacy instruction for a child with multiple disabilities. *Focus on Autism and Other Developmental Disabilities, 12,* 142–150.

Fullan, M. (2001). *The new meaning of educational change* (3rd ed.). New York: Teachers College Press.

Fullan, M., & Miles, M. (1992). Getting reform right: What works and what doesn't. *Phi Delta Kappan, 73*(10), 744–752.

Garmston, R., & Wellman, B. (1999). *The adaptive school: A sourcebook for developing collaborative groups.* Norwood, MA: Christopher-Gordon Publishers.

Giangreco, M.F. (2000). Related services research for students with low-incidence disabilities: Implications for speech-language pathologists in inclusive classrooms. *Language, Speech, and Hearing Services in Schools, 31,* 230–239.

Giangreco, M.F., Cloninger, C.J., Dennis, R., & Edelman, S. (1994). Problem-solving methods to facilitate inclusive education. In J.S. Thousand, R.A. Villa, & A.I Nevin (Eds.), *Creativity and cooperative learning: A practical guide to empowering students and teachers* (pp. 321–346). Baltimore: Paul H. Brookes Publishing Co.

Giangreco, M.F., Cloninger, C.J., & Iverson, V.S. (1998). *Choosing outcomes and accommodations for children (COACH): A guide to educational planning for students with disabilities* (2nd ed.). Baltimore: Paul H. Brookes Publishing Co.

Giangreco, M.F., Prelock, P.A., Reid, R.R., Dennis, R.E., & Edelman, S.W. (2000). Role of related service personnel in inclusive schools. In R.A. Villa & J.S. Thousand (Eds.), *Restructuring for caring and effective education: Piecing the puzzle together* (2nd ed., pp. 360–388). Paul H. Brookes Publishing Co.

Goossens', C. (1989). Aided communication intervention before assessment: A case study of a child with cerebral palsy. *Augmentative and Alternative Communication, 5,* 14–26.

Harrower, J., & Dunlap, G. (2001). Including children with autism in general education classrooms: A review of effective strategies. *Behavior Modification, 25,* 762–784.

Hunt, P., Soto, G., Maier, J., Muller, E., & Goetz, L. (2002). Collaborative teaming to support students with augmentative and alternative communication needs in general education classrooms. *Augmentative and Alternative Communication, 18,* 20–35.

Jorgensen, C.M. (1998). *Restructuring high school for all students: Taking inclusion to the next level.* Baltimore: Paul H. Brookes Publishing Co.

Jorgensen, C.M. (2005a). The least dangerous assumption: A challenge to create a new paradigm. *Disability Solutions, 6,* 1–15.

Jorgensen, C.M. (2005b). An inquiry-based instruction planning model that accommodates student diversity. *International Journal of Whole Schooling, 1,* 5–14.

Jorgensen, C.M., Fisher, D., Sax, C., & Skoglund, K. (1998). Innovative scheduling, new roles for teachers, and heterogeneous grouping: The organizational factors related to student success in inclusive, restructuring schools. In C.M. Jorgensen (Ed.), *Restructuring high schools for all students: Taking inclusion to the next level* (pp. 29–48). Baltimore: Paul H. Brookes Publishing Co.

Jorgensen, C.M., McSheehan, M., & Sonnenmeier, R. (2002). *Best practices that promote the learning of the general education curriculum content by students with significant disabilities.* Durham, NH: Institute on Disability, University of New Hampshire.

Jorgensen, C.M., McSheehan, M., & Sonnenmeier, R.M. (2007). Presumed competence reflected in students' educational programs before and after the Beyond Access professional development intervention. *Journal of Intellectual and Developmental Disabilities, 32,* 248–262.

Jorgensen, C.M., McSheehan, M., & Sonnenmeier, R.M. (in press). *Beyond Access: Promoting membership, participation, and learning of the general education curriculum in the general education classroom by students with intellectual and other developmental disabilities.* Baltimore: Paul H. Brookes Publishing Co.

Jorgensen, C.M., Schuh, M., & Nisbet, J. (2005). *The inclusion facilitator's guide.* Baltimore: Paul H. Brookes Publishing Co.

Kaner, S. (1996). *Facilitator's guide to participatory decision-making.* Gabriola Island, British Columbia, Canada: New Society Publishers.

Kasa-Hendrickson, C. (2005). "There's no way this kid's retarded": Teachers' optimistic construction of students' ability. *International Journal of Inclusive Education, 9,* 55–69.

Kent-Walsh, J., & Light, J.C. (2003). General education teachers' experiences with inclusion of students who use augmentative and alternative communication. *Augmentative and Alternative Communication, 19,* 104–124.

Kleinert, H., & Kearns, J. (2001). *Alternate assessment: Measuring outcomes and supports for students with disabilities.* Baltimore: Paul H. Brookes Publishing Co.

Kliewer, C., & Biklen, D. (2001). "School's not really a place for reading": A research synthesis of the literate lives of students with severe disabilities. *Journal of The Association for Persons with Severe Handicaps, 26,* 1–12.

Kluth, P. (2003). *You're gonna love this kid: Teaching students with autism in the inclusive classroom.* Baltimore: Paul H. Brookes Publishing Co.

Koppenhaver, D., Spadorcia, S., & Erickson, K. (1998). How do we provide inclusive literacy instruction for children with disabilities? In S.B. Neuman & K.A. Roskos (Eds.), *Children achieving: Best practices in early literacy* (pp. 77–98). Newark, DE: International Reading Association.

Light, J.C. (1989). Toward a definition of communicative competence for individuals using augmentative and alternative communication systems. *Augmentative and Alternative Communication, 5,* 137–144.

McCarthy, C., McLean, L., Miller, J., Paul-Brown, D., Romski, M., Rourk, J., et al. (1998). *Communication Supports Checklist for programs serving individuals with severe disabilities.* Baltimore: Paul H. Brookes Publishing Co.

McGregor, G., & Vogelsberg, R.T. (1998). *Inclusive schooling practices: Pedagogical and research foundations. A synthesis of the literature that informs best practices about inclusive schooling.* Baltimore: Paul H. Brookes Publishing Co.

McSheehan, M., Sonnenmeier, R.M., Jorgensen, C.M., & Turner, K. (2006). Promoting learning of the general education curriculum by students with significant disabilities. *Topics in Language Disorders, 26,* 266–290.

Mirenda, P. (2003). "He's not really a reader…": Perspectives on supporting literacy development in individuals with autism. *Topics in Language Disorders, 23,* 271–282.

Mirenda, P., & Erickson, K.A. (2000). Augmentative communication and literacy. In S.F. Warren & J. Reichle (Series Eds.) & A.M. Wetherby & B.M. Prizant (Vol. Eds.), *Communication and language intervention series: Vol. 9. Autism spectrum disorders: A transactional developmental perspective* (pp. 333–367). Baltimore: Paul H. Brookes Publishing Co.

National Staff Development Council. (2001). *NSDC's standards for staff development, revised: Advancing student learning through staff development.* Oxford, OH: National Staff Development Council.

Olson, L. (1994, May 4). Critical friends. *Education Week, 13*(31), 20–27.

Rainforth, B., York, J., & Macdonald, C. (1992). *Collaborative teams for students with severe disabilities: Integrating therapy and educational services.* Baltimore: Paul H. Brookes Publishing Co.

Robertson, K., Chamberlain, B., & Kasari, C. (2003). General education teachers' relationships with included students with autism. *Journal of Autism & Developmental Disorders, 33,* 123–130.

Ryndak, D., Morrison, A., & Sommerstein, L. (1999). Literacy before and after inclusion in general education settings: A case study. *Journal of The Association for Persons with Severe Handicaps, 24,* 5–22.

Simpson, R., de Boer-Ott, S., & Smith-Myles, B. (2003). Inclusion of learners with autism spectrum disorders in general education settings. *Topics in Language Disorders, 23,* 116–133.

Snell, M., Chen, L., & Hoover, K. (2006). Teaching augmentative and alternative communication to students with severe disabilities: A review of intervention research 1997–2003. *Research and Practice for Persons with Severe Disabilities, 31,* 203–214.

Snell, M.E., & Janney, R. (2005). *Teachers' guides to inclusive practices: Collaborative teaming* (2nd ed.). Baltimore: Paul H. Brookes Publishing Co.

Sonnenmeier, R.M., McSheehan, M., & Jorgensen, C.M. (2005). A case study of team supports for a student with autism's communication and engagement within the general education curriculum: Preliminary report of the Beyond Access model. *Augmentative and Alternative Communication, 21,* 101–115.

Soto, G., Muller, E., Hunt, P., & Goetz, P. (2001a). Critical issues in the inclusion of students who use augmentative and alternative communication: An educational team perspective. *Augmentative and Alternative Communication, 17,* 62–72.

Soto, G., Muller, E., Hunt, P., & Goetz, P. (2001b). Professional skills for serving students who use AAC in general education classrooms: A team perspective. *Language, Speech, and Hearing Services in Schools, 32,* 51–56.

Stainback, S., & Stainback, W. (1996). *Inclusion: A guide for educators.* Baltimore: Paul H. Brookes Publishing Co.

Thousand, J.S., & Villa, R.A. (1992). Collaborative teams: A powerful tool in school restructuring. In R.A. Villa, J.S. Thousand, W. Stainback, & S. Stainback (Eds.), *Restructuring for caring and effective education: An administrative guide to creating heterogeneous schools* (pp. 73–108). Baltimore: Paul H. Brookes Publishing Co.

U.S. Department of Education. (2007). *To assure the free appropriate public education of all children with disabilities: 27th annual report to Congress.* Washington, DC: Author.

Villa, R.A., & Thousand, J.S. (Eds.). (1995). *Creating an inclusive school.* Alexandria, VA: Association for Supervision and Curriculum Development.

Villa, R.A., Thousand, J.S., Stainback, W., & Stainback, S. (1992). *Restructuring for caring and effective education: An administrative guide to creating heterogeneous schools.* Baltimore: Paul H. Brookes Publishing Co.

Wagner, M., Newman, L., Cameto, R., & Levine, P. (2006). *The academic achievement and functional performance of youth with disabilities. A report of findings from the National Longitudinal Transition Study-2 (NLTS2).* Menlo Park, CA: SRI International. Retrieved on January 2, 2008, from http://www.nlts2.org/reports/2006_07/nlts2_report_2006_07_complete.pdf

Wehmeyer, M., Lattin, D., Lapp-Rincker, G., & Agran, M. (2003). Access to the general curriculum of middle school students with mental retardation: An observational study. *Remedial and Special Education, 24,* 262–272.

Williams, L.J., & Downing, J.E. (1998). Membership and belonging in inclusive classrooms: What do middle school students have to say? *Journal of The Association for Persons with Severe Handicaps, 23,* 98–110.

Beyond Access Model Best Practices

HIGH EXPECTATIONS
AND THE LEAST DANGEROUS
ASSUMPTION OF PRESUMED COMPETENCE

All students with ASDs pursue the same learner outcomes as students without disabilities. When students do not currently demonstrate content knowledge or skills, the least dangerous assumption principle (Donnellan, 1984) of presumed competence (Biklen, 1999) applies and all aspects of their educational programs reflect high expectations.

GENERAL EDUCATION CLASS
MEMBERSHIP AND FULL PARTICIPATION

Students with ASDs are members of age-appropriate general education classes in their neighborhood school and have access to the full range of learning experiences and environments offered to students without disabilities (Jorgensen, 1998; McGregor & Vogelsberg, 1998).

QUALITY AUGMENTATIVE
AND ALTERNATIVE COMMUNICATION

Students with ASDs are provided with accurate and reliable AAC supports and services that enable them to communicate about the content of the academic curriculum and in social situations with adults and age-appropriate classmates (Beukelman & Mirenda, 2005; McCarthy et al., 1998; Snell, Chen, & Hoover, 2006).

CURRICULUM, INSTRUCTION, AND SUPPORTS

Curriculum and instruction are designed to accommodate the full range of student diversity. Individualized supports are provided to enable students to fully participate and make progress within the general education curriculum (Jorgensen, 1998; Kleinert & Kearns, 2001).

ONGOING AUTHENTIC ASSESSMENT

Authentic, performance-based assessments are conducted within typical activities in inclusive environments for the purpose of identifying students' learning and communication styles, preferences and interests, academic strengths and weaknesses, and need for support (Beukelman & Mirenda, 2005; Goossens', 1989).

FAMILY-SCHOOL PARTNERSHIPS

Families and schools are engaged in partnership to create quality inclusive educational experiences for students with ASDs (Giangreco et al., 2000).

TEAM COLLABORATION

General and special education teachers and related service providers demonstrate shared responsibility by collaborating in the design, implementation, and evaluation of students' educational programs and their IEPs (Giangreco et al., 2000; Rainforth et al., 1992).

SPECIAL AND GENERAL EDUCATION REFORM

Administrators provide leadership to align general and special education reform and improvement with respect to the creation of a community of learners that is inclusive of students with significant disabilities (Kleinert & Kearns, 2001).

PROFESSIONAL DEVELOPMENT

Professional development for general and special education staff is linked to improved educational outcomes for students with ASDs (Danielson, 1996; National Staff Development Council, 2001).

For the list of best practice indicators, see Jorgensen, C.M., McSheehan, M., & Sonnenmeier, R.M. (2002). *Best practices that promote the learning of the general education curriculum content by students with significant disabilities.* Accessed May 12, 2008, at http://iod.unh.edu/beyond-access/best_practice.pdf

16

Supporting the Participation of Adolescents and Adults with Complex Communication Needs

TERESA IACONO, HILARY JOHNSON, AND SHERIDAN FORSTER

The focus of this chapter is on adolescents and adults with autism spectrum disorders (ASDs) and complex communication needs who have not developed functional speech and have been determined at some point in their lives to have moderate to profound levels of intellectual disability (ID). For this group, the distinction between ASDs and ID is often blurred. In addition, the extent of their autism may be unclear, with many described as having autistic features or being on the autism spectrum without a formal diagnosis as such. In other cases, a formal autism diagnosis may have been assigned by professionals but was not communicated to those who provide the person with daily support or act as key communication partners. The relevance of considering the potential for people with ID to be on the autism spectrum relates to developing an understanding of their profiles of skills, behaviors, and preferences.

The personal histories of many adults with ASDs and ID are likely to be characterized by broken connections, limited and changing social networks, and limited and changing support systems as a result of their movement from institutions to community-supported accommodations. In many cases, these adults have experienced the outcomes of government and educational policy changes motivated by a desire to embrace the principles of normalization, functional skill development, social participation, and community inclusion. On the other hand, they are likely to have experienced limited communication support, limited opportunities for self-determination, and behavioral interventions that reflect more traditional than contemporary practices.

The aim of this chapter is to explore 1) what is known about adolescents and adults with ASDs and ID and 2) the role of AAC in facilitating their communication, social networks, and participation. Such exploration provides clinical implications and directions for research.

ASD, INTELLECTUAL DISABILITY, AND COMPLEX COMMUNICATION NEEDS

The presence of ID, particularly at more severe levels, is likely to result in people with ASDs having complex communication needs and thus requiring augmentative and alternative communication (AAC). Prevalence data provide some insights into the extent to which people with ID with complex communication needs demonstrate features that are also suggestive of ASDs. In addition, outcome studies of young children with ASDs indicate the extent to which IQ scores appear to remain stable from childhood to adulthood and the impact of ID on adult outcomes.

Researchers have suggested that the potential for multiple associated disabilities is higher for people with more severe levels of ID than those with milder levels (McLean, Brady, & McLean, 1996). For example, Arvio and Sillanpää (2003) found that, among 461 people with severe and profound ID aged between 1 and 71 years, 92% had between one and six associated impairments. Most common was a "speech handicap" (not defined), followed by a seizure disorder. "Autistic features" (although again not defined) were identified in 72 individuals (16%). Of course, the extent of a person's level of ID becomes somewhat controversial when considering the concerns expressed by people with ASDs themselves about problems with intelligence testing, especially in people with ASDs and severe communication impairments (Autism Rights Movement, n.d.).

Data from the Australian Institute of Health and Welfare (2006) indicated that 26% of people with ID (at any level) and 25% of people with ASDs had no effective means of communication. Hence, for people with identified ASDs who also have the label of ID, the potential for having complex communication needs appears high. A recent demographic study of 3,759 individuals with complex communication needs conducted in the State of Victoria, Australia, indicated that 10% of the individuals had a primary diagnosis of autism; of these, 81% also had a diagnosis of ID (Perry, Reilly, Cotton, Bloomberg, & Johnson, 2004).

These data indicate that people with ASDs who are most likely to require and potentially benefit from AAC are those who also have an apparent ID, particularly at severe to profound levels. Care is needed in extrapolating from these data; complex communication needs do not necessarily imply the presence of ID, but lack of the ability to communicate certainly has the potential to confound judgments of underlying cognitive capacity. In this chapter, the potential for misdiagnosis of ID is recognized. The focus here is on the experience of people who have lived their lives with the label of ID and who also are on the autism spectrum. Hence, research relating to both disabilities is relevant to any attempt to understand this experience.

Implications of Deinstitutionalization and Inclusion

The normalization movement has been the impetus for the integration and community inclusion of people with developmental disabilities (in particular, those with ID) in the Western world (Cambridge et al., 2002; Young, Sigafoos, Suttie, Ashman, & Grevell, 1998). Integration and community inclusion have been driven largely by attitude changes brought about by the application of social role valorization principles (Wolfensburger, 1983) to enhance roles for devalued and marginalized people. It was hoped that such efforts would offer people with ID the opportunity to form meaningful relationships and social networks. These movements have resulted in policy initiatives in Western countries motivated by a desire to ensure the rights, independence, choices, and inclusion of people with disabilities, as articulated in documents such as a U.K. White Paper (Department of Health, 2001), the Montreal Declaration on Intellectual Disabilities (Lecompt & Mercier, 2007), the Convention on the Rights of Persons with Disabilities (United Nations, 2006), and the Australian State of Victoria's Disability Plan (Department of Human Services, 2002). Such policy documents acknowledge the problems that people with disabilities face in terms of social connectedness. For adults with ASDs, achieving social connectedness is likely to present a particular challenge in light of their social impairments, which in turn are likely to have an impact on the quality of their social networks.

Social Networks

According to Scott (1991), the construct of social networks and attempts to measure them originated in the discipline of sociometric analysis and combined the fields of gestalt theory and mathematics. The theoretical portions that are especially applicable to people with disabilities are in the domain of personal social networks (Antonucci, 1985; Reindeers, 2002), which comprise two main aspects. First, the quantitative aspect involves measuring the size of a social network; the strength of the bond between two people (i.e., ties); how closely people are related to one another (i.e., density); the length of and frequency of interactions in relationships (i.e., stability); and the interconnectedness of people in relationships (i.e., multiplexity). Second, but equally important, is the qualitative aspect of the social support that is provided in the relationships. This quality relies on the reciprocity of physical and emotional support provided within social networks, which can be considered "vehicles through which social support is distributed or exchanged" (Antonucci, 1985, p. 96).

Autism Spectrum Disorders Information about the social networks of adults with ASDs comes largely from interviews with family members. Howlin, Goode, Hutton, and Rutter (2004), for example, explored friendships among a group of 68 adults with ASDs. They found that only 26% of participants had relationships with peers that involved participation in a range of activities or interests; those who had such acquaintances typically shared activities through arranged social groups. Over half the participants were reported to have no friends or acquaintances, whereas 19% were reported to have at least one relationship that "involved some degree of selectivity and sharing" (p. 217). Other researchers have reported similar paucity in reciprocal relationships with larger groups of adults (Orsmond, Krauss, & Seltzer, 2004; Seltzer et al., 2003). These studies have indicated the difficulty that adults with ASDs appear to have in sustaining friendships compared to younger individuals. Orsmond et al. (2004) found that being young and relatively less impaired in social skills was predictive of whether people had peer relationships, but findings by other researchers (e.g., Beadle-Brown et al., 2002) suggest that living in the community, even for long periods, does not appear to ameliorate social impairments.

Intellectual Disability In comparison with research involving people with ASDs, more research has been conducted into the size and mix of the social networks of people with ID alone, although with the potential for ASD as an associated condition often unknown. Some of this research has focused on the potential benefits of deinstitutionalization. Researchers, particularly in the United Kingdom, have tracked changes in the relationships and behaviors of people who have moved from large congregate care institutions to smaller hostels/houses located with the rest of the community (Cambridge et al., 2002; Stancliffe & Lakin, 2006). This change in location does not always ensure that individuals meet new people or form new social relationships (Donnelly et al., 1996). In fact, they may even have reduced contacts and broken connections, depending on the place of relocation and their proximity to people who previously shared their residences (de Kock, Saxby, Thomas, & Felce, 1988). Although some research suggests an initial increase in social contacts when people move from institutions into the community (e.g., Stancliffe & Lakin, 2006; Young et al., 1998), some has also found that people who have been in the community longer may have reduced social networks (Bigby, 2008; Stancliffe & Lakin, 2006).

In general, research has shown that people with ID tend to have quite small social networks (Forrester-Jones et al., 2006; Kennedy, 2004; Renblad, 2002; Robertson et al., 2001). Although relatively large social networks comprising up to 46 people were reported by Forrester-Jones, Jones, and Heason (2004), much smaller networks of only one or two people seem to be more common (Bigby, 2008; Donnelly et al., 1996). When individuals have complex communication needs, information about their networks is usually provided by parents (Krauss, Seltzer, & Goodman, 1992) or staff (Robertson et al., 2001), but there is some evidence that such reporting underestimates social network size (e.g., Landesman-Dwyer, Berkson, & Romer, 1979). Parker, Sprague, Flannery, Niess, and Zumwait (1991), for example, found that even people who knew adolescents with moderate and severe ID quite well were often unaware of how they indicated their friendships. This difficulty may be especially true for adults with ASDs and ID, who may exhibit idiosyncratic communicative behaviors.

People with both ASDs and ID would appear to be especially vulnerable to having small social networks because of their social impairments and limited communication skills. Robertson et al. (2001) included this group in a study of 500 residents with ID (mild to severe) drawn from various-sized residential options; 38% of the residents were also diagnosed with ASDs and 24% were identified as having concurrent mental health issues. The two criteria for including someone as a member of a resident's social network were that the person was important to the resident and had been seen by him or her during the last month. The overall size of the networks varied from 0 to 20 people, with a median of five. Staff members comprised 44% of the total network members; when they were excluded, the median network size was reduced to 2 people (range, 0–13).

Reciprocity of social supports remains a less-reported aspect of social networks, but may be integral to sustaining relationships. Krauss et al. (1992), in one of few qualitative studies in this area, conducted structured interviews with the mothers of 418 adults with ID who lived at home. Almost half of the adults were reported to have no friends. Social support was described according to six types: serving as a confidante, providing reassurance, providing respect, providing care when ill, listening when upset, and discussing health matters. Network members were reported to provide four types of support to persons with ID, but to receive only two types of support in return. Robertson et al. (2001) also found that social and emotional supports were provided mostly by staff and family; it was unusual for adults with ID to provide such supports to others or to demonstrate reciprocity. This result might reflect, at least in part, the large proportion of residents with ASDs or mental health problems, as noted previously.

Newton and Horner (1995) provided a contrasting pattern to reports of poor reciprocity on the basis of in-depth interviews of 14 community members who had friendships with people with severe ID. All participants reported receiving reciprocity of affirmation ("unconditional love... complete acceptance," p. 389), but they noted that more tangible reciprocity was lacking. Tangible reciprocity relied on staff members, who did things such as sending birthday cards or presents on behalf of the person with ID.

The differences reported across studies of social networks and reciprocity, in all likelihood, are attributable to some extent to differences in data collection strategies and proxy reports, as well as to other differences in methodology. Also, network size variations may arise from differences in definitional criteria such as including people who are important or who the central participant really likes (Forrester-Jones et al., 2004; Kennedy, Horner, & Newton, 1990) and excluding paid workers (Dagnan & Ruddick, 1997). A further potential cause of different results across studies may be the fact that informants often vary widely in their knowledge about the individuals they support. An increased use of direct observations in data collection may lead to more accurate indicators of social networks.

Summary   Despite differences across studies in terms of methodology and findings, it is apparent that social networks of people with ID are limited in size and tend to be comprised largely of family members and paid support staff. The addition of social impairments, as occurs for people with ASDs, appears to contribute to difficulties in forming friendships and sustaining social networks, particularly in terms of reciprocity in relationships. The extent to which ASD affects a person's ability to form friendships and to develop social networks may result not only from the social impairment itself, but also from other characteristics that continue from childhood or develop in adolescence or adulthood. As a result, social reciprocity may remain limited throughout the lifespan.

OUTCOMES FOR ADOLESCENTS AND ADULTS WITH ASD AND INTELLECTUAL DISABILITY

In this section, we provide an overview of long-term follow-up studies that have examined various outcomes for adolescents and adults with ASDs and, in most cases, diagnoses of ID as well. In particular, we focus on behavior and psychiatric problems, communication concerns, and social outcomes. We also examine the scant literature on the long-term impact of various types of intervention for individuals with ASD.

Long-Term Follow-Up Studies

In a number of studies, changes in individuals with ASDs over time have been documented (e.g., Ballaban-Gil, Rapin, Tuchman, & Shinnar, 1996; Kobayashi, Murata, & Yoshinaga, 1992; Larsen & Mourisden, 1997), often in comparison to the outcomes documented for other groups of people with disabilities (e.g., Mawhood, Howlin, & Rutter, 2000; Rutter & Lockyer, 1967). Studies by Mawhood et al. (2000) and Howlin et al. (2004), which focused on individuals with ASDs and measured IQs above 50, demonstrated that most of these individuals remained dependent on others for support throughout their lives. In addition, Howlin et al. noted that people with formal IQ test scores in the range of 50–70 had the poorest outcomes overall.

Other long-term studies have included individuals with severe levels of ID. For example, Kobayashi et al. (1992) reported on 201 Japanese children who had been involved in early intervention, 33% with moderate and 16% with severe ID. The follow-up durations ranged from 5 to 28 years. Ballaban-Gil et al. (1996) reported on 99 adolescents and adults in the United States, over half of whom had moderate or severe ID. These participants' initial diagnoses occurred between 9.5 months to 20 years of age, with follow-up data collected an average of 12 years after the time of each participant's diagnosis. Larsen and Maurisden (1997) reported on 18 Danish children 30 years after their original diagnoses of autism ($n = 9$) or Asperger syndrome ($n = 9$). Seven children in the autism group were reported to have ID, ranging from mild to severe.

Despite the use of indirect data sources, including reliance on patient registers (Larsen & Mourisden, 1997) and informant reports (Ballaban-Gil et al., 1996; Kobayashi et al., 1992), similar outcomes were reported across all of these studies. The outcomes indicated a persistence of numerous problems into adolescence and adulthood (e.g., receptive and expressive language, social skills, problem behavior). The gains that were noted tended to be for children with higher formal IQ scores and better communication skills at initial assessment. The results of these studies reflect those of an early seminal and comprehensive study conducted by Rutter and Lockyer (1967) that examined the outcomes for children with ASD who attended a clinic in the United Kingdom between 1950 and 1958. In this study, children with IQ scores less than 60 had the poorest outcomes, with the majority remaining unable to speak, living in institutions, and developing epilepsy as adults (Lockyer & Rutter, 1969; Rutter, Greenfeld, & Lockyer, 1967).

Behavior and Psychiatric Problems

A large proportion of people with ASDs show evidence of behavior problems in adolescence and adulthood, although reports vary with regard to whether these problems persist from childhood or originate later on in life. Kobayashi et al. (1992), for example, reported an overall deterioration in 31.5% of the individuals in their study, especially with regard to behavior problems (e.g., aggression and self-injury) and obsessive or repetitive behaviors, with the greatest increase occurring after the age of 10 years. However, Ballaban-Gil et al. (1996) reported that behavior problems persisted from childhood in 69% of their adolescents and adults.

In the ID literature, much has been written about challenging (i.e., problem) behavior, but it is not clear whether such behaviors are more likely in people who also have ASDs. One exception is a U.K. population study by Bhaumik, Branford, McGrother, and Thorp (1997), who examined the relationship between the presence of autistic traits and challenging behavior in 2,201 adults with ID. They found that the number of autistic traits was associated with severe and profound ID and with many challenging behaviors, including physical aggression, property destruction, self-injury, temper tantrums, uncooperative behavior, and excessive activity.

The presence of challenging behaviors appears to result in a high usage of medications, usually psychotropic in nature, in an effort to control them (e.g., Ballaban-Gil et al., 1996; Tsakanikos et al., 2006). Unfortunately, the use of these drugs for mere behavior control versus for bona fide treatment of one or more psychiatric conditions is not always clear in research reports (e.g., Tsakanikos et al., 2006). Researchers such as La Malfa et al. (2007) have argued that people with ID are especially vulnerable to mental health disorders resulting from a wide range of interactive factors, including those that are biological, relational, and social in origin. Certainly, a number of studies have indicated variable rates of mental health problems in people with ASDs that are generally higher than in the general population, although it is often unclear whether behavior problems are included in these studies as symptoms of various psychiatric conditions (e.g., Cooper & Bailey, 2001) or as separate entities unto themselves (e.g., Deb, Thomas, & Bright, 2001).

The extent to which the presence of ASD places people with ID at a higher risk of psychiatric disorders has been the focus of recent research. For example, Bradley, Summers, Wood and Bruson (2004) compared 12 adults with ASDs and ID to 12 adults with ID only, matched according to age, sex, and nonverbal IQ score (less than 40) on a tool designed to screen for psychiatric disorders in people with ID. The proportion of participants for whom scores reached clinical significance was greater in the ASD/ID group on a number of scales, including anxiety and depression. The overall rate of comorbidity was four times higher in the ASD/ID than the ID only group. Based on a review of several long-term outcome studies, Howlin (2004) noted that psychiatric disorders are more likely in adults with ASD who are at the severe end of the ID continuum.

Language and Social Impairment

Persistent problems in communication have also been found to be characteristic of people with ASDs who also appear to have severe ID (e.g., Ballaban-Gil et al., 1996; Rutter & Lockyer, 1967). However, Howlin et al. (2004) reported data indicating that even those with moderate to mild levels of ID are at risk of persistent difficulties in both linguistic and social aspects of communication. Mawhood et al. (2000) examined communication outcomes in 19 men with ASDs in comparison with 20 men with language disorders at 23–24 years after their original diagnoses. Of the 19 men with ASDs, 6 lacked spontaneous functional language; of these, 4 men were unable to speak and 2 men demonstrated only echolalic speech. At follow-up, the men with ASD, who were more likely to have improved verbal IQ and receptive language scores overall, were nonetheless significantly more impaired in all areas of language (including social communication skills) than those in the language-disordered group. Unlike those in the language-disordered group, their formal receptive language scores from childhood were strongly associated with their overall outcome measures.

The relationship between language and social skills is evident in people with ASDs from early childhood. Typically, young children with ASDs communicate for the purpose of behavioral regulation more than for the purposes of either social interaction or joint engagement (see Chapter 3). Such early difficulties may be ameliorated as cognitive skills and social responsiveness develops as a result of early intervention (Howlin, 2004). However, as noted previously, difficulties in forming social relationships with adults and peers often endure regardless (Howlin, Mawhood, & Rutter, 2000; Rutter & Lockyer, 1967). Howlin et al. (2000) found large associations between receptive vocabulary skills and friendships ($r = 0.89$) and between receptive vocabulary skills and social competence ($r = 0.88$). These findings, in conjunction with those from other follow-up studies, suggest that enduring problems reflect the compounding effects of ongoing cognitive, language, and social impairments. The result is poor outcomes in terms of forming friendships, lack of employment, and continued dependence on family and support services (Howlin et al., 2004).

Results of Intervention

Rutter et al. (1967) argued that the likelihood of poor outcomes for people with ASDs, including those with low IQ scores, can be ameliorated by opportunities for appropriate schooling and communication interventions. However, research into the long-term impact of such factors and of the movement toward deinstitutionalization is sorely lacking. Howlin (2004), in a comparison of studies conducted before and after the 1980s, attempted to capture the potential influence of greater educational opportunities and the closure of institutions. She found that the proportions of adults with good outcomes increased from 11% to 20% in this analysis; for those with poor outcomes, the proportions decreased from 65% to 50%.

Given the rise in early intervention opportunities that occurred in the mid-1980s and thereafter, there is surprisingly little research into their long-term effects. In a review of intervention efficacy studies, Howlin (2004) found limited outcome data to indicate the long-term effects of early childhood intervention programs or to evaluate different forms of education. She noted that even fewer intervention studies have addressed outcomes for adults with ASD, perhaps because of a lack of services for adults overall. Hamm and Mirenda (2006), in one of the few published studies examining long-term outcomes for adults with developmental disabilities who used AAC while at school, noted the lack of access to AAC services after graduation. Six of their eight participants were reported to have ID and/or ASDs.

Although the study by Hamm and Mirenda (2006) was conducted in Canada, the findings may reflect a similar situation in other Western countries and may extend beyond AAC services to more general supports. For example, Stancliffe (2006) noted that there is a substantial shortage of specialist disability services in Australia. Partly as a result of such shortages, there has been a trend in Australia and the United Kingdom to provide speech pathology interventions by training residential or vocational staff to work with clients with developmental disabilities and communication impairments (e.g., Bloomberg, West, & Iacono, 2003; Money, 2002). Using this model, services are often provided to groups of clients rather than to individuals. This strategy is more time efficient but may fail to address individual needs, which have been identified in government policy documents as one of the goals of service provision (e.g., Department of Human Services, 2002). On the other hand, such an approach may be more effective in the long run because it insures that communication supports are provided by a person's most frequent communication partners. Clearly, research is needed to examine the impact of such service provision models.

Summary

Although improvements across various areas of functioning have been demonstrated from childhood to adulthood in individuals with ASDs, these are primarily limited to individuals with IQ scores above 70. Those with IQ scores lower than 50 and concurrent severe communication delays, including a lack of functional speech, appear to demonstrate the poorest outcomes. This pattern appears evident even with the increased educational opportunities and closure of institutions in Western countries that have occurred since the 1980s. In addition, the persistence of behavior problems into adulthood and a high incidence of psychiatric disorders, which often go undiagnosed or are masked by behavior problems, contribute to poor outcomes for people with ASDs and ID. There is little to indicate that the needs of this group are met through access to appropriate services either in the communication domain or in other areas. Such lack of access to services may exacerbate problem behaviors or mental health issues as they deprive these adolescents and adults with a means to facilitate the development of social networks.

FACILITATING POSITIVE
OUTCOMES FOR ADULTS WITH ASD

Given the apparently bleak outlook for adults with ASDs and ID that is evident from outcome studies, there is an urgent need for documentation of strategies that will enhance their quality of life. The relationship between communication and social skills—and hence social networks—points to the potential of AAC as a starting point. In this section, we review the research base on the outcomes of AAC interventions for adolescents and adults with ASDs. We then present information on areas that have received limited research attention, but which may provide some direction on how AAC may supplement or be integrated with other strategies to enhance both friendships and community inclusion for this group.

AAC Interventions

Research addressing AAC in adolescents and adults with ID, including those with ASDs, has focused largely on the use of functional communication training to reduce problem behavior (see Chapter 12, this volume). Research on the use of AAC to enhance more general communication skills for individuals in this age group has been quite limited in comparison to research concerning children. A representative sample of AAC studies focusing on adolescents and adults are summarized in Table 16.1.

A literature search was conducted using key words that included *adolescents, adults, intellectual disability, mental retardation, learning disability, autism, autism spectrum disorder, AAC,* and *communication.* Studies with a focus on functional communication training or problem behaviors were excluded, as were those with little or no data and those in which the participant description was insufficient to determine whether or not ASD was present.

Inspection of Table 16.1 indicates that participants older than 23 years of age are not represented. Most of the seven studies used experimental single-subject designs to examine the effectiveness of AAC on a narrow range of outcomes (e.g., learning to request desired items using one or more graphic symbols). In a longitudinal descriptive study by Romski and Sevcik (1996), more comprehensive outcomes were obtained, including receptive and productive use of symbols on a speech generating device, increased communicative interactions with adults and peers, use of symbol combinations, printed word recognition, improved speech intelligibility, and maintenance of gains over several years. In this study, improvements in all

Table 16.1. Studies demonstrating effective teaching of AAC to adolescents and adults with autism spectrum disorders (ASDs)

Study	Participants with ASDs	Design	Intervention targets and strategies	Outcomes
Reichle & Brown (1986)	23-year-old man with severe ID and ASD	Series of A-B case studies	The participant was taught to use symbols in a multipage wallet. Object names, a generalized WANT symbol, discriminant use of the symbols for commenting versus naming, and locating symbols were taught, using systematic fading of physical prompts. Spontaneous and meaningful use of the symbols was also assessed.	The participant learned all targets, with generalized requests most rapidly acquired (in 80 trials). The participant required 260 trials to learn to locate symbols. He was observed to use the symbols for spontaneous requesting but not for commenting within appropriate contexts.
Rotholz, Berkowitz, & Burberry (1989)	John: 17-year-old boy with ID and ASD Sam: 18-year-old boy with ID and ASD	A-B-A-B reversal design and multiple baseline across participants	Participants were taught to request items in a fast-food restaurant using manual signs and symbols in a communication book. Interaction success was compared between manual signs and the book. Treatment consisted of a four-step process to teach receptive and productive naming and use of symbols to request, using a progressive time-delay strategy.	Participants demonstrated more successful ordering (up to 100%) with the communication book compared with manual signs. The number of requests varied from 0 to 4 across sign and communication book conditions.

(Continued)

455

Table 16.1. *(Continued)*

Study	Participants with ASDs	Design	Intervention targets and strategies	Outcomes
Hamilton & Snell (1993)	Carl: 15-year-old boy with severe ID and ASD	Changing criterion design with a multiple probe across settings	Carl was taught to use a communication book across four settings using a milieu approach. The settings included his classroom and surrounding area, the school cafeteria with nondisabled peers, various locations in the community, and at home.	Carl increased his use of the communication book in response to naturalistic opportunities in all four settings. Data collected 12 months later indicated Carl had maintained his use of the communication book, including to express multiword phrases, in all settings except home.
Romski & Sevcik (1996)	K.H.: boy (age 10 years 8 months) with severe ID and autistic behaviors

E.C.: boy (age 16 years 7 months) with severe ID and ASD

J.A.: boy (age 13 years 3 months) with moderate ID and autistic behaviors (One other child participant with autism; nine others with various developmental disabilities) | Longitudinal descriptive study, with participants grouped according to whether they were taught in home or school settings | The System for Augmenting Language (SAL) was used to teach the use of symbolic communication. Key elements of the intervention were 1) use of an aided AAC system with speech output; 2) use of lexigrams as graphic symbols and the gradual increase of target vocabulary; 3) teaching during natural communication exchanges; 4) encouraging active partner use of participant's AAC devices; and 5) monitoring ongoing participant and partner use, from the partner's perspective. | Overall results indicated that over the 2-year period of data collection, compared with the use of informal methods (e.g., gestures and vocalizations), communication using SAL was more successful in terms of gaining a response from partners and more effective in terms of resulting in continued communication. Of the participants with ASD, J.A. demonstrated improvements in all of 10 domains measured, E.C. in 7 domains, and K.H. showed modest gains across domains. |

456

| Cafiero (2001) | Timothy: 13-year-old boy with ID and ASD | Descriptive case study (A-B) | The use of activity boards was taught using natural aided language stimulation. Techniques used in settings in the school and community were milieu teaching, creative sabotage, and interrupted behavior chains. | Timothy increased his use of picture communication symbols from 16 to 64. Data across the baseline and intervention phases also indicated a reduction in a problem behavior. His curriculum and individualized education programs were reworked to make them more complex, challenging and academic as a result of the classroom staff members' changed perceptions about him. |
| Sigafoos & Drasgow (2001) | Shane: 14-year-old boy with moderate-severe ID and autism-like behaviors | Experimental single-case: A-B-C-D | Shane was taught to use sign and then a VOCA to gain and maintain access to preferred objects. He was then taught the conditional use of these modalities. | Shane rapidly learned to use sign or the VOCA to request items. When the VOCA was present, he always used that modality, and when not, he used signs. |

(Continued)

457

Table 16.1. *(Continued)*

Study	Participants with ASDs	Design	Intervention targets and strategies	Outcomes
Chambers & Rehfeldt (2003)	Brian: 19-year-old boy with severe ID and autistic behaviors (plus three other participants).	Experimental single-case: alternating treatments	Two mands (requests for reinforcer items) were taught in each of PECS and sign conditions. Ability to request items out of view and generalization to participants' residences were also tested.	Brian learned mands in the PECS condition more rapidly than the mands taught in the sign condition. Performance in sign was also more variable. He was more likely to request items out of view using PECS than sign, but there was no difference in performance on generalization probes.
Sigafoos, Didden, & O'Reilly (2003)	Michael: 13-year-old boy with profound/severe ID and ASD (plus two other child participants).	Experimental single-case: multiple baseline across participants for an acquisition phase with a postacquisition comparison phase	Participants were taught to request preferred items using a switch (SGD) within a rapid acquisition phase. This phase was followed by a postacquisition phase in which having the speech turned off or on was compared to determine whether requesting was maintained and whether vocalizations occurred during requests.	Results for Michael were inconclusive. He demonstrated a low rate of requesting postacquisition, and it was not clear if his vocalizations functioned as requests.

Sigafoos, Drasgow, et al. (2004)	Jason: 16-year-old boy with ID, PDD-NOS Megan: 20-year-old woman with ID, ASD, and hearing impairment	Experimental single-case: Multiple probe within an A-B	Participants were taught to use a VOCA to request preferred items. To teach repair when the initial request was not successful, trainers feigned not hearing the request, then used a least-to-most prompts hierarchy to prompt use of the VOCAs to repair the conversational break-down.	Both participants demonstrated an increase in the use of the VOCA, including in combination with behavioral indicators, to request items following intervention. Correct repairs using the VOCA increased from 0 to 100%, stabilizing at 80% following intervention.
Sigafoos, O'Reilly, Seely-York, & Edrisinha (2004)	Megan: 20 year-old woman with ID, ASD, and hearing impairment Jason: 16-year-old boy with ID, PDD-NOS Ryan: 12-year-old boy with ID and ASD	Experimental single case: multiple baseline across participants	Participants were taught to use their VOCAs to request items. Then they were taught to search for their VOCAs when they were not present, using a least-to-most prompts hierarchy.	Following intervention, participants showed a significant increase in their searching for the VOCA, which was used instead of reaching, leading the trainer's hand, or tantrums.

Key: ID, intellectual disability; PDD-NOS, pervasive developmental disorder-not otherwise specified; VOCA, voice output communication device; SGD, speech-generating device; PECS, Picture Exchange Communication Symbols.

areas were demonstrated for participants both with and without ASDs. Additional information about this study and the outcomes are available in Chapter 8.

Social Networks Inventory

Blackstone and Hunt Berg (2003) noted that people may show preferences with regard to communication modes according to their relationships with various communication partners. They developed a Social Networks Inventory (SNI) to provide a systematic strategy for documenting the modes used by a person with complex communication needs when interacting with people in each of five circles of communication partners (CCPs), which range from partners or close family members to people encountered regularly in the community. The SNI also facilitates documentation of the effectiveness and efficiency of various modes of communication, as well as the strategies that are used by communication partners to enhance both receptive and expressive communication.

A study by Iacono, Forster, Bryce, and Bloomberg (2004) indicated that the SNI was useful in profiling the communication skills, modality preferences, and learning styles of three adults with ID, including two with ASDs (Craig and Mark). They also found the inventory to be useful in documenting changes over a 1-year period during which the three adults, who had moved into shared supported accommodation (i.e., a community house) shortly before the study was initiated, became more familiar with one another and with their support workers. During this period, communication supports were introduced through a consultative service provided by two speech pathologists to the support workers.

An SNI interview with both Craig's and Mark's parents and key support workers indicated that they both used mainly informal modes of communication (e.g., facial expressions, vocalizations, gestures) with limited use of echolalic phrases and communication displays. Craig's support workers also reported that he used manual signs, but this was not reported by his mother. Changes in the men's communication profiles were determined by asking five speech pathologists to compare SNIs that were completed at both the beginning and the end of a 12-month period. They were provided with information from the summary profiles on the SNIs but information about when the inventories were completed was removed. Both men were judged to have made improvements over 12 months. Changes for Craig included more communication partners in all five CCPs, but particularly in the good friends circle; use of a greater range of effective communication modes, with an increased use of typing for communication noted most frequently; increased use of representational strategies, especially photographs and alphabetic systems; use of a broader range of and more complex strategies to support interactions; and introduction of a greater range of conversational topics that reflected Craig's perspective rather than that of his partners.

Changes for Mark included an increase in the number of people with whom he interacted, particularly unfamiliar communication partners in community settings; increased use of various communication modes with community partners and with close friends; increased use of specific representational strategies such as community request cards; and a broader range of conversational topics that focused on Mark's needs and wants.

An unanticipated outcome of the study by Iacono et al. (2004) was that the structured interview format of the SNI allowed the informants (i.e., parents and key support workers) to discuss their concerns, attitudes, and roles in supporting the adults. A case study specifically focused on Mark's experience (Forster & Iacono, 2007) revealed how these in-depth interviews resulted in a comprehensive picture of Mark as a person rather than as an individual with limited communication skills and problem behaviors. It became evident that Mark's most positive communication interactions were with people with whom he was very familiar and who most readily understood and accepted his informal modes of communication (gestures, vocalizations, and facial expressions). He rejected the use of graphic symbols in his home but, through a process of trial and error, appeared happy to use them to request goods and services at local shops. It also became evident that he enjoyed the company of two other adults who were living in his house; his parents enjoyed the fact that he was becoming less reliant on them as communication partners as he gained increased access to his community.

Intensive Interaction

Intensive Interaction (Nind & Hewett, 2001, 2006) is a communication intervention that has become popular in both the United Kingdom and Australia (see Chapter 3). Intensive Interaction targets the strategies used by communication partners to support the social and communication abilities of individuals with complex communication needs. As such, the approach has particular relevance to adults with ASDs and severe ID who demonstrate social withdrawal—people for whom truly interactive relationships, even with familiar partners, are often very difficult to achieve because of their high levels of self-engagement.

Intensive Interaction was developed from a model of care giver–infant interaction and involves "an intellectualization of a naturally occurring social phenomenon that pays attention to both the qualities inherent in that phenomenon and to the particular learning needs of the [person] with autism" (Nind & Powell, 2000, p. 10). A combination of techniques is used, such as pausing, playful dramatization, imitation, physical contact, and imputing intentionality (Nind & Hewett, 2006) to enhance the quality of interactions (Nind, 1999). As such, this intervention may use behaviors that are considered preintentional or intentional but informal.

Nind and Powell (2000) examined how areas of difficulty for people with ASDs and ID could be addressed through Intensive Interaction. For example, some people with ASDs appear to experience anxiety during social interactions. In an Intensive Interaction approach, a partner will attempt to both avoid and alleviate this anxiety by using a responsive interaction style that involves careful watching and waiting throughout the interaction. According to Nind and Powell, Intensive Interaction takes into consideration many so-called autistic patterns of behavior by using a person's interests—including those that may be considered to be self-stimulatory in nature—as potential sources of interactive play. Hence, a person's behavior may be imitated to engage his or her interest. Caldwell (2006) described such a strategy as learning the language of the person, in which a person recognizes another person's language as familiar yet different because it comes from someone other than him- or herself.

Proponents of Intensive Interaction stress that the technique does not involve a robotic type of imitation, but rather a style of responding such that the original behavior is reflected back to the person with very small modifications (Nind & Hewett, 2006). Of particular note is that Intensive Interaction sessions are not preplanned; rather, interactions involve following the interest of the person and responding empathetically to all of his or her nonverbal signals, such as slowing down the interaction in response to signals of distress or increasing the pace of an interaction if the person is losing interest (Nind & Hewett, 2001).

Case studies on the use of Intensive Interaction (e.g., Leaning & Watson, 2006; Nind, 1999) have demonstrated its potential as an effective strategy for engaging people with ASDs in social interactions. For example, Nind (1999) reported on a man with ASD who was withdrawn and showed no interest in people. Measures of self-involvement, the duration of interaction behaviors, and the man's engagement in interactions were taken biweekly over a 5-month period during baseline. This was followed by 13 months of Intensive Interaction observations. Among other improvements, Nind reported increases in vocalizing and smiling contingent on teacher activity, as well as increases in joint attention and turning towards the teacher.

Similarly, Leaning and Watson (2006) reported on the use of Intensive Interaction with three adults with profound ID; the descriptions of two of these adults were also indicative of ASDs. Momentary time sampling techniques were used throughout baseline, group intervention, and follow-up sessions. Improvements were observed in both smiling and eye contact, with concomitant reductions in self-stimulatory and avoidant behaviors. Unfortunately, the latter two reductions reverted to baseline levels for one adult following a disruption in the intervention. In addition to these studies, anecdotal written and videotaped case studies of Intensive Interaction have been presented in training materials (Caldwell, 2000, 2002; Hewett, 2006).

Person-Centered Planning

Person-Centered Planning (PCP) is an approach that concentrates on the perspectives of the person with a disability. PCP is a process for engaging a person and the people that matter most to him or her in working toward ways of increasing choice, honoring the desires of the person and those that know him or her best, and building relationships with other people (Lyle O'Brien & O'Brien, 2000). The people involved in PCP may include family, friends, acquaintances, and paid support workers. The process involves rich discussions and ongoing observations to ascertain the effectiveness of existing supports. Such an approach would appear to have much to offer in gaining insights into what friendships mean to people with ASDs and ID because it is designed to focus on their dreams, preferences, and social networks.

Although PCP has been practiced and discussed in the literature for over 20 years, there has been limited research examining its outcomes (Holburn, Jacobson, Schwartz, Flory, & Vietze, 2004). In recognition of the absence of robust evidence for the impact of PCP, the Department of Health in England commissioned a study to evaluate the impact of the introduction of PCP on the life experiences of people with ID and the nature and costs of supports provided to them (Robertson et al., 2007). The study included 93 people from four different sites who were followed for an average of 1.5 years. Results of questionnaires that were completed by key informants indicated positive associations between the PCP process and a number of outcomes, including having contact with friends. On the other hand, features such as diagnoses of ASDs, behavior problems, or psychiatric disorders were associated with either nonparticipation in PCP or failure to benefit from a plan designed within this model.

Summary

The striking lack of research addressing the social communication needs of adults with ASDs and ID suggests that these individuals often have few opportunities to receive intervention in this area. Only a few AAC intervention studies that go beyond teaching basic requesting have focused on adults with ASDs and complex communication needs. In particular, there is a paucity of data on how AAC may influence the development of friendships, social networks, and—perhaps more fundamentally—the quality of social interactions.

Strategies such as the Social Networks Inventory approach or Person-Centered Planning, which focus on social networks and aim to enhance the nature of interactions across settings and partners—may hold promise for addressing the needs of adults whose social impairments arise as a result of ASDs in association with ID. Approaches such as Intensive Interaction, which address the quality of interactions rather than communication itself, may function either as a preliminary step toward formal communication, including AAC, or as a means of engaging and interacting with individuals who may never achieve intentional communication.

CLINICAL IMPLICATIONS

Adults with ASDs and complex communication needs seem to have little presence in the literature beyond studies that address the prevalence of behavior problems and strategies to reduce them (including those that incorporate AAC). Nonetheless, a subgroup of people with ASDs are also identified as having ID, resulting in a need to extrapolate from that literature to draw clinical implications. In Chapter 2, Iacono and Caithness noted a similar pattern in the assessment literature, resulting in a need to use assessment strategies that were originally developed for people with severe ID in order to examine potential profiles indicative of ASDs.

There is a need to acknowledge the implications of continued social impairments and ritualistic behaviors in addition to persistent communication impairments in this group of individuals. Howlin (2004) noted that people with ASD may experience particular difficulties with regard to attempts to include them in the community. The study by Forster and Iacono (2007) suggested that, at least for one adult with ASD and ID, considerable time was needed to develop a routine that involved repeated experiences within controlled community settings, to allow both the settings and the people within them to become familiar. A failure to take into consideration such need for incremental exposure or introduction of new experiences may result in failed attempts at inclusion and may trigger problem behaviors or social withdrawal as a result.

Adults with complex communication needs associated with ID and ASDs often use informal communication modes (e.g., gestures and vocalization), although not necessarily for intentional communication (Mirenda & Schuler, 1988), or they may use symbolic communication in the form of single symbols or limited symbol combinations (Mirenda & Schuler, 1988; Romski & Sevcik, 1996). The extent to which their communications can be enhanced may be limited by a lack of appropriate support services and lack of access to communication interventions. One strategy for dealing with this is to develop the communication skills of the adults who are often their primary communication partners, although the long-term effectiveness of this approach is still unknown.

For people who live in community-supported group homes and attend day services or programs, their key communication partners are usually paid support workers, who also play significant roles in their social networks (Bloomberg et al., 2003; Iacono et al., 2004). However, little information is available about the extent of these workers' knowledge about how to support social interactions, communication, or the use of AAC. An exception is a recent study conducted by Tulloch (2007), who surveyed support workers from 15-day services for adults with ID in Victoria, Australia. The results indicated familiarity with 10 different AAC strategies across support workers, although the workers were unable to indicate whether any of these strategies were particularly relevant to people with ASDs. This finding appeared to be related to lack of awareness about their clients' diagnoses and limited knowledge of AAC.

Recently, a training package (i.e., manual and videotape) was developed to support such workers to enhance the communication skills of adults with severe ID. The InterAACtion training assessment and intervention materials (Bloomberg, West, & Johnson, 2004) provide strategies that correspond to five levels of communication that range from unintentional to intentional/informal to early symbolic. Strategies include those that help persons with disabilities to understand the world around them (e.g., teaching support workers to use manual signs, gestures, and timetables to communicate and to depict daily routines); provide a reason to communicate and something to communicate about (e.g., photograph menu plans and picture-based shopping lists); and provide a method of communication (e.g., key word signs, gestures, and chat books). In addition, for some adults whose extensive social impairments preclude social interactions, an approach that focuses on preintentional behaviors to encourage awareness of and desire to interact with others may be warranted. One such approach, Intensive Interaction, may provide a first step in intervention, even prior to developing informal methods of communication.

The apparently limited success in achieving true community inclusion for adults with ASDs and ID, despite government policies that have highlighted this as a goal, may result (at least in part) from a failure to address the communication needs of these adults. Advocates, family members, and service providers often request interventions that focus on social relationships because these are essential to personal connectedness and to being part of a community (e.g., McIntyre, Kramer, Blacher, & Simmerman, 2004). Given the central role of communication to such connectedness, especially in terms of reciprocal interactions, the focus of such interventions should include an emphasis on assisting communication partners to provide communication opportunities, to recognize and respond to communication attempts, and to maintain interactions. Romski and Sevcik (1996) demonstrated that these outcomes can be achieved using symbolic communication systems for youth with ID, including those with ASDs.

For people who are presymbolic or who use idiosyncratic gestures, strategies such as personal communication dictionaries (i.e., gesture dictionaries) may be more effective. A personal communication dictionary provides a record of a person's informal and formal communication modes (e.g., facial expressions, gestures, signs), what they mean, and how the communication partner might respond to their use (Beukelman & Mirenda, 2005; Bloomberg et al., 2004). In addition, augmented input in the form of touch cues (i.e., specific touches paired consistently with words or short phrases), object calendars to represent routines and changes in routines, and scripted routine strategies can be used to assist individuals to understand and predict upcoming events, thereby alleviating anxiety (Beukelman & Mirenda, 2005; Bloomberg et al., 2004). A community request card consisting of a partial object attached to a card with a written message for the communication partner may be useful in community venues. For example, a few pieces of popcorn glued to a card and accompanied by the message *I would like a regular popcorn; my friend who is with me will pay* can be used to involve the person with a disability in a brief but important social interaction at a movie theater (Beukelman & Mirenda, 2005; Bloomberg et al., 2004). Longer interactions can be encouraged by developing chat or remnant books, which include items of interest that are accompanied by text for literate communication partners (Bloomberg et al., 2004). In addition, obtaining information about how people communicate with individuals in their social networks can provide a basis for individualizing communication modes that best fit specific settings and partners (Iacono et al., 2004).

RESEARCH IMPLICATIONS

Given the paucity of research evidence in this area, most of the clinical work with adolescents and adults with ASDs and ID draws on research pertaining to similar-age individuals with ID alone. Missing from the research is information on the long-term outcomes of the introduction of AAC during childhood, especially with regard to communication success and effectiveness within social interactions. Hamm and Mirenda (2006) provided some such information for a few individuals, but much more is needed to facilitate an understanding of how AAC can be used to address the persistent communication, social, and behavior impairments of adults with ASDs and ID. There is also a need to evaluate the extent to which AAC can be used to support individuals to demonstrate latent cognitive capabilities that may, in fact, challenge diagnoses of ID.

What is not clear from the research literature addressing social networks of people with ASDs and ID is the perspective of these individuals themselves with regard to challenges such as friendship development and social network expansion. Much of the current information on this issue comes from personal accounts. For example, Howlin et al. (2000) canvassed the perspectives of 19 participants with ASDs (age 21–26 years) who were able to report on their experiences and noted that, despite the fact that others described their lives as solitary, few saw themselves as being lonely. Wendy Lawson (2006)—an Australian counselor, trainer, and writer with ASD—provided additional insights into what friendship means for people with Asperger syndrome and noted that, contrary to some reports, many people with this label do desire friendships. Lawson described a number of close friendships that were developed as a result of her own efforts to learn about the assumptions made by others and how to interpret their behaviors. Conversely, she noted that the ability and willingness of others to learn the same about her has contributed to her lasting friendships.

Along the same lines, Autism Network International convenes *Autreat,* an annual retreat-style conference for people with ASDs. A key component of their philosophy is that "autistic people have characteristically autistic styles of relating to others, which should be respected and appreciated rather than modified to make them 'fit in'" (Autism Network International, 2002). Qualitative research strategies that allow the voice of people with ASDs to be heard may assist professionals and the community to develop such understanding and provide respect.

Whether or not the insights into friendship and social network development that are provided through self-reports and self-advocacy are relevant to those who also have ID and complex communication needs is unknown. Information is lacking about the extent to which these individuals desire friendships and social contacts, as well as the role(s) they wish such relationships to play in their lives. In addition, there is a lack of information about the role of communication supports, particularly AAC, in facilitating friendships and social networks. Such information may come from both person-centered approaches and from people with whom these individuals have close relationships, which allow them to contribute information about preferences and desires in relation to communication modes and strategies, among other variables. Again, qualitative approaches may be best suited to addressing these areas.

Intensive Interaction, which was developed specifically for people with ASDs and those with profound ID, would appear to hold some promise as a means of addressing the fundamental social impairment. Research is needed into the efficacy of this approach, as well as how it might be used to develop communication skills and communicative interactions with various partners. Another area that holds promise but requires research is an examination of interactions with various communication partners within a person's social networks—that is, their CCPs as defined by Blackstone and Hunt Berg (2003). Such an examination may provide a means of profiling the communication skills and preferences of adults with ASDs and of identifying strategies that enhance communication. Similarly, research is needed to examine the impact of training and AAC interventions that are developed with paid support staff in mind, such as the InterAACtion approach.

Another challenge for researchers is ensuring that people with complex communication needs and ASD are involved as much as possible in the research process (Bersani, 1999). Engaging the participation of autism self-advocacy groups might provide a means of gaining the perspectives of adults who, through AAC, have effectively challenged the labels that have been assigned to them by others, such as mental retardation or ID (e.g., Rubin, n.d.). Use of PCP principles within research may also assist to ensure that individuals' perspectives are considered and actualized.

CONCLUSION

The striking lack of literature on adults with ASDs and complex communication needs that are associated with ID is indicative that this group has largely been forgotten. The focus of existing literature on behavior problems and psychiatric disorders suggests that these adults come to professionals' attention primarily when their needs cannot be ignored by the people around them. This bleak outcome, combined with the underlying social impairment inherent in ASDs, means that most of these individuals have few opportunities to form meaningful friendships or to extend their social networks beyond close family members or people who are paid to provide them with care. AAC has much to offer people with ASDs and complex communication needs in terms of enhancing social interactions, the development of social networks, community inclusion, and their overall quality of life. In addressing this potential, there is an urgent need for research about how to tailor AAC interventions to address these adults' needs, preferences, and desires.

REFERENCES

Antonucci, T.C. (1985). Personal characteristics, social support and social behavior. In R.H. Binstock, E. Shanas, G.L. Maddox, G.C. Myers, & J.H. Schulz (Eds.), *Handbook of aging and the social sciences* (pp. 94–128). New York: Van Nostrand Reinhold.

Arvio, M., & Sillanpää, M. (2003). Prevalence, aetiology and comorbidity of severe and profound intellectual disability in Finland. Journal of Intellectual Disability Research, 47, 108–112.

Australian Institute of Health and Welfare. (2006). *Disability support services 2004–2005: National data on services provided under the Commonwealth State/ Territory Disability Agreement.* Retrieved February 22, 2007, from http:// www.aihw.gov.au/publications/dis/dss04-05/dss04-05.pdf

Autism Network International. (2002). Introducing ANI. Retrieved September 1, 2007, from http://ani.autistics.org/intro.html

Autism Rights Movement. (n.d.). Retrieved June 11, 2008, from http:// www.autism-help.org/points-autism-rights-movement.htm

Ballaban-Gil, K., Rapin, I., Tuchman, R., & Shinnar, S. (1996). Longitudinal examination of the behavioral, language, and social changes in a population of adolescents and young adults with autistic disorder. *Pediatric Neurology, 15,* 877–900.

Beadle-Brown, J., Murphy, G.H., Wing, L., Gould, J., Shah, H., & Holmes, N. (2002). Changes in social impairment for people with intellectual disabilities: A follow up of the Camberwell cohort. *Journal of Autism and Developmental Disabilities, 32,* 195–206.

Bersani, H., Jr. (1999). Nothing about me without me: A proposal for participatory action research. In F. Lonke, J. Clibbens, H. Arvidson, & L. Lloyd (Eds.), *Augmentative and alternative communication: New directions in research and practice* (pp. 262–277). London: Whurr.

Beukelman, D.R., & Mirenda, P. (2005). *Augmentative and alternative communication: Supporting children and adults with complex communication needs* (3rd ed.). Baltimore: Paul H. Brookes Publishing Co.

Bhaumik, S., Branford, D., McGrother, C., & Thorp, C. (1997). Autistic traits in adults with learning disabilities. *British Journal of Psychiatry, 170*, 502–506.

Bigby, C. (2008). Known well by no one: Trend of the informal social networks of people with intellectual disability five years after moving into the community. *Journal of Intellectual and Developmental Disabilities, 33*(2), 148–157.

Blackstone, S., & Hunt Berg, M. (2003). *Social networks: A communication inventory for individuals with complex communication needs and their communication partners. Manual.* Monterey, CA: Augmentative Communication.

Bloomberg, K., West, D., & Iacono, T. (2003). PICTURE IT: An evaluation of a training program for carers of adults with severe and multiple disabilities. *Journal of Intellectual and Developmental Disability, 28*, 260–282.

Bloomberg, K., West, D., & Johnson, H. (2004). *InterAACtion: Strategies for intentional and unintentional communicators.* Melbourne, Australia: Scope.

Bradley, E., Summers, J., Wood, H., & Bruson, S. (2004). Comparing rates of psychiatric and behavior disorders in adolescents and young adults with and without autism. *Journal of Autism and Developmental Disorders, 34*, 151–161.

Cafiero, J. (2001). The effect of an augmentative communication intervention on the communication, behavior, and academic program of an adolescent with autism. *Focus on Autism and Other Developmental Disabilities, 16*, 179–189.

Caldwell, P. (2000). *You don't know what it's like: Finding ways of building relationships with people with severe learning disabilities, autistic spectrum disorder, and other impairments.* Brighton, East Sussex, England: Pavilion.

Caldwell, P. (2002). Learning the language: Building relationships with people with severe learning disability, autistic spectrum disorder and other challenging behaviours [videotape]. Brighton, East Sussex, England: Pavilion.

Caldwell, P. (2006). Speaking the other's language: Imitation as a gateway to relationship. *Infant and Child Development, 15*, 275–282.

Cambridge, P., Carpenter, J., Beecham, J., Hallam, A., Knapp, M., Forrester-Jones, R., et al. (2002). Twelve years on: The long-term outcomes and costs of deinstitutionalisation and community care for people with learning disabilities. *Tizard Learning Disability Review, 7*, 34–42.

Chambers, M., & Rehfeldt, R.A. (2003). Effects of rules on preference for reliable reinforcement in a 5-year-old child. *North American Journal of Psychology, 5*, 67–74.

Cooper, S., & Bailey, N. (2001). Psychiatric disorders amongst adults with learning disabilities—prevalence and relationship to ability level. *Irish Journal of Psychiatric Medicine, 18*, 45–53.

Dagnan, D., & Ruddick, L. (1997). The social networks of older people with learning disabilities living in staffed community based homes. *British Journal of Developmental Disabilities, 43*, 43–53.

de Kock, U., Saxby, H., Thomas, M., & Felce, D. (1988). Community and family contact: An evaluation of small community homes for severe and profound mental handicaps. *Mental Handicap Research, 1*, 127–140.

Deb, S., Thomas, M., & Bright, C. (2001). Mental disorder in adults with intellectual disability. 1: Prevalence of functional psychiatric illness among a community-based population aged between 16 and 64 years. *Journal of Intellectual Disability Research, 45*, 495–505.

Department of Health. (2001). *Valuing people: A new strategy for learning disability for the 21st century.* Retrieved April 5, 2007 from http://www.archive. official-documents.co.uk/document/cm50/5086/5086.htm.

Department of Human Services. (2002). *Victorian state disability plan 2002–2012.* Melbourne, Australia: Disability Services, Department of Human Services.

Donnelly, M., McGilloway, S., Mays, N., Knapp, M., Kavanagh, S., Beecham, J., & Feny, A. (1996). One and two year outcomes for adults with learning disabilities discharged to the community. *British Journal of Psychiatry, 168,* 598–606.

Forrester-Jones, R., Carpenter, J., Coolen-Schrijner, P., Cambridge, P., Tate, A., Beecham, J., et al. (2006). The social networks of people with intellectual disability living in the community 12 years after resettlement from long-stay hospitals. *Journal of Applied Research in Intellectual Disabilities, 19,* 741–751.

Forrester-Jones, R., Jones, S., & Heason, S. (2004). Supported employment: A route to social networks. *Journal of Applied Research in Intellectual Disabilities, 17,* 199–208.

Forster, S., & Iacono, T. (2007). Perceptions of communication before and after a speech pathology intervention for an adult with intellectual disability. *Journal of Intellectual and Developmental Disability, 32,* 302–314.

Hamm, B., & Mirenda, P. (2006). Post-school quality of life for individuals with developmental disabilities who use AAC. *Augmentative and Alternative Communication, 22,* 134–147.

Hamilton, B., & Snell, M. (1993). Using the milieu approach to increase spontaneous communication book use across environments by an adolescent with autism. *Augmentative and Alternative Communication, 9,* 259–272.

Hewett, D. (2006). *Intensive Interaction* [DVD]. Puckeridge, England: Author.

Holburn, S., Jacobson, J.W., Schwartz, A.A., Flory, M.J., & Vietze, P.M. (2004). The Willowbrook Futures Project: A longitudinal analysis of person-centered planning. *American Journal on Mental Retardation, 109,* 63–76.

Howlin, P. (2004). *Autism and Asperger syndrome.* London: Routledge.

Howlin, P., Goode, S., Hutton, J., & Rutter, M. (2004). Adult outcomes for children with autism. *Journal of Child Psychology and Psychiatry, 45,* 212–229.

Howlin, P., Mawhood, L., & Rutter, M. (2000). Autism and developmental receptive language disorder: A follow-up comparison in early adult life. II: Social, behavioural, and psychiatric outcomes. *Journal of Child Psychology and Psychiatry, 41,* 561–578.

Iacono, T., Forster, S., Bryce, R., & Bloomberg, K. (2004, October). *Perspectives on communication in adults with severe intellectual disability according to a social networks inventory.* Paper presented at the International Society for Augmentative and Alternative Communication Biennial Conference, Brazil.

Kennedy, C.H. (2004). Research on social relationships. In E. Emerson, C. Hatton, T. Thompson, & T.R. Parmenter (Eds.), *The international handbook of applied research in intellectual disabilities* (pp. 298–309). Chichester, England: Wiley & Sons.

Kennedy, C.H., Horner, R.H., & Newton, S. (1990). The social networks and activity patterns of adults with severe disabilities: A correlational analysis. *Journal of the Association for Persons with Severe Handicaps, 15,* 86–90.

Kobayashi, R., Murata, T., & Yoshinaga, K. (1992). A follow-up study of 201 children with autism in Kyushu and Yamagachi areas, Japan. *Journal of Autism and Developmental Disorders, 22,* 395–411.

Krauss, M.W., Seltzer, M.M., & Goodman, S.J. (1992). Social support networks of adults with mental retardation who live at home. *American Journal of Mental Retardation, 96,* 432–441.

La Malfa, G., Lassi, S., Salvini, R., Giganti, C., Bertelli, M., & Albertini, G. (2007). The relationship between autism and psychiatric disorders in intellectually disabled adults. *Research in Autism Spectrum Disorders, 1,* 218–228.

Landesman-Dwyer, S., Berkson, G., & Romer, D. (1979). Affiliation and friendship of mentally retarded residents in group homes. *American Journal on Mental Deficiency, 83,* 571–580.

Larsen, F.W., & Mourisden, S.E. (1997). The outcome in children with childhood autism and Asperger syndrome originally diagnosed a psychotic: A 30-year follow-up study of subjects hospitalized as children. *European Child and Adolescent Psychiatry, 6,* 181–190.

Lawson, W. (2006). *Friendships the Aspie way.* London: Jessica Kingsley.

Leaning, B., & Watson, T. (2006). From the inside looking out: An Intensive Interaction group for people with profound and multiple learning disabilities. *British Journal of Learning Disabilities, 34,* 103–109.

Lecompt, J., & Mercier, C. (2007). The Montreal Declaration on Intellectual Disabilities of 2004: An important first step. *Journal of Policy and Practice in Intellectual Disabilities, 4,* 66–69.

Lockyer, L., & Rutter, M. (1969). A five to fifteen year follow-up study of infantile psychosis: III. Psychological aspects. *British Journal of Psychiatry, 115,* 865–882.

Lyle O'Brien, C., & O'Brien, J. (2000). *The origins of Person-Centered Planning: A community of practice perspective.* Atlanta: Responsive Systems Associates.

Mawhood, L., Howlin, P., & Rutter, M. (2000). Autism and developmental language disorder: A comparative follow-up in early adult life. I: Cognitive and language outcomes. *Journal of Child Psychology and Psychiatry, 41,* 547–559.

McIntyre, L.L., Kraemer, B.R., Blacher, J., & Simmerman, S. (2004). Quality of life for young adults with severe intellectual disability: Mothers' thoughts and reflections. *Journal of Intellectual & Developmental Disability, 29,* 131–146.

McLean, L.K., Brady, N.C., & McLean, J.E. (1996). Reported communication abilities of individuals with severe mental retardation. *American Journal of Mental Retardation, 100,* 580–589.

Mirenda, P., & Schuler, A. (1988). Augmenting communication for persons with autism: Issues and strategies. *Topics in Language Disorders, 9,* 24–43.

Money, D. (2002). Speech and language therapy management models. In S. Abudarham & A. Hurd (Eds.), *Management of communication needs in people with learning disability* (pp. 82–102). London: Whurr.

Newton, J.S., & Horner, R.H. (1995). Feedback to staff on resident lifestyle. A descriptive analysis. *Behavior Modification, 19,* 95–117.

Nind, M. (1999). Intensive Interaction and autism: A useful approach? *British Journal of Special Education, 26,* 96–102.

Nind, M., & Hewett, D. (2001). *A practical guide to Intensive Interaction.* Kidderminster, England: British Institute of Learning Disabilities.

Nind, M., & Hewett, D. (2006). *Access to communication: Developing basic communication with people who have severe learning difficulties* (2nd ed.). London: David Fulton.

Nind, M., & Powell, S. (2000). Intensive Interaction and autism: Some theoretical concerns. *Children & Society, 14,* 98–109.

Orsmond, G.I., Krauss, M.W., & Seltzer, M.M. (2004). Peer relationships and social recreational activities among adolescents and adults with autism. *Journal of Autism and Developmental Disabilities, 34,* 245–256.

Parker, R., Sprague, J., Flannery, K.B., Niess, J., & Zumwait, L. (1991). Measuring the social perceptions of persons with moderate and severe disabilities to construct social network maps. *Journal of Developmental & Physical Disabilities, 3,* 23–45.

Perry, A., Reilly, S., Cotton, S., Bloomberg, K., & Johnson, H. (2004). A demographic survey of people who have a disability and complex communication needs in Victoria, Australia. *Asia-Pacific Journal of Speech, Language and Hearing, 9,* 259–271.

Reindeers, J.S. (2002). The good life for citizens with intellectual disability. *Journal of Intellectual Disability Research, 46,* 1–5.

Renblad, K. (2002). People with intellectual disabilities: Activities, social contacts and opportunities to exert influence (an interview study with staff). *International Journal of Rehabilitation Research, 4,* 279–286.

Reichle, J., & Brown, L. (1986). Teaching the use of a multipage direct selection communication board to an adult with autism. *Journal of the Association for Persons with Severe Handicaps, 11,* 68–73.

Robertson, J., Emerson, E., Gregory, N., Hatton, C., Kessissoglou, S., Hallam, A., & Linehan, C. (2001). Social networks of people with mental retardation in residential settings. *Mental Retardation, 39,* 201–214.

Robertson, J., Emerson, E., Hatton, C., Elliott, J., McIntosh, B., Swift, P., et al. (2007). Person-centred planning: Factors associated with successful outcomes for people with intellectual disabilities. *Journal of Intellectual Disability Research, 51,* 232–243.

Romski, M., & Sevcik, R. (1996). *Breaking the speech barrier: Language development through augmented means.* Baltimore: Paul H. Brookes Publishing Co.

Rotholz, D., Berkowitz, S., & Burberry, J. (1989). Functionality of two modes of communication in the community by students with cerebral palsy and mental retardation. *The Journal of the Association for Persons with Severe Handicaps, 14,* 227–233.

Rubin, S. (n.d.). Sue Rubin: Living and thoroughly enjoying life in spite of autism. Retrieved June 11, 2008, from http://www.sue-rubin.org/

Rutter, M., Greenfeld, D., & Lockyer, L. (1967). A five to fifteen year follow-up study of infantile psychosis: II. Social and behavioural outcome. *British Journal of Psychiatry, 113,* 1183–1199.

Rutter, M., & Lockyer, L. (1967). A five to fifteen year follow-up study of infantile psychosis: I. Description of sample. *British Journal of Psychiatry, 113,* 1169–1182.

Scott, J. (1991). *Social network analysis*. London: Sage Publications.

Seltzer, M.M., Krauss, M.W., Shattuck, P.T., Orsmond, G., Sew, A., & Lord, C. (2003). The symptoms of autism spectrum disorders in adolescence and adulthood. *Journal of Autism and Developmental Disorders, 33,* 565–581.

Sigafoos, J., Didden, R., & O'Reilly, M. (2003). Effects of speech output on maintenance of requesting and frequency of vocalizations in three children with developmental disabilities. *Augmentative and Alternative Communication, 19,* 37–47.

Sigafoos, J., & Drasgow, E. (2001). Conditional use of aided and unaided AAC. *Focus on Autism and Other Developmental Disabilities, 16,* 152–161.

Sigafoos, J., Drasgow, E., Halle, J., O'Reilly, M., Seely-York, S., Edrisinha, C., et al. (2004). Teaching VOCA use as a communication repair strategy. *Journal of Autism and Developmental Disorders, 34,* 411–422.

Sigafoos, J., O'Reilly, M., Seely-York, S., & Edrisinha, C. (2004). Teaching students with developmental disabilities to locate their AAC device. *Research in Developmental Disabilities, 25,* 371–383.

Stancliffe, R. (2006). Services, availability, issues and models. In I. Dempsey & K. Nankervis (Eds.), *Community disability services: An evidence-based approach to practice* (pp. 272–295). Sydney, Australia: UNSW Press.

Stancliffe, R.J., & Lakin, K.C. (2006). Longitudinal frequency and stability of family contact in institutional and community living. *Mental Retardation, 44,* 418–429.

Tsakanikos, E., Costello, H., Holt, G., Bouras, N., Sturmey, P., & Newton, J. (2006). Psychopathology in adults with autism and intellectual disability. *Journal of Autism and Development Disorders, 36,* 1123–1129.

Tulloch, J. (2007). *The use of augmentative and alternative communication (AAC) techniques with adults with autism in adult training and support services: Is there a difference between techniques used with adults with autism and other adults with communication difficulties?* Unpublished master's thesis, Latrobe University, Melbourne, Australia.

United Nations. (2006). *Convention on the rights of persons with disabilities.* Retrieved September 1, 2007, from http://www.un.org/esa/socdev/enable/rights/convtexte.htm

Wolfensburger, W. (1983). Social role valorization: A proposed new term for the principle of normalisation. *Mental Retardation, 21,* 234–239.

Young, L., Sigafoos, J., Suttie, J., Ashman, A., & Grevell, P. (1998). Deinstitutionalisation of persons with intellectual disabilities: A review of Australian studies. *Journal of Intellectual & Developmental Disability, 23,* 155–170.

Index

Page numbers followed by *f* indicate figures; those followed by *t* indicate tables.